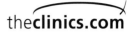

EMERGENCY MEDICINE CLINICS OF NORTH AMERICA

Endocrine and Metabolic Emergencies

GUEST EDITORS
Mary Jo Wagner, MD, FACEP and
Kathleen Cowling, DO, MS, FACEP

August 2005 • Volume 23 • Number 3

SAUNDERS

An Imprint of Elsevier, Inc.
PHILADELPHIA   LONDON   TORONTO   MONTREAL   SYDNEY   TOKYO

W.B. SAUNDERS COMPANY
A Division of Elsevier Inc.

1600 John F. Kennedy Boulevard, Suite 1800 • Philadelphia, Pennsylvania 19103-2899

http://www.theclinics.com

EMERGENCY MEDICINE CLINICS   Volume 23, Number 3
OF NORTH AMERICA   ISSN 0733-8627
August 2005   ISBN 1-4160-2712-2
Editor: Karen Sorensen

The ideas and opinions expressed in *Emergency Medicine Clinics of North America* do not necessarily reflect those of the Publisher. The Publisher does not assume any responsibility for any injury and/or damage to persons or property arising out of or related to any use of the material contained in this periodical. The reader is advised to check the appropriate medical literature and the product information currently provided by the manufacturer of each drug to be administered to verify the dosage, the method and duration of administration, or contraindications. It is the responsibility of the treating physician or other health care professional, relying on independent experience and knowledge of the patient, to determine drug dosages and the best treatment for the patient. Mention of any product in this issue should not be construed as endorsement by the contributors, editors, or the Publisher of the product or manufacturers' claims.

Emergency Medicine Clinics of North America (ISSN 0733-8627) is published quarterly by W.B. Saunders Company. Corporate and Editorial Offices: 1600 John F. Kennedy Boulevard, Suite 1800, Philadelphia, PA 19103-2899. Accounting and Circulation Offices: 6277 Sea Harbor Drive, Orlando, FL 32887-4800. Periodicals postage paid at Orlando, FL 32862, and additional mailing offices. Subscription prices are $170.00 per year (US individuals), $263.00 per year (US institutions), $225.00 per year (international individuals), $312.00 per year (international institutions), $205.00 per year (Canadian individuals), and $312.00 per year (Canadian institutions). International air speed delivery is included in all *Clinics'* subscription prices. All prices are subject to change without notice. POSTMASTER: Send address changes to *Emergency Medicine Clinics of North America*, W.B. Saunders Company, Periodicals Fulfillment, Orlando, FL 32887-4800. **Customer Service: 1-800-654-2452 (US). From outside of the US, call 1-407-345-4000. E-mail: hhspcs@harcourt.com.**

Emergency Medicine Clinics of North America is covered in *Index Medicus, Current Contents/Clinical Medicine, EMBASE/Excerpta Medica, BIOSIS, SciSearch, CINAHL, ISI/BIOMED,* and *Research Alert.*

Printed in the United States of America.

GUEST EDITORS

MARY JO WAGNER, MD, FACEP, Program Director, Synergy Medical Education Alliance/Michigan State University Emergency Medicine Residency, Saginaw; Program in Emergency Medicine, Michigan State University College of Human Medicine, Lansing, Michigan

KATHLEEN COWLING, DO, MS, FACEP, Assistant Clinical Professor, Program in Emergency Medicine, Michigan State University College of Human Medicine, Lansing; Emergency Physician, Emergency Care Center, Covenant HealthCare, Saginaw, Michigan

CONTRIBUTORS

MARY LYNN ARVANITIS, DO, FACOEP, Attending Physician, Emergency Medicine, Covenant HealthCare, Saginaw; Clinical Assistant Professor, Emergency Medicine, Michigan State University College of Human Medicine, East Lansing, Michigan

ANDREW M. BAZAKIS, MD, FACEP, Assistant Residency Director, Synergy Medical Education Alliance; Michigan State University Emergency Medicine Residency Program, Saginaw, Michigan

RICHARD BOLES, MD, Associate Professor of Pediatrics, Children's Hospital Los Angeles; Keck School of Medicine at the University of Southern California, Los Angeles, California

JAMES T. BROWN, MD, Clinical Assistant Professor, Emergency Medicine, University of Illinois, College of Medicine; OSF Saint Francis Medical Center, Peoria, Illinois

JENNIFER J. CASALETTO, MD, Attending Physician, Department of Emergency Medicine, Maricopa Medical Center, Phoenix, Arizona

MICHELLE A. CHARFEN, MD, Clinical Instructor, Department of Medicine, David Geffen School of Medicine at University of California-Los Angeles; Research Fellow, Department of Emergency Medicine, Harbor-University of California-Los Angeles Medical Center, Torrance, California

ILENE CLAUDIUS, MD, Assistant Professor, Department of Emergency and Transport Medicine, Children's Hospital Los Angeles; Assistant Professor of Pediatrics, Keck School of Medicine at the University of Southern California, Los Angeles, California

TEAGUE A. DOMBECK, MD, Clinical Instructor/Resident, Program in Emergency Medicine, Michigan State University College of Human Medicine, East Lansing; Emergency Medicine Resident, Synergy Medical Education Alliance/Michigan State University Emergency Medicine Residency Program, Saginaw, Michigan

BERNARD H. EISENGA, PHD, MD, Medical Director, DeVos Children's Hospital Regional Poison Center and Assistant Clinical Professor, Department of Medicine/MERC, Michigan State University College of Human Medicine, Grand Rapids, Michigan

MADONNA FERNÁNDEZ-FRACKELTON, MD, FACEP, Assistant Professor of Medicine, David Geffen School of Medicine at University of California-Los Angeles; Director, Adult Emergency Department, Harbor-University of California-Los Angeles Medical Center Department of Emergency Medicine, Torrance, California

COLLEEN FLUHARTY, MD, Emergency Medicine Attending and Pediatric Resident Physician at Children's Hospital Los Angeles, Los Angeles, California

SCOTT C. GIBSON, MD, FACEP, Clinical Associate Professor, Emergency Medicine, Michigan State University College of Human Medicine; Core faculty member, MSU-Kalamazoo Center for Medical Studies, Emergency Medicine Residency; Associate Medical Director, Trauma and Emergency Center, Bronson Methodist Hospital, Kalamazoo, Michigan

VED V. GOSSAIN, MD, FACP, FACEP, Professor of Medicine; Chief, Division of Endocrinology, Department of Medicine, Michigan State University, Lansing, Michigan

DAVID A. HARTMAN, MD, FACEP, Clinical Assistant Professor, Emergency Medicine, Michigan State University College of Human Medicine; Core faculty member, MSU-Kalamazoo Center for Medical Studies, Emergency Medicine Residency, Kalamazoo, Michigan

BRYAN S. JUDGE, MD, Associate Medical Director, DeVos Children's Hospital Regional Poison Center and Assistant Clinical Professor, Department of Emergency Medicine/MERC, Michigan State University College of Human Medicine, Grand Rapids, Michigan

CATHERINE KUNZLER, DO, Clinical Instructor, Program in Emergency Medicine, Michigan State University College of Human Medicine, East Lansing, Michigan

INGRID T. LIM, MD, Stanford-Kaiser Emergency Medicine Residency Program, Palo Alto, California

MICHELLE LIN, MD, San Francisco General Hospital Emergency Services; Assistant Clinical Professor of Medicine, University of California San Francisco, San Francisco, California

STEPHEN J. LIU, MD, Stanford-Kaiser Emergency Medicine Residency Program, Palo Alto, California

NATHANAEL J. McKEOWN, DO, Clinical Instructor, College of Osteopathic Medicine, Emergency Medicine Residency Program, Michigan State University, Lansing, Michigan

BRUCE W. NUGENT, MD, Associate Clinical Professor, Grand Rapids MERC/Michigan State University Program in Emergency Medicine, Grand Rapids, Michigan

JULIA L. PASQUALE, MD, Resident Physician, Emergency Medicine, Synergy Medical Education Alliance, Saginaw; Clinical Instructor, Michigan State University College of Human Medicine, East Lansing, Michigan

JOHN SARKO, MD, Clinical Attending Physician, Department of Emergency Medicine, Maricopa Medical Center, Phoenix, Arizona

ROBERT C. SATONIK MD, FACEP, Clinical Assistant Professor, Program in Emergency Medicine, Michigan State University College of Human Medicine, East Lansing; Associate Program Director, Synergy Medical Education Alliance/Michigan State University Emergency Medicine Residency Program, Saginaw, Michigan

TIMOTHY J. SCHAEFER, MD, Clinical Associate Professor and Associate Residency Director, Section of Emergency Medicine, Department of Surgery, University of Illinois College of Medicine at Peoria; Attending Physician, Department of Emergency Medicine OSF-Saint Francis Medical Center, Peoria, Illinois

JASON M. SCHENCK, MD, Clinical Instructor, Emergency Medicine, Michigan State University College of Human Medicine; Resident, MSU-Kalamazoo Center for Medical Studies, Emergency Medicine Residency, Kalamazoo, Michigan

SID M. SHAH, MD, FACEP, Attending Physician, Ingham Regional Medical Center and Michigan State University, Emergency Medicine Residency; Associate Clinical Professor, Program in Emergency Medicine, Michigan State University College of Human Medicine, Lansing, Michigan

MATTHEW C. TEWS, DO, Emergency Medicine Resident, Michigan State University, Emergency Medicine Residency; Clinical Instructor/Resident, Program in Emergency Medicine, Michigan State University College of Osteopathic Medicine, Lansing, Michigan

SUSAN P. TORREY, MD, Associate Professor of Emergency Medicine, Tufts University School of Medicine; Associate Residency Director, Department of Emergency Medicine, Baystate Medical Center, Springfield, Massachusetts

ROBERT W. WOLFORD, MD, MMM, Associate Professor, Program in Emergency Medicine, Michigan State University College of Human Medicine; Attending Physician, Emergency Care Center, Covenant HealthCare, Saginaw, Michigan

CONTENTS

are discussed, with special emphasis on the role medications play in the etiologies of each.

Disorders of water imbalance manifest as hyponatremia and hypernatremia. To diagnose these disorders, emergency physicians must maintain a high index of suspicion, especially in the high-risk patient, because clinical presentations may be nonspecific. With severe water imbalance, inappropriate fluid resuscitation in the emergency department may have devastating neurological consequences. The rate of serum sodium concentration correction should be monitored closely to avoid osmotic demyelination syndrome in hyponatremic patients and cerebral edema in hypernatremic patients.

Metabolic acidosis is defined as an acidemia created by one of three mechanisms: increased production of acids, decreased excretion of acids, or loss of alkali. This article addresses the identification and correct diagnosis of metabolic acidosis by reviewing important historical factors, pathophysiological principles, clinical presentation, and laboratory findings accompanying common high and normal anion gap metabolic acidoses in emergency department patients.

Disorders of fuel metabolism as they relate to abnormal fuel intake, abnormal fuel expenditure, and dietary supplements are the focus of this article. The emergency physician should be aware of the medical complications that can occur as a result of starvation states, eating disorders, fad diets, hypermetabolic states, and ergogenic aids. Knowledge and understanding of the complications associated with these disorders will facilitate the diagnosis and management of patients who present to the emergency department with any of the disorders reviewed.

Anabolic steroids have not currently made their way into the daily practice of emergency physicians. The patients that use and abuse them have. In addition, those patients that are suffering from the consequences of illnesses that have excess levels of androgens are commonly evaluated in the emergency department. Clinicians should familiarize themselves with the practices of anabolic steroid users, so they can provide more beneficial council to their patients. As research continues, the emergency physician may find uses for androgens within the emergency department.

who present with lethargy, anxiety, psychosis, and seizures should be considered. Using the complaint-based approach, this article discusses some of the often less obvious etiologies for these presentations related to endocrine and metabolic disease states.

This review will provide an updated overview of the neuroendocrine response to critical illness. Specifically, the current evidence for "stress steroid" administration will be examined, as well as interventional glucose control during critical illness. The emergency physician will also find relevance in the alterations of thyroid hormones that occur in the face of severe illness or trauma.

FORTHCOMING ISSUES

RECENT ISSUES

GOAL STATEMENT

The goal of Emergency Medicine Clinics of North America is to keep practicing physicians up to date with current clinical practice in emergency medicine by providing timely articles reviewing the state of the art in patient care.

ACCREDITATION

The Emergency Medicine Clinics of North America is planned and implemented in accordance with the Essential Areas and Policies of the Accreditation Council for Continuing Medical Education (ACCME) through the joint sponsorship of the University Of Virginia School Of Medicine and Elsevier. The University Of Virginia School of Medicine is accredited by the ACCME to provide continuing medical education for physicians.

The University of Virginia School of Medicine designates this educational activity for a maximum of 60 category 1 credits per year, 15 category 1 credits per issue, toward the AMA Physician's Recognition Award. Each physician should claim only those credits that he/she actually spent in the activity.

The American Medical Association has determined that physicians not licensed in the US who participate in this CME activity are eligible for AMA PRA category 1 credit.

Category 1 credit can be earned by reading the text material, taking the CME examination online at http://www.theclinics.com/home/cme, and completing the evaluation. After taking the test, you will be required to review any and all incorrect answers. Following completion of the test and evaluation, your credit will be awarded and you may print your certificate.

FACULTY DISCLOSURE

As a provider accredited by the Accreditation Council for Continuing Medical Education (ACCME), the Office of Continuing Medical Education of the University of Virginia School of Medicine must ensure balance, independence, objectivity, and scientific rigor in all its individually sponsored or jointly sponsored educational activities. All authors/editors participating in a sponsored activity are expected to disclose to the readers any significant financial interest or other relationship (1) with the manufacturer(s) of any commercial product(s) and/or provider(s) of commercial services discussed in an educational presentation and (2) with any commercial supporters of the activity (significant financial interest or other relationship can include such things as grants or research support, employee, consultant, stock holder, member of speakers bureau, etc.) The intent of this disclosure is not to prevent authors/editors with a significant financial or other relationship from writing an article, but rather to provide readers with information on which they can make their own judgments. It remains for the readers to determine whether the author's/editor's interest or relationships may influence the article with regard to exposition or conclusion.

The authors/editors listed below have identified no professional or financial affiliations related to their article:
Mary Lynn Arvantis, DO; James T. Brown, MD; Jennifer J. Casaletto, MD; Michelle A. Charfen, MD; Ilene Claudius, MD; Teague A. Dombeck, MD; Bernard H. Eisenga, PhD, MD; Madonna Fernandez-Frackelton, MD, FACEP; Colleen Fluharty, MD; Scott C. Gibson, MD, FACEP; Ved V. Gossain, MD, FACP, FACE; David A. Hartman, MD, FACEP; Bryan S. Judge, MD; Ingrid T. Lim, MD; Michelle Lin, MD; Stephen J. Liu, MD; Nathan J. McKeown, DO; Bruce W. Nugent, MD; Julia L. Pasquale, MD; John Sarko, MD; Robert C. Satonik, MD; Jason M. Schenck, MD; Karen Sorensen, Acquisitions Editor; Matthew C. Tews, DO; Susan P. Torrey, MD, FACEP; Mary Jo Wagner, MD, FACEP; and, Robert W. Wolford, MD, MMM.

Disclosure of discussion of non-FDA approved uses for pharmaceutical products and/or medical devices: The University of Virginia School of Medicine, as an ACCME provider, requires that all authors/editors identify and disclose any "off label" uses for pharmaceutical products and/or for medical devices. The University of Virginia School of Medicine recommends that each reader fully review all the available data on new products or procedures prior to instituting them with patients.

All authors who provided disclosures have indicated that they will not be discussing off-label uses except:
Ilene Claudius, MD will discuss the use of ammonia lowering productes for organic acidemias.
Colleen Fluharty, MD will discuss the use of bisphosphonates in the treatment of Vit D toxicity & PTH-mediated hypercalemia. This has not been well studied and is likely not FDA approved (in the article it is mentioned for discussion, not recommended).
John Sarko, MD - Furosemide: used to lower serum calcium levels in hypercalcemic patients. Etidronate: used to lower serum calcium levels in hypercalcemic patients. Pamidronate: used to lower serum calcium levels in hypercalcemic patients who do not have hypercalcemia of malignancy. Mithramycin: used to lower serum calcium levels in hypercalcemic patients who do not have hypercalcemia of malignancy.

The following authors have not provided disclosure or off-label information.
Andrew M. Bazakis, MD, FACEP; Kathleen Cowling, DO, MS, FACEP; Catherine Kunzler, DO; Timothy J. Schaefer, MD; and, Sid M. Shah, MD, FACEP.

TO ENROLL

To enroll in the Emergency Medicine Clinics of North America Continuing Medical Education program, call customer service at 1-800-654-2452 or visit us online at www.theclinics.com/home/cme. The CME program is available to subscribers for an additional fee of $165.00

ELSEVIER
SAUNDERS

EMERGENCY
MEDICINE
CLINICS OF
NORTH AMERICA

Emerg Med Clin N Am 23 (2005) xv–xvi

Preface

Endocrine and Metabolic Emergencies

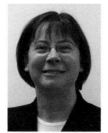 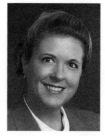

Mary Jo Wagner, MD, FACEP   Kathleen Cowling, DO, MS, FACEP
Guest Editors

Endocrinology and metabolism often have been viewed as just biochemistry topics, more theoretical than practical, that were to be memorized in medical school. In fact, mastery of this field is essential for the effective practice of emergency medicine. This issue is designed to make the knowledge of this field become more pertinent and accessible to emergency physicians. While including the pathophysiology that is necessary for understanding basic details, each article emphasizes the emergency department presentation, diagnostic evaluation, and immediate therapeutic approach to the patient who presents with a metabolic problem.

One of the goals of the editors was to address topics not often covered in emergency medicine textbooks. Original subjects like the approach to anabolic steroids and fuel metabolism in light of today's fitness and diet crazes are two timely topics in emergency medicine. Some articles challenge long-standing dogma in emergency medicine, such as the conventional practice of using sodium bicarbonate for every patient with hyperkalemia. The current emphasis on monitoring and treating hyperglycemia in critical care patients also is examined.

Finally, the editors have tested these articles in their own practice in the emergency department. For instance, while caring for a 3-day-old infant with hypoglycemia, the editors followed the step-by-step list in the newborn and childhood metabolic crisis article. This clear, concise guide helped differentiate the concerns raised about this patient who was treated appropriately. The simplified logical work-up of a patient with hyponatremia is also comprehensive and efficient. The editors have put an emphasis on the use of reference tables for critical areas, to make it easy to use the text as a bedside resource.

This issue of *Emergency Medicine Clinics of North America* will provide some interesting reading and many useful tips for treating patients in the emergency department. The editors would like to thank the article authors for their time, dedication, and interest in this collaborative effort. The editors would especially like to thank their families for their patience and support of this work, with extra gratitude given to Diane Wagner for her many helpful suggestions.

Mary Jo Wagner, MD, FACEP
Program Director
Synergy Medical Education Alliance/
Michigan State University Emergency Medicine Residency
1000 Houghton Avenue
Saginaw, Michigan 48602, USA

Program in Emergency Medicine
Michigan State University College of Human Medicine
Lansing, Michigan

E-mail address: mjwagner@synergymedical.org

Kathleen Cowling, DO, MS, FACEP
Assistant Clinical Professor
Program in Emergency Medicine
Michigan State University College of Human Medicine
Lansing, Michigan

Emergency Physician
Emergency Care Center
Covenant HealthCare
900 Cooper Avenue
Saginaw, Michigan 48602, USA

E-mail address: cowling911@yahoo.com

ELSEVIER
SAUNDERS

EMERGENCY
MEDICINE
CLINICS OF
NORTH AMERICA

Emerg Med Clin N Am 23 (2005) 609–628

Diabetic Ketoacidosis

Michelle A. Charfen, MD[a,b],
Madonna Fernández-Frackelton, MD, FACEP[a,b],*

[a]David Geffen School of Medicine at University of California-Los Angeles,
405 Hilgard Avenue Los Angeles, CA 90095, USA
[b]Department of Emergency Medicine,
Harbor-University of California-Los Angeles Medical Center,
1000 West Carson Street, Box 21, Torrance CA, 90509, USA

Diabetic ketoacidosis (DKA) and hyperosmolar hyperglycemic syndrome (HHS) are the most serious and life-threatening complications of diabetes. Although significant overlap exists between these two entities, this article addresses issues specific to DKA. DKA is a syndrome characterized by hyperglycemia, ketosis, and acidosis. It occurs as the result of a relative or absolute insulin deficiency and an excess of insulin counter-regulatory hormones (ICRH) [1].

History and epidemiology

The earliest documented description of diabetes was found in a 1552 BC Egyptian papyrus [2]. In 1886, Dreschfeld provided the first description of diabetic ketoacidosis in the modern medical literature [3]. In 1971, Roger Unger described DKA as a bihormonal disorder involving insulin deficiency and glucagon excess [4].

Before the discovery of insulin by Dr. Frederick Banting in 1921, the mortality of DKA was 100%. After this landmark discovery and the institution of insulin therapy, the mortality began to decrease significantly. Currently, mortality is approximately 4% to 10% [5,6]. The incidence of DKA is between 4.6 and 8.0 per 1000 person-years among patients with diabetes [6]. DKA most commonly occurs in patients with insulin-dependent diabetes but may also occur in patients with noninsulin-dependent diabetes. The treatment of DKA episodes accounts for more than 25% of all health

---

* Corresponding author.
E-mail address: fernandez@emedharbor.edu (M. Fernández-Frackelton).

0733-8627/05/$ - see front matter © 2005 Elsevier Inc. All rights reserved.
doi:10.1016/j.emc.2005.03.009
emed.theclinics.com

care dollars spent on direct medical care for patients with type I diabetes, and for 50% of every $2 for patients experiencing multiple episodes of DKA [7]. Annually, approximately 100,000 hospitalizations for DKA occur in the United States [6], with overall costs that exceed $1 billion per year [7].

Emergency department presentation

Precipitating factors

The most common precipitating factor in DKA is infection [8], with pneumonia and urinary tract infections accounting for 30% to 50% of cases [7]. Recent studies suggest that omission of insulin or undertreatment with insulin may be the most important precipitating factor in urban African-American populations [7,9,10]. New-onset diabetics account for up to 30% of patients presenting in DKA [6]. Other precipitating factors include cerebrovascular accident, alcohol abuse, pancreatitis, gastrointestinal (GI) bleeding, myocardial infarction, trauma, or drugs [11]. Medications that affect carbohydrate metabolism such as corticosteroids, thiazide diuretics, and sympathomimetic agents may precipitate DKA [8]. Psychological stress also causes an increase in insulin counter-regulatory hormones, and may precipitate DKA. In 2% to 10% of patients, no precipitating cause is identified [1].

History

Patients with DKA often complain of nonspecific symptoms such as fatigue and malaise. Complaints of polyuria, polydipsia, polyphagia, and weight loss are more characteristic of DKA. Nausea, vomiting and abdominal pain are also common complaints and are caused by either the acidosis itself, or to decreased mesenteric perfusion. Up to 25% of patients in DKA have emesis, which may have a coffee ground appearance. Endoscopic studies have related this finding to hemorrhagic gastritis [8]. Patients may present with depressed mental status or coma, and in these cases, the physician should attempt to illicit a history of antecedent symptoms from a family member when possible. A thorough review of systems should be performed, as specific complaints suggesting a possible source of infection or other precipitating factors may be elucidated.

The use of prescription and illicit drugs should be noted. Insulin omission or underdosing and the use of drugs that affect carbohydrate metabolism such as corticosteroids, thiazide diuretics, terbutaline, and cocaine can contribute to DKA [12,13].

Pathophysiology

The basic metabolic derangements in DKA arise secondary to a relative lack of insulin and an excess in insulin counter-regulatory hormones (ICRH).

Even in the absence of changes in insulin administration, ICRHs are elevated during times of stress and may outweigh the effects of insulin. This leads to catabolic disturbances in the metabolism of carbohydrates, protein, and fat, which collectively culminate in the two cardinal features of diabetic ketoacidosis, hyperglycemia, and ketogenesis (Fig. 1).

Hyperglycemia

The hyperglycemia seen in DKA results from a combination of glucose underuse and overproduction. Insulin promotes the uptake and storage of glucose in the liver through glycogenesis (incorporation of glucose into glycogen) and lipogenesis (formation of fatty acids). Insulin is necessary for the uptake of glucose into muscle and fat cells. In the absence of adequate insulin, the body is unable to use or store circulating glucose, and ICRH levels increase. The ICRHs include glucagon, catecholamines, cortisol, and growth hormone. In DKA, glucagon becomes the primary hormone driving carbohydrate metabolism, stimulating hepatic glycogenolysis (breakdown of glycogen to glucose) and gluconeogenesis (glucose production from noncarbohydrate precursors). Although both increased hepatic glucose production and decreased peripheral glucose use occur in DKA, the major cause of the hyperglycemia is increased hepatic gluconeogenesis [5]. Hyperglycemia leads to glycosuria, osmotic diuresis, and dehydration. As a result of the osmotic diuresis, large amounts of sodium, chloride, and potassium are lost in the urine, resulting in the dehydration and electrolyte abnormalities commonly seen in DKA [5].

Ketogenesis

In the presence of insulin, triglycerides are incorporated into fat cells, and breakdown and release of triglycerides from fat cells are inhibited. In DKA, the combined relative insulin deficiency and ICRH excess promote the breakdown of triglycerides and the release of free fatty acids into the blood. Insulin deficiency is primarily responsible for the mobilization of free fatty acids, while the presence of glucagon is primarily responsible for accelerated fatty acid oxidation. Glucagon exerts its effects by acting on the carnitine palmitoyltransferase system of enzymes responsible for the transport of fatty acids into the mitochondria [14] and by inhibiting conversion of acetyl CoA to malonyl CoA by acetyl CoA carboxylase, the first intermediate in the lipogenesis pathway. Because lipogenesis is blocked, fatty acids are unable to enter the citric acid cycle and instead enter the mitochondria, where they are oxidized further to ketone bodies [7]. The major ketone bodies are acetoacetate and β-hydroxybutyrate, with acetone contributing a minor component. Ketone bodies are weak acids, but as they accumulate, they overwhelm the body's buffering capacity, and metabolic acidosis ensues [1].

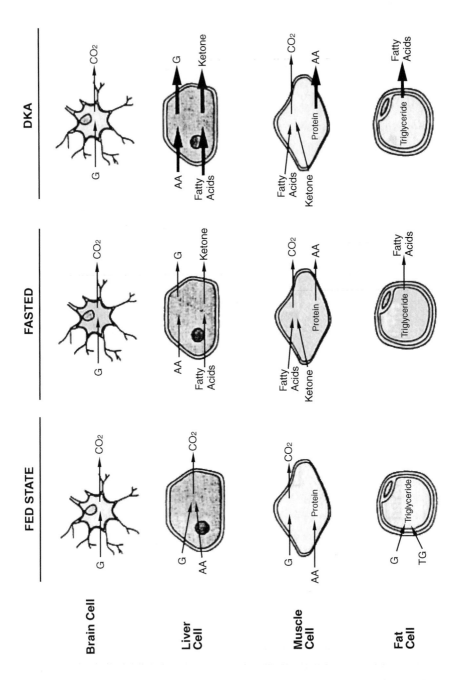

Differential diagnosis

Other causes of ketosis and acidosis should be considered in patients presenting with DKA. Both starvation ketosis and alcoholic ketoacidosis (AKA) can be distinguished from DKA by clinical history and a blood glucose that ranges from mildly elevated (rarely greater than 250 mg/dL) to hypoglycemic. In patients with starvation ketosis, the serum bicarbonate level is usually not lower than 18 mEq/L, while patients with AKA may exhibit a profound acidosis [8]. AKA usually is seen in the setting of alcohol abuse with recent decreased consumption of alcohol [15].

Other causes of elevated anion gap metabolic acidosis should be considered, including lactic acidosis, chronic renal insufficiency, and ingestion of drugs such as salicylate, methanol, ethylene glycol, and paraldehyde [8] (Fig. 2). Drug ingestion history should be sought, including use of metformin, which, in rare cases, may cause lactic acidosis [16]. Some authors question the causality of the relationship of metformin use with lactic acidosis [17,18]. In the appropriate clinical situation, measurement of serum lactate, salicylate, and blood methanol level may be helpful. If concern for ethylene glycol (antifreeze) ingestion exists, the urine can be examined for calcium oxalate and hippurate crystals. Paraldehyde ingestion is suggested by characteristic strong unpleasant odor on the breath [8].

In the hyperglycemic patient, the diagnosis of HHS always must be considered. Table 1 shows a comparison of the laboratory findings in HHS and DKA.

Emergency department evaluation

Physical exam findings

The general appearance of patients with DKA is one of fatigue and dehydration. Tachycardia and hypotension may be present as a result of volume depletion, sepsis or both. The patient may be tachypneic with Kussmaul respirations. This pattern of deep, sighing respirations is an attempt to compensate for the metabolic acidosis and may or may not be accompanied by an increased respiratory rate. Patients may be normothermic or hypothermic despite accompanying infection. Hypothermia is caused primarily by peripheral vasodilation [8]. A fruity odor often is appreciated on the patient's breath because of the presence of exhaled acetone. Patients may have a depressed sensorium, and, in severe cases, may present

Fig. 1. Substrate utilization in the fed and fasting states and in diabetic ketoacidosis in insulin-insensitive tissue (brain cells) and in insulin-sensitive tissue (live, muscle, and fat). *Abbreviations:* G, glucose; AA, amino acid; TG, triglyceride. (*Adapted from* Cahill GF. Pathophysiology of diabetes. In: Hanwi GJ, Danowski TS, editors. Diabetes mellitus: diagnosis and treatment. New York: American Diabetes Association; 1967. p. 1–6; with permission.)

Other Hyperglycemic States
Diabetes Mellitus
Non-Ketotic Hyperosmolar Coma
Impaired Glucose Tolerance
Stress Hyperglycemia

Other Ketotic States
Ketotic Hypoglycemia
Alcoholic Ketosis
Starvation Ketosis

Other Metabolic Acidotic States
Lactic Acidosis
Hyperchloremic Acidosis
Salicylism
Uremic Acidosis
Drug-Induced Acidosis

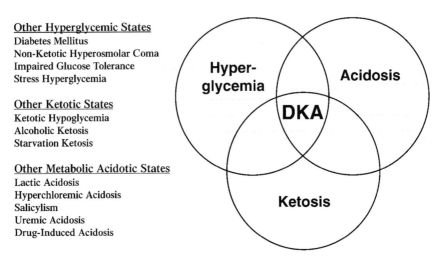

Fig. 2. The triad of DKA (hyperglycemia, acidemia, and ketonemia) and other conditions with which the individual components are associated. (*From* Kitabchi AE, Wall BM. Diabetic ketoacidosis. Med Clin North Am 1995;70(1):9–37; with permission.)

comatose. Skin examination reveals <u>poor turgor</u>, and mucous membranes are typically dry secondary to dehydration. The abdomen is often diffusely tender. Careful palpation for localizing tenderness should be performed, as an intra-abdominal pathology may be the precipitating factor for DKA.

The physical examination should include a thorough attempt to find a precipitating cause. Fewer than 10% of patients with DKA have no identifiable precipitant of the disease [1]. The sinuses should be palpated for

Table 1
Diagnostic criteria for diabetic ketoacidosis and hyperosmolar hyperglycemic syndrome

| | DKA | | | |
	Mild	Moderate	Severe	HHS
Plasma Glucose (mg/dL)	> 250	> 250	> 250	> 600
Arterial pH	7.25–7.30	7.00–7.24	< 7.00	< 7.30
Serum bicorbonate (mEq/L)	15–18	10 to < 15	< 10	> 15
Urine ketones[a]	Positive	Positive	Positive	Small
Serum ketones[a]	Positive	Positive	Positive	Small
Effective serum osmolality (mOsm/kg)[b]	Variable	Variable	Variable	> 320
Anion gap[c]	> 10	> 12	> 12	Variable
Alteration in sensorial or mental obtundation	Alert	Alert/drowsy	Stupor/coma	Stupor/coma

[a] Nitroprusside reaction method.
[b] Calculation: 2 [measured Na (mEq/L)] + glucose (mg/dL)/18.
[c] Calculation: (Na) – (Cl + HCO₃) (mEq/L).
From Kitabchi AE, Umpierrez GE, Murphy MB, et al. Hyperglycemic crisis in diabetes. Diabetes Care 2004;27:S94–102; with permission.

tenderness and the oral cavity explored for signs of dental infection. The ears should be examined for signs of otitis media or externa. The skin should be examined thoroughly for signs of infection such as abscess, cellulitis, or decubitus ulcers. A rectal examination should be performed looking for possible perirectal abscess or occult GI hemorrhage. In the female patient with abdominal pain, pelvic examination should be performed. A complete neurological examination should be performed on patients with altered mental status or localizing neurological complaints.

Laboratory evaluation

Serum glucose, ketones, electrolytes, serum urea nitrogen (BUN), and creatinine always should be ordered in suspected DKA. Although the serum glucose usually is elevated above 250 mg/dL, euglycemic DKA has been reported in up to 18% of cases [19]. Normoglycemia also may occur in patients who took insulin before presentation or have impaired gluconeogenesis caused by liver failure or alcohol abuse [1].

Hyperglycemia exerts an osmotic affect in the serum, shifting water from the intracellular to the extracellular space, creating a dilutional effect and resultant hyponatremia. The serum sodium therefore may be low despite total body water loss. The corrected serum sodium can be calculated by adding 1.6 mEq/L to the sodium for every 100 mg/dL glucose over the norm. (Table 2) Lipids also dilute the blood in a similar fashion, causing pseudohyponatremia [7,8]. Newer autoanalyzers remove triglycerides before this assay, eliminating this artifact in hyperlipidemia, but not hyperglycemia [19].

Initial serum potassium values are usually normal to high despite significant total body potassium depletion. There is a shift of intracellular potassium to the extracellular space as a result of insulin deficiency, hypertonicity, and acidemia [8]. Insulin carries glucose intracellularly with potassium and magnesium. Therefore, insulin deficiency contributes to the serum hyperkalemia. To buffer the serum acidosis, hydrogen ions move from the extracellular space to the intracellular space in exchange for

Table 2
Useful formulas in diabetic ketoacidosis

Anion gap	$[Na - (CL + HCO_3)]$
Correction of serum sodium	Measured $[Na] + \dfrac{[1.6 \text{ glucose (mg/dL)} - 100]}{100}$
Serum osmolality (mOsm/L)	$2\,[Na + K]\,(mEq/L) + glucose\,(mg/dL)/18 + BUN(mg/dL)/2.8$
Effective serum osmolality	$2\,[Na\,(mEq/L)] + glucose\,(mg/dL)/18$
Total body water deficit (L)	$0.6 \times wt(kg) \times [1 - 140/\text{serum sodium}]$
Correction of serum potassium during acidemia	$[K] + (0.6 \text{ mEq/L per } 0.1 \text{ drop in pH})$

potassium ions. To correct for the effects of acidemia on serum potassium, add 0.6 mEq/L to the measured serum potassium for every 0.1 drop in pH on the arterial blood gas (ABG) (see Table 2) [20,21].

The serum bicarbonate level is decreased to varying degrees depending on the severity of the DKA: (see Table 1) 15 to 18 mmol/L in mild DKA, 10 to 14 mmol/L in moderate and less than 10 mmol/L in severe DKA [8].

Diabetic ketoacidosis causes an elevated anion gap metabolic acidosis secondary to increased β-hydroxybutyrate and acetone levels. Rarely, a well-hydrated patient with DKA may have a pure hyperchloremic acidosis and no anion gap [19]. To calculate the anion gap, subtract the serum chloride and bicarbonate from the measured serum sodium (see Table 2). A superimposed metabolic alkalosis from vomiting or diuretic use may obscure the severity of ketoacidosis. Traditionally, an ABG has been considered part of the standard initial work-up. Recent studies have shown that the ABG rarely influences emergency department (ED) management and that the venous pH correlates sufficiently with the arterial pH [22].

Leukocytosis is often present and may be secondary to hemoconcentration, ketosis, or infection. This is a nonspecific finding and may be associated with other precipitating factors of DKA such as pancreatitis and myocardial infarction. The total white blood cell count is generally less than $25,000/mm^3$ in the absence of bacterial infection [5]. An elevation in band form neutrophils has been demonstrated to indicate infection with 100% sensitivity and 80% specificity [23].

Amylase is elevated in most patients with DKA. In one study, 79% of patients in DKA had hyperamylasemia, with 48% having pancreatic type amylase [24]. This is typically subclinical and may represent effects of hypertonicity or hypoperfusion [25]. If patients have persistent abdominal pain after the treatment of DKA, consider further evaluation. Most laboratories are not equipped to differentiate between pancreatic and salivary isoenzymes [19]. Lipase is a more sensitive and specific indicator of pancreatitis, although this also may be elevated in DKA [8].

A urinalysis should be performed on all patients to screen for urinary tract infection. Urine ketones and glucose will be present.

A pregnancy test should be performed on all females of childbearing age. Other laboratory evaluation should be performed based on the review of systems and physical examination findings.

Emergency department management

The management of DKA should include intravenous fluid hydration, insulin administration, and electrolyte replacement. The presence of infection or other precipitating factors will determine whether other specific treatments are necessary. Admission and frequent monitoring are indicated to minimize the possibility of iatrogenic complications from the treatment of

DKA. Serum glucose should be checked hourly, and serum electrolytes should be repeated every 2 to 4 hours to assess the efficacy of therapy.

Intravenous fluids

The primary goal in the initial management of DKA is to restore intravascular volume and improve tissue perfusion. This will decrease ICRH levels and glucose concentration [1]. Fluid replacement alone may decrease serum glucose concentration by as much as 23% through increased renal perfusion and loss of glucose in the urine [1,26].

The use of intravenous fluid replacement in the management of DKA is supported by well-designed trials that have adequate power, and meta-analysis of the literature further supports the conclusion [11]. Although all authors agree that fluid replacement is essential in DKA, there is no uniformly accepted formula for administration. Initial intravenous fluids should be given rapidly to achieve hemodynamic stability, then decreased to a rate that allows for replacement of the total deficit over a 24-hour period. The total body water (TBW) deficit in these patients is usually 5 to 8 L. See Table 2 for TBW deficit calculation. The goal in fluid administration is to replace approximately 50% of the TBW deficit in the first 8 hours and the remainder in the subsequent 16 hours. The initial fluid of choice is normal saline (0.9% sodium chloride) with 1 to 2 L administered in the first hour. The subsequent choice for fluid replacement depends on the patient's hydration status, serum electrolytes levels, and urinary output [8]. The 2004 Position Statement of the American Diabetes Association (ADA) recommends that, after the initial fluid bolus, the corrected serum sodium should be calculated and used to determine further fluid replacement. If the corrected serum sodium is high or normal, replacement with 0.45% NaCl, 4 to 14 mL/kg per hour (depending on the state of hydration), is recommended. If the corrected serum sodium is low, continued replacement with 0.9% NaCl, 4-14 mL/kg/h, (depending on the hydration status) is recommended [8].

One approach is to start with 0.9% NaCl 1 to 2 L bolus, followed by an infusion rate of 0.9% NaCl 500 mL per hour until hemodynamically stable. Then the rate is decreased to 250 mL per hour and can be switched to half-normal saline to replace the large free water deficit [1].

When the blood glucose level falls below 250 mg/dL, a solution of 5% dextrose should be added to the intravenous fluids. This allows for continued administration of insulin to treat the ketosis and acidosis without causing hypoglycemia. The serum glucose should be maintained between 150 and 200 mg/dL until the ketoacidosis has resolved [8]. Dextrose combinations may be increased to 10% or 20% if glucose levels remain below 100 mg/dL. One efficient and cost-effective method is to use two bags of fluid with the same electrolyte content but different glucose concentrations [1,27]. One bag contains no dextrose, and the other contains

20% dextrose. The rates of infusion can be adjusted to deliver anywhere from 0% to 20% dextrose.

Special care should be taken to avoid overhydration in children, patients with cardiac or renal compromise, and elders with DKA. The lung sounds and oxygenation should be assessed frequently. In children, mental status should be evaluated frequently, as deterioration in mental status may be the first sign of cerebral edema [8]. This will be discussed further in the section on complications.

Insulin

Insulin therapy will improve the hyperglycemia, ketosis, and acidosis that occur in DKA [1]. Insulin therapy inhibits gluconeogenesis and ketone production in the liver and decreases lipolysis. The use of insulin by intravenous infusion is supported by randomized, controlled trials that have adequate power, and meta-analysis of the data further supports this conclusion [11].

Insulin therapy is secondary to intravenous fluid replacement and should be withheld initially in patients with hypotension and hypokalemia. In hypotensive patients, the administration of insulin can lead to vascular collapse secondary to rapid shifts of fluid into the intracellular space. Insulin should not be initiated until the blood pressure is stabilized with fluid administration [1]. Hypokalemic patients should not receive insulin until potassium has been administered, as the insulin-mediated movement of potassium into the intracellular compartment will worsen the hypokalemia. Insulin therapy should not be initiated until serum potassium is over 3.3 mEq/L [8].

A standard insulin regimen consists of regular insulin intravenous drip at 0.1 U/kg per hour. Some authors recommend an initial intravenous bolus of regular insulin 0.10 to 0.15 U/kg [8], but there are no data to support any clinical benefit [11]. Because insulin adsorbs to intravenous tubing, 50 mL of the infusion should be run through the pump before beginning the infusion [28]. The blood glucose level should be monitored hourly, with a goal of decreasing the glucose by approximately 50 to 75 mg/dL per hour [8]. If serum glucose does not decrease appropriately, and adequate hydration has been ensured, the insulin drip may be doubled every hour [8]. If serum glucose is not falling appropriately, consider inadequate intravascular volume replacement or the development of renal failure as potential causes.

Once the blood sugar falls below 250 mg/dL, glucose should be added to the intravenous fluids as previously discussed. The insulin drip should be continued until resolution of ketosis and improvement in the acidosis. Ketosis should be monitored by serum β-hydroxybutyrate. Urinary ketones are measured by the nitroprusside reaction, which measures acetoacetate and acetone but not β-hydroxybutyrate [1]. With treatment of DKA, β-hydroxybutyrate is converted to acetoacetate, and urinary measurements may give the false impression that ketosis is worsening [8]. Criteria for the resolution of DKA also includes glucose less than 200 mg/dL, serum bicarbonate at least 18 mmol/L, and a venous pH greater than 7.3 [8]. In a study using an extended insulin regimen, all patients had complete resolution of their ketosis by 7 hours after achieving normoglycemia [29]. This suggests that using 7 hours of continuous insulin infusion after normoglycemia would allow for complete resolution of ketosis [1].

Once ketosis has resolved, the patient should be given his or her first dose of subcutaneous insulin. Two hours after this first dose, the insulin drip may be discontinued. It is important that the insulin drip be continued for 2 hours after the initiation of subcutaneous insulin, because hyperglycemia may recur rapidly with interruptions in insulin administration [1].

In mild DKA, regular insulin can be given subcutaneously or intramuscularly every hour. Patients should first receive a priming dose of regular insulin 0.4 to 0.6 U/kg, half as an intravenous bolus and half as either subcutaneous or intramuscular injection [8]. This should be followed by 0.1 U/kg per hour subcutaneously or intramuscularly. In the critically ill patient with DKA, insulin never should be given subcutaneously because of decreased medication absorption in the hypotensive patient [7].

Potassium

The use of electrolyte replacement in the management of DKA is supported by well-designed trials that have adequate power, and meta-analysis of the data further support the conclusion [11].

Potassium is the major electrolyte lost in DKA. Despite total body potassium depletion, mild-to-moderate hyperkalemia is common. This is secondary to an extracellular shift of potassium caused by insulin deficiency, hypertonicity, and acidemia [8]. During the treatment of DKA, serum potassium levels are decreased by insulin-mediated movement of potassium into the intracellular compartment and to a lesser extent by volume expansion and resolution of acidemia [5]. There is also ongoing potassium loss through a continued osmotic diuresis. The potential development of significant hypokalemia is the most life-threatening electrolyte abnormality that may occur during the treatment of DKA [8]. Before potassium administration, adequate urine output must be ensured. To prevent hypokalemia, the ADA recommends potassium replacement once serum levels fall below 5.5 mEq/L [5,8]. Generally, 20 to 30 mEq potassium in each liter of fluid is sufficient to maintain the serum potassium in the goal range of 4.0 to 5.0 mEq/L [5,8]. Others recommend withholding potassium until serum levels drop below 5.0, then giving 20 mEq/L if serum potassium is between 4 and 5 mEq/L, 30 to 40 mEq/L if serum potassium is between 3 and 4 mEq/L, and 40 to 60 mEq/L if serum levels are less than 3 mEq/L [1]. Tables 3 and 4 summarize approaches to potassium replacement in adult and pediatric patients, respectively.

Table 3
Potassium replacement in adult diabetic ketoacidosis

Initial potassium	Replacement

K < 3.3 mEq/L hold insulin until
  K ≥ 3.3 mEq/L
	*KCl 40 mEq in first hour, then 20–30 mEq/h
	  to keep serum K between 4–5 mEq/L

K ≥ 3.3 but <5.0 mEq/L	*KCl 20–30 mEq/L of IVF to keep serum K between 4–5 mEq/L
K > 5.0 mEq/L	Do not give K but check potassium levels every 2 hours

Abbreviations: K, potassium; KCl, potassium chloride; mEq, milliequivalents; IVF, intravenous fluids.

* Kitabchi et al recommend replacing one third of the potassium as potassium phosphate to avoid excessive chloride administration and to prevent severe hypophosphatemia.

Adapted from Kitabchi AE, Umpierrez GE, Murphy MB, et al. Management of hyperglycemic crises in patients with diabetes. Diabetes Care 2001:24(1):131–53.

Bicarbonate

The use of bicarbonate for managing DKA is not well supported in the literature [11]. The potential disadvantages of bicarbonate therapy include worsening hypokalemia, production of paradoxical central nervous system (CNS) acidosis, worsening of intracellular acidosis owing to increased carbon dioxide production, and prolongation of ketoanion metabolism [5].

Studies have shown no benefit of bicarbonate therapy for managing DKA [30–32]. These studies have looked at patients with serum pH ranging from 6.9 to 7.1. Because studies have not been done in patients with a pH of less than 6.9, some authors continue to advocate the use of bicarbonate in these severely acidemic patients. If acidosis is severe (pH less than 7.0), bicarbonate may be used to treat the possible adverse hemodynamic effects caused by severe acidemia. These include negative inotropism, CNS

Table 4
Potassium replacement in pediatric diabetic ketoacidosis

Initial potassium	Replacement

K < 2.5 mEq/L, hold insulin until
  K ≥ 3.3 mEq/L
	[a]KCl 10 mEq in first hour, recheck serum
	  K after one hour

K 2.5–3.5 mEq/L	[b]KCl 40–60 mEq/L of IVF until K > 3.5 mEq/L
K 3.5–5.5 mEq/L	[b]KCl 30–40 mEq/L of IVF to keep serum K between 3.5–5 mEq/L
K > 5.5 mEq/L	Do not give K, but check potassium levels every hour until < 5.5 mEq/L

Abbreviations: K, potassium; KCl, potassium chloride; mEq, milliequivalents; IVF, intravenous fluids.

[a] Kitabchi et al recommend replacing one third of the potassium as potassium phosphate to avoid excessive chloride administration and to prevent severe hypophosphatemia.

[b] Fluid should be run at 1.5 times maintenance for smooth rehydration.

Adapted from Kitabchi AE, Umpierrez GE, Murphy MB, et al. Management of hyperglycemic crises in patients with diabetes. Diabetes Care 2001:24(1):131–53.

depression, peripheral vasodilation, and insulin resistance [1]. If bicarbonate is used, it should be given as an isotonic solution over a 1-hour period. This can be done by adding 1 to 2 ampules (44 to 88 mEq sodium bicarbonate) to a liter of 0.45% NaCl [1,5,8].

Phosphate

Phosphate replacement has no benefit for most patients with DKA [5]. In certain groups of patients, phosphate replacement may be indicated to avoid cardiac dysfunction, skeletal muscle weakness, and respiratory depression [8]. These include patients with cardiac dysfunction, anemia, respiratory depression, and those with serum phosphate levels less than 1.0 g/dL [8]. Hypophosphatemia causes the depletion of 2,3-diphosphoglycerate (2,3-GPD), resulting in a left shift of the oxyhemoglobin curve, resulting in decreased tissue oxygenation [33]. Replacement of phosphate in patients with impaired oxygen carrying capacity may enhance tissue oxygen delivery. When phosphate replacement is indicated, 20 to 30 mEq/L potassium phosphate can be added to fluids [8]. Replacement of phosphate in patients with levels less than 1.0 g/dL is indicated and supported by randomized controlled trials with adequate power [11].

Emergency department management of diabetic ketoacidosis in the pediatric population (younger than 20 years of age) [8]

Intravenous fluids

Caution must be used with fluid replacement in pediatric DKA patients given the possible risk for cerebral edema associated with rapid fluid administration. In the first hour, intravenous fluid should be isotonic saline at a rate of 10 to 20 mL/kg per hour. This may need to be repeated in the severely dehydrated patient, but initial re-expansion should not exceed 50 mL/kg over the first 4 hours of therapy. Further fluid replacement should be calculated to replace the fluid deficit over 48 hours. In general 0.45 to 0.9% NaCl (depending on serum sodium concentration) at a rate of 1.5 times maintenance requirements (approx 5 mL/kg per hour) will accomplish a safe rehydration. Once serum glucose reaches 250 mg/dL, fluid should be changed to 5% dextrose and 0.45 to 0.75% NaCl with potassium [8].

Insulin

An initial intravenous insulin bolus is not recommended in pediatric patients. Regular insulin infusion at a dose of 0.1 U/kg per hour is recommended. Insulin therapy should not be started until adequate potassium levels are ensured to avoid cardiac arrhythmias associated with hypokalemia [8].

Bicarbonate

There are no randomized studies assessing the use of bicarbonate in pediatric patients with DKA with a pH of less than 6.9. Caution should be used when administering bicarbonate, as an association between bicarbonate use and cerebral edema has been reported [34]. Despite the decrease in use of bicarbonate in pediatric patients with DKA over the last 10 years, however, there has not been a corresponding reduction in the incidence of cerebral edema [35]. The use of bicarbonate should be reserved for children with severe circulatory failure caused by profound acidosis. The ADA recommends the use of bicarbonate if the pH remains less than 7.0 after the initial hour of hydration. If given, bicarbonate can be administered as 1 to 2 mEq/kg added to NaCl with any required potassium to produce a solution that does not exceed 155 mEq/L [8].

Complications of diabetic ketoacidosis

Most complications of DKA are related to the treatment. The most common complications include hypoglycemia, hypokalemia, hyperglycemia, and hyperchloremia [8]. Less common complications include cerebral edema, fluid overload, acute respiratory distress syndrome, thromboembolism, and acute gastric dilation.

Hypoglycemia

Hypoglycemia may occur secondary to overzealous administration of insulin [8]. The occurrence of hypoglycemia during the treatment of DKA often is associated with high-dose (1 U/kg per hour) insulin therapy but not with low-dose (0.1 U/kg per hour) insulin therapy. The risk of hypoglycemia can be reduced by adding dextrose to the intravenous fluid therapy when the blood glucose falls below 250 mg/dL [1,8]. This allows the continued administration of insulin to resolve ketoacidosis while decreasing the risk of hypoglycemia.

Hypokalemia

Hypokalemia may develop secondary to treatment with insulin and bicarbonate [8]. The occurrence of hypokalemia is less common with low-dose insulin regimens [5].

To avoid hypokalemia, insulin should not be administered until the serum potassium level is known. Potassium should be replaced as discussed in the treatment section.

Hyperglycemia

Hyperglycemia often occurs secondary to interruption or discontinuation of intravenous insulin therapy without proper administration of subcutaneous doses of insulin [8].

Hyperchloremia

Patients may develop a nonanion gap metabolic acidosis as a result of excessive saline administration. Chloride replaces ketoanions lost as sodium and potassium salts during osmotic diuresis. These abnormalities are usually transient and clinically insignificant except in cases of acute renal failure or extreme oliguria [8].

Cerebral edema

Cerebral edema is a rare but frequently fatal complication of DKA that primarily occurs in pediatric patients. In the largest reported series, 95% of cases occurred in patients younger than 20 years, with one third occurring in patients younger than 5 years [36]. The incidence of cerebral edema in children with DKA is between 0.7% and 1% [8,34,37]. It is more common in patients with newly diagnosed diabetes [36,37] and is the most common cause of death in young children with diabetes [38]. The mortality rate according to different series has varied widely, with reports between 24% and 90% [37,39].

The clinical presentation of cerebral edema is characterized by deterioration in the level of consciousness, with lethargy, decrease in arousal, and headache [1,8]. The timing of the development of cerebral edema is variable, with most cases occurring 4 to 12 hours after starting treatment. There have been several case reports of cerebral edema occurring before the initiation of therapy [39].

The pathophysiology of cerebral edema is understood poorly. Many mechanisms have been proposed, but a clear understanding remains elusive. Possible contributing factors include: (1) hypoxia, (2) the osmotically driven movement of water into the CNS when plasma osmolality declines too rapidly during the treatment of DKA, and (3) the direct effect of insulin on the plasma membrane of brain cells, which may promote cellular edema [1,8,39].

When cerebral edema develops, the treatment is aimed at reducing intracranial pressure. The data on effective treatments are limited to case reports. In these reports, mannitol has been used to lower intracranial pressure, and the authors recommend that it be administered within 5 to 10 minutes of initial neurological deterioration for maximum effect [39–41]. The dose of mannitol is 1 to 2 g/kg over 15 minutes. Intracranial pressure monitoring and hypoventilation started immediately after cerebral edema is suspected have been reported to improve outcome [39,42–44]. The role of dexamethasone and diuretics has not been established [11,39]. Further study is needed in this area.

Preventive measures that might decrease the risk of cerebral edema in high-risk patients are:

- Gradual replacement of sodium and water deficits in patients who are hyperosmolar (maximal reduction in osmolality of 3 mOsm/kg H_2O per hour)
- Avoidance of bicarbonate administration unless absolutely necessary
- The addition of dextrose to the intravenous fluid therapy once blood glucose reaches 250 mg/dL [8]

Fluid overload

Patients with underlying cardiac disease or renal insufficiency who receive excess fluid or excessively rapid administration of fluid may develop congestive heart failure. Administer intravenous fluids at a slower rate and frequently monitor fluid input and output in patients with underlying cardiac disease or renal insufficiency [1].

Acute respiratory distress syndrome

During the course of treatment for DKA, patients may develop cardiogenic and noncardiogenic pulmonary edema from excessive fluid replacement. ARDS is a rare but potentially fatal complication of DKA [1,5]. Patients with pulmonary rales and increased alveolar-to-arterial gradient may be at an increased risk of developing pulmonary edema and ARDS and should have continuous pulse oximetry monitoring [1,5,8,45]. In high-risk patients, lower rates of fluid administration should be used [5].

Thromboembolism

Diabetes mellitus is a hypercoagulable state. Subclinical endothelial injury, hypofibrinolysis, and platelet hyperaggregation are the main factors responsible for coagulation activation in diabetes mellitus [46–48]. In DKA, this hypercoagulable state is enhanced. In a study of 34 patients with DKA, hemostatic markers were measured during DKA and 1 week after resolution of DKA. During DKA patients were found to have coagulation system and platelet activation and endothelial injury. There was also a relative hypofibrinolysis during DKA [47].

Acute gastric dilation

Acute gastric dilation is a relatively uncommon but potentially lethal complication of DKA. In the patient with abdominal distension, other causes of intra-abdominal pathology should be excluded. A nasogastric tube can be placed as a diagnostic and therapeutic tool. Metoclopramide 10 mg intravenously every 6 hours may be helpful [1].

Disposition

No randomized prospective studies have evaluated the optimal site of care for patients with DKA. The decision concerning the site of care should be based on clinical prognostic indicators and availability of hospital resources [7].

Select patients with mild DKA may be discharged after treatment and observation in the ED. A study in the pediatric population found that 94% of patients with an initial pH of at least 7.20 or a bicarbonate concentration of at least 10 mEq/L had resolution of their metabolic acidosis within 3 hours of initiating therapy and were able to be discharged from the ED [49,50]. Patients must be alert and able to tolerate oral intake to be discharged from the ED.

Patients with moderate-to-severe DKA require admission to a bed where frequent monitoring is possible, hourly glucose measurements can be obtained, there is a rapid turnaround time for laboratory services, and nurses are able to administer intravenous insulin infusions. In most cases this requires admission to a step-down or intensive care unit (ICU). Admission to a ward bed may be possible if the hospital has a general ward unit where the following are in place:

- A protocol for managing DKA
- An on-site blood glucose monitoring system
- Available nursing coverage that allows for frequent patient monitoring and hourly glucose measurements
- A rapid turnaround of laboratory values [5,7]

Indications for admission to a step-down or ICU include: (1) pregnancy, (2) hypotension refractory to initial rehydration, (3) oliguria refractory to initial rehydration, (4) mental obtundation, and (5) sepsis [7].

Summary

In summary, DKA is a common complication of diabetes, and patients frequently present to the ED. The care of patients with DKA requires frequent and intensive monitoring. The following points should be remembered when assessing and treating these patients.

1. Perform a thorough history and physical examination in search of a precipitating cause.
2. A patient may present with DKA with a near normal glucose. This is more common in patients who have taken insulin recently, have

decreased food intake or impaired gluconeogenesis as can be seen in liver disease.

3. Consider other causes of anion gap metabolic acidosis.
4. Initial therapy consists of intravenous fluid administration. It is prudent to wait for adequate rehydration and serum potassium levels before starting insulin or potassium replacement therapy.
5. Frequent monitoring of glucose and electrolytes should guide further treatment.
6. Caution should be used in fluid administration in patients with cardiovascular and renal disease.
7. If abdominal pain does not resolve with initial treatment, consider evaluating for intra-abdominal pathology.
8. Treatment of rare complications such as cerebral edema requires further studies before the development of standards of care.

References

[1] Magee MF, Bankim AB. Management of decompensated diabetes. Diabetic ketoacidosis and hyperosmolar hyperglycemic syndrome. Crit Care Clin 2001;17(1):75–106.
[2] Canadian Diabetes Association. The history of diabetes. Available at: http://www.diabetes. ca/Section_About/timeline.asp. Accessed June 29, 2004.
[3] Dreschfeld J. The Bradshaw lecture on diabetic coma. BMJ 1886;2:358–63.
[4] Fleckman AM. Diabetic ketoacidosis. Endocrinol Metab Clin North Am 1993;22(2): 181–207.
[5] Kitabchi AE, Wall BM. Diabetic ketoacidosis. Med Clin North Am 1995;70(1):9–37.
[6] Fishbein H, Palumbo PJ. Acute metabolic complications in diabetes. Bethesda (MD): National Institutes of Health; 1995 #NIH 95–1468.
[7] Kitabchi AE, Umpierrez GE, Murphy MB, et al. Management of hyperglycemic crises in patients with diabetes. Diabetes Care 2001;24(1):131–53.
[8] Kitabchi AE, Umpierrez GE, Murphy MB, et al. American Diabetes Association. Hyperglycemic crises in diabetes. Diabetes Care 2004;27(Suppl 1):S94–102.
[9] Musey VC, Lee JK, Crawford R, et al. Diabetes in urban African-Americans. I. Cessation of insulin therapy is the major precipitating cause of diabetic ketoacidosis. Diabetes Care 1995; 18(4):483–9.
[10] Umpierrez GE, Kelly JP, Navarrete JE, et al. Hyperglycemic crises in urban blacks. Arch Intern Med 1997;157(6):669–75.
[11] Stewart C. Diabetic emergencies: diagnosis and management of hyperglycemic disorders. Emergency Medicine Practice 2004;6(2):1–24.
[12] Warner EA, Greene GS, Buchsbaum MS, et al. Diabetic ketoacidosis associated with cocaine use. Arch Intern Med 1998;14:158(16):1799–802.
[13] Chiasson JL, Aris-Jilwan N, Belanger R, et al. Diagnosis and treatment of diabetic ketoacidosis and the hyperglycemic hyperosmolar state. CMAJ 2003;168(7):859–66.
[14] Foster DW. Diabetes mellitus. In: Fauci AS, Braunwald E, editors. Harrison's principles of internal medicine. New York: McGraw-Hill; 1998. p. 2061–81.
[15] Israel RS. Diabetic ketoacidosis. Emerg Med Clin North Am 1989;7(4):859–71.
[16] von Mach MA, Sauer O, Sacha Weilemann L. Experiences of a poison center with metformin-associated lactic acidosis. Exp Clin Endocrinol Diabetes 2004;112(4): 187–90.

[17] Stades AM, Heikens JT, Erkelens DW, et al. Metformin and lactic acidosis: cause or coincidence? A review of case reports. J Intern Med 2004;255(2):179–87.

[18] Salpeter SR, Greyber E, Pasternak GA, et al. Risk of fatal and nonfatal lactic acidosis with metformin use in type 2 diabetes mellitus: systematic review and meta-analysis. Arch Intern Med 2003;163(21):2594–602.

[19] Cydulka RK, Jonathon S. Diabetes mellitus and disorders of glucose homeostasis. In: Marx JA, Hockberger RS, editors. Emergency medicine: concepts and clinical practice. 5th edition. St. Louis (MO): Mosby; 2002. p. 1744–62.

[20] Adrogue HJ, Madias NE. Changes in plasma potassium concentration during acute acid–base disturbances. Am J Med 1981;71(3):456–67.

[21] Adrogue HJ, Lederer ED, Suki WN, et al. Determinants of plasma potassium levels in diabetic ketoacidosis. Medicine 1986;65(3):163–72.

[22] Ma OJ, Rush MD, Godfrey MM, et al. Arterial blood gas results rarely influence emergency physician management of patients with suspected diabetic ketoacidosis. Acad Emerg Med 2003;10(8):836–41.

[23] Slovis CM, Mork VG, Slovis RJ, et al. Diabetic ketoacidosis and infection: leukocyte count and differential as early predictors of serious infection. Am J Emerg Med 1987;5(1):1–5.

[24] Vinicor F, Lehrner LM, Karn RC, et al. Hyperamylasemia in diabetic ketoacidosis: sources and significance. Ann Intern Med 1979;91:200–4.

[25] Fontaine P, Hautefeuille P, Mathieu C, et al. Blood amylase and lipase in diabetic ketoacidosis. Presse Med 1987;16(18):895–8.

[26] West ML, Marsden PA, Singer GG, et al. Quantitative analysis of glucose loss during acute therapy for hyperglycemic hyperosmolar syndrome. Diabetes Care 1986;9(5):465–71.

[27] Grimberg A, Cerri RW, Satin-Smith M, et al. The two bag system for variable intravenous dextrose and fluid administration: benefits in diabetic ketoacidosis management. J Pediatr 1999;134(3):376–8.

[28] Petty C, Cunningham NL. Insulin adsorption by glass infusion bottles, polyvinylchloride infusion containers, and intravenous tubing. Anesthesiology 1974;40(4):400–4.

[29] Wiggam MI, O'Kane MJ, Harper R, et al. Treatment of diabetic ketoacidosis using normalization of blood 3-hydroxybutyrate concentration as the endpoint of emergency management. A randomized controlled study. Diabetes Care 1997;20(9):1347–52.

[30] Green SM, Rothrock SG, Ho JD, et al. Failure of adjunctive bicarbonate to improve outcome in severe pediatric diabetic ketoacidosis. Ann Emerg Med 1998;31(1):41–8.

[31] Viallon A, Zeni F, Lafond P, et al. Does bicarbonate therapy improve the management of severe diabetic ketoacidosis? Crit Care Med 1999;27(12):2690–3.

[32] Lever E, Jaspan JB. Sodium bicarbonate therapy in severe diabetic ketoacidosis. Am J Med 1983;75(2):263–8.

[33] Gibby OM, Veale KE, Hayes TM, et al. Oxygen availability from the blood and the effect of phosphate replacement on erythrocyte 2,3-diphosphoglycerate and haemoglobin-oxygen affinity in diabetic ketoacidosis. Diabetologia 1978;15(5):381–5.

[34] Glaser N, Barnett P, McCaslin I, et al. Risk factors for cerebral edema in children with diabetic ketoacidosis. The Pediatric Emergency Medicine Collaborative Research Committee of the American Academy of Pediatrics. N Engl J Med 2001;344(4):264–9.

[35] Dunger DB, Edge JA. Predicting cerebral edema during diabetic ketoacidosis. N Engl J Med 2001;344(4):302–3.

[36] Rosenbloom AL. Intracerebral crisis during the treatment of diabetic ketoacidosis. Diabetes Care 1990;13:22–33.

[37] Edge JA, Hawkins MM, Winter DL, et al. The risk and outcome of cerebral oedema developing during diabetic ketoacidosis. Arch Dis Child 2001;85:16–22.

[38] Edge JA, Ford-Adams ME, Dunger DB. Causes of death in children with insulin dependent diabetes. Arch Dis Child 1999;81:318–23.

[39] Edge JA. Cerebral oedema during treatment of diabetic ketoacidosis: are we any nearer finding a cause? Diabetes Metab Res Rev 2000;16:316–24.

[40] Duck SC, Kohler E. Cerebral edema in diabetic ketoacidosis. J Pediatr 1981;98(4):674–6.

[41] Franklin B, Liu J, Ginsberg-Fellner F. Cerebral edema and ophthalmoplegia reversed by mannitol in a new case of insulin-dependent diabetes mellitus. Pediatrics 1982;69(1):87–90.

[42] McAloon J, Carson D, Crean P. Cerebral oedema complicating diabetic ketoacidosis. Acta Paediatr Scand 1990;79(1):115–7.

[43] Greene SA, Jefferson IG, Baum JD. Cerebral oedema complicating diabetic ketoacidosis. Dev Med Child Neurol 1990;32(7):633–8.

[44] Wood EG, Go-Wingkun J, Luisiri A, et al. Symptomatic cerebral swelling complicating diabetic ketoacidosis documented by intraventricular pressure monitoring: survival without neurologic sequela. Pediatr Emerg Care 1990;6(4):285–8.

[45] Carroll P, Matz R. Adult respiratory distress syndrome complicating severely uncontrolled diabetes mellitus: report of nine cases and a review of the literature. Diabetes Care 1982;5(6): 574–80.

[46] Kitchens CS. Concept of hypercoagulability: a review of its development, clinical application, and recent progress. Semin Thromb Hemost 1985;11(3):293–315.

[47] Ileri NS, Buyukasik Y, Karaahmetoglu S, et al. Evaluation of the haemostatic system during ketoacidotic deterioration of diabetes mellitus. Haemostasis 1999;29(6):318–25.

[48] Matsuda T, Morishita E, Jokaji H, et al. Mechanism on disorders of coagulation and fibrinolysis in diabetes [review]. Diabetes 1996;45(Suppl 3):S109–10.

[49] Bonadio WA, Gutzeit MF, Losek JD, et al. Outpatient management of diabetic ketoacidosis. Am J Dis Child 1988;142(4):448–50.

[50] Bonadio WA. Pediatric diabetic ketoacidosis: pathophysiology and potential for outpatient management of selected children. Pediatr Emerg Care 1992;8(5):287–90.

ELSEVIER
SAUNDERS

EMERGENCY
MEDICINE
CLINICS OF
NORTH AMERICA

Emerg Med Clin N Am 23 (2005) 629–648

Hyperosmolar Hyperglycemic State

Bruce W. Nugent, MD*

*Division of Emergency Medicine, Spectrum Health-Butterworth,
100 Monroe NW, MC-49,
Grand Rapids, MI 49503, USA*

As the prevalence of diabetes mellitus escalates, emergency medicine practitioners will continue to see increasing numbers of patients with complications of uncontrolled hyperglycemia. Hyperosmolar hyperglycemic state (HHS) represents one of the two most serious acute metabolic complications of diabetes mellitus and is a life-threatening emergency. HHS is the end result of a sustained osmotic diuresis, and is characterized by severe hyperglycemia, hyperosmolarity, and dehydration, but without significant ketoacidosis. Less common than the other critical hyperglycemic diabetic emergency, diabetic ketoacidosis (DKA), HHS carries a higher mortality rate, associated with serious concurrent illness. It is usually seen in older type 2 diabetics, but can present at any age, and in patients with type 1 diabetes mellitus.

Hyperosmolar hyperglycemic state first was described in 1957, and the literature since has referred to this syndrome by many terms, including hyperosmolar nonketotic state, hyperosmolar coma, hyperglycemic hyperosmolar syndrome, or nonketotic hyperosmolar syndrome [1]. Hyperosmolar hyperglycemic state is the nomenclature recommended by the American Diabetes Association (ADA), used here to emphasize that varying alterations in sensorium less than coma are usually present and that HHS may occur with some degree of ketosis and acidosis [1–3]. Diagnostic features of HHS include the following [2]:

- Plasma glucose level of 600 mg/dL or greater
- Effective serum osmolality of 320 mOsm/kg or greater
- Profound dehydration (typically 8 to 12 L) with elevated serum urea nitrogen (BUN):creatinine ratio
- Small ketonuria, absent to low ketonemia
- Bicarbonate greater than 15 mEq/L
- Some alteration in consciousness

---

* 1792 Tahoe Pine Drive Southwest, Grand Rapids, MI 49509, USA.
E-mail address: nugentbw@cs.com

0733-8627/05/$ - see front matter © 2005 Elsevier Inc. All rights reserved.
doi:10.1016/j.emc.2005.03.006   *emed.theclinics.com*

Hyperosmolar hyperglycemic state often is reviewed together with DKA because of similarities in pathogenesis and treatment approach. Many experts view these as two extremes on the spectrum of decompensated diabetes, differing from each other by the magnitude of hyperglycemia, the severity of acidosis/ketonemia, and the degree of dehydration [4–7]. Both disorders can occur in type 1 and type 2 diabetes mellitus, and up to one third of patients with decompensated diabetes share features of both DKA and HHS [4,5]. Important distinctions, however, exist in pathogenesis, clinical presentation, and treatment between these disease states. This article focuses on the emergency department (ED) evaluation and management of HHS.

Emergency department presentation

Epidemiology

In 2002, an estimated 6.3% of the US population (about 18.2 million people) had diabetes. Type 2 diabetes mellitus accounts for 90% to 95% of cases, and people 65 years or older make up almost 40% of all persons with diabetes [8]. The prevalence of type 2 diabetes mellitus is increasing dramatically and parallels the epidemic of obesity. Blacks, Hispanics, and Native Americans are affected disproportionately. Type 2 diabetes mellitus now accounts for as much as half of newly diagnosed diabetes in children ages 10 to 21 years, depending on the socioeconomic and ethnic composition of the population [9,10].

Hyperosmolar hyperglycemic state occurs primarily in patients with type 2 diabetes mellitus, although that diagnosis may not have been known previously. In 30% to 40% of cases, HHS is the initial presentation of a patient's diabetes [11,12]. HHS is significantly less common than DKA. The incidence of HHS is less than 1 case per 1000 person-years, compared with DKA, which occurs at a rate of 4.6 to 8 cases per 1000 person-years [13]. The mean age of patients with HHS is 60 years, yet cases in pediatric patients are reported [14]. Elderly people, especially those dependent on others for their daily care, are at greatest risk, and many patients are direct admissions from nursing homes [15]. There is a small female predominance [1,16].

Mortality rates continue to be high, even with proper treatment, and are higher than those associated with DKA. Precise mortality rates are not available because of the prevalence of comorbid illnesses that may be listed as the main cause of death, rather than HHS [12]. HHS historically has had reported mortality rates reaching as high as 50%; however, the most recently quoted average mortality is 15% [2,12,15]. In contrast, the mortality rate for DKA is usually less than 2% to 5% [2]. Mortality in HHS increases with increasing age and increases with higher levels of serum osmolality [1,16,17]. Patients with HHS usually do not die because of the hypertonicity, but rather succumb to a comorbid illness that may have precipitated or developed during the treatment of HHS [16]. Prognosis is worsened substantially in the presence of a coma or hypotension [2,16,18]. Higher mortality also may be associated with a delay in diagnosis and failure to aggressively treat HHS [19,20]. Mortality may occur as a complication of treatment.

Despite the increasing incidence of type 2 diabetes mellitus, HHS is rare in childhood. Recent reports, however, highlight a disturbing trend in the epidemiology of pediatric-type 2 diabetes mellitus, including complications (eg, DKA and HHS). Although DKA is most common in type 1 diabetes mellitus and may be its initial presentation in children, DKA also may occur at the time of diagnosis in up to 25% of pediatric patients presenting with type 2 diabetes mellitus [14]. In contrast, it is estimated that 4% of newly diagnosed type 2 diabetes mellitus cases in children are associated with HHS, and that 12% of these cases will be fatal, often caused by cerebral edema and dehydration [14]. Before 2002, HHS had been reported in only 12 children, 10 of whom were 9 months to 7 years old, two 12 and 13 years old; none were overweight [14]. A more recent report, however, describes six male adolescent patients with HHS complicated by malignant hyperthermia and rhabdomyolysis [21]. Another report documents seven obese African American youths who were considered to have died from DKA caused by type 1 diabetes mellitus, but actually met the criteria for HHS and not DKA, and who had previously unrecognized type 2 diabetes mellitus [14]. Common findings in these patients include disease onset in early adolescence, positive family history of type 2 diabetes mellitus, and physical findings of insulin resistance including obesity, and acanthosis nigricans, a velvety hyperpigmented thickened skin patch most prominent in intertriginous areas (eg, neck and groin) [14,21]. More timely diagnosis and treatment could have prevented some of these complications and deaths. Physicians need to have a high index of suspicion for type 2 diabetes mellitus in children. When discovered, this diagnosis should be considered as much an emergency as recognition of type 1 diabetes mellitus, and appropriate referral for urgent initiation of diabetic education and treatment should take place [10].

Predisposing and precipitating factors

Patients with known or unknown diabetes progress from poor glucose control to overt HHS typically over a period of days to weeks, and the process may be initiated or sustained by serious underlying illness and other factors. Infection (eg, pneumonia, urinary tract infection, and sepsis) is the most common precipitating illness, occurring in up to 60% of cases [4,11,22]. Other acute conditions that may provoke release of counter regulatory hormones and precipitate HHS include silent myocardial infarction, cerebrovascular accident, pulmonary embolism, and mesenteric thrombosis [13]. Acute pancreatitis, gastrointestinal (GI) bleeding, heat illness, and procedures with glucose loading (eg, peritoneal dialysis and recent surgical operation) have been identified as precipitants [4,12,22]. Patients with underlying renal insufficiency and congestive heart failure (CHF) are at greater risk. Many different medications have been identified that may contribute to the development of HHS by their affect on carbohydrate metabolism. These include glucocorticoids, thiazide diuretics, phenytoin, and beta blockers [4]. More recently, the antipsychotic drugs clozapine and olanzapine have been associated with the development of hyperglycemia, and cases of DKA and HHS have been reported [23,24]. Use of alcohol and cocaine also has been implicated in the development of HHS [11,25].

In general, any medical illness that predisposes to dehydration may contribute to development of HHS. Disorders that affect mental function, impair means of communication, or limit mobility, and therefore create dependence on others for providing access to and ensuring adequate fluid intake can precipitate HHS [12]. One of the most common predisposing factors is under-recognition of the signs and symptoms of uncontrolled diabetes, especially when the patient is not known to be diabetic, and underestimation of fluid needs by caregivers in nursing homes and other settings [6]. Replacement with high glucose containing fluids, poor diabetic education, not monitoring blood sugars, and noncompliance with insulin or oral therapy also may contribute [2].

For the emergency medicine practitioner, identification of any underlying acute illness precipitating HHS is critical, and treatment must be initiated concurrent with that of HHS. The search for hidden precipitants should continue even in the presence of one or more obvious causes. Box 1 summarizes common precipitating factors.

Clinical presentation

Despite the profound metabolic abnormalities that are present, HHS may not be clinically obvious. The classical picture of HHS includes a history of first the signs and symptoms of uncontrolled hyperglycemia (eg, polyuria, polydipsia, fatigue, and visual disturbances), and then subsequent de-hydration (including weakness, anorexia, weight loss, leg cramps, dizziness, confusion, and lethargy). The average duration of symptoms is 12 days in HHS versus less than 1 to 2 days in DKA [20]. In some cases, however, the clinical presentation of HHS is similar to DKA, and a definite diagnosis must be confirmed through laboratory investigation [13]. Because significant acidosis is absent, abdominal pain is much less common in HHS than in DKA, and nausea and vomiting may not be present [26]. When abdominal pain is a prominent symptom, it should be investigated as either a precipitating cause or complication (eg, mesenteric ischemia) of the HHS.

The most common reason caretakers seek medical attention for the patient is concern related to a change in level of cognition [20]. Despite the previous nomenclature, less than 20% of patients with HHS present in coma [6,27]. Some patients may present alert with a near normal mental status, but a gradual clouding of consciousness is typical [6]. The degree of alteration in mental status tends to correlate with the degree of hyperosmolarity, and

Box 1. Precipitating factors to development of hyperosmolar hyperglycemic state

Infection
Pneumonia
Sepsis (particularly gram-negative)
Urinary Tract Infection

Concurrent medical illness
Vascular occlusive illness
  - Cerebral vascular accident
  - Mesenteric thrombosis
  - Myocardial infarction
  - Pulmonary embolus
Metabolic illness
  - Acute pancreatitis
  - Heat illness
  - Hypothermia
  - Intestinal obstruction
  - Renal failure
Endocrine causes
  - Acromegaly
  - Cushing's syndrome
  - Previously undiagnosed diabetes mellitus
  - Thyrotoxicosis
Other
  - Alcohol abuse
  - Burns
  - Cocaine abuse
  - GI bleeding
  - Neuroleptic malignant syndrome
  - Peritoneal or hemodialysis
  - Rhabdomyolysis
  - Trauma

Medications
Beta-blockers
Calcium channel blockers
Carbamazepine
Chlorpromazine
Cimetidine
Corticosteroids
Didanosine
Glucocorticoids
Immunosuppressants
Lithium
Mannitol
Neuroleptics
Olanzapine
Pentamidine
Phenytoin
Thiazide and loop diuretics
Total parenteral nutrition or enteral nutrition
Noncompliance with diabetes mellitus therapy

Postoperative
Coronary artery bypass graft
Neurosurgery
Orthopedic surgery
Renal transplant

Sociodemographic factors
Dependent on others for self-care (unable to meet fluid needs)
Elderly
Female

Reference
1,2,4–7,10,11,13,15,16

serious alteration in consciousness is uncommon with osmolarities less than 340 mOsm/L [22]. Coma is associated with severe hypertonicity, with serum osmolarity at 350 mOsm/L or greater, and usually more significant hypernatremia than hyperglycemia [12,28]. The absence of hyperosmolarity or hypoglycemia in an obtunded patient with diabetes mellitus suggests an etiology other than a direct complication of diabetes [6,22,29].

Many neurologic changes can occur in HHS, including unilateral or bilateral focal motor or sensory deficits, aphasia, myoclonic jerks, chorea, nystagmus, and Babinski's signs [27]. Seizures occur in 15% of cases, and are often focal seizures, either intermittent or continuous (epilepsia partialis continuum) [5,12,27]. It is important to note that the neurologic changes seen as a result of HHS typically reverse completely with appropriate treatment and correction of the metabolic abnormalities [22]. Focus solely on the neurologic deficits (eg, seizures, hemiparesis, and coma) can delay diagnosis and appropriate treatment unless a glucose level is obtained early in the presentation. Especially in the era of thrombolytic reperfusion therapy for acute ischemic stroke, evaluation of new focal neurologic deficits always must include a glucose level to exclude a stroke mimic from either hypoglycemia or, in the case of HHS, extreme hyperglycemia [30,31]. Hyperglycemia is common in patients with acute stroke, and it is associated with a worse outcome in reperfused and non-reperfused stroke patients. The level, however, will not be to the extremes seen with HHS [32].

Patients with HHS typically present with a debilitated weakened general appearance and show physical signs of dehydration including dry mucous membranes, poor skin turgor, and sunken eyes, although these changes can often be subtle in the elderly. Tachycardia and tachypnea (not Kussmaul respirations) are common, as are hypotension and signs of decreased perfusion in advanced cases. Although some authors suggest that patients may have a low-grade fever because of dehydration and lack of sweating, in general any degree of fever suggests infection [33]. Signs of localized infection (eg, pneumonia or cellulitis) may be present. Finally, the physical exam may show evidence of insulin resistance, including obesity, acanthosis nigricans, and diabetic dermatopathy.

Pathophysiology

In a diabetic patient with pre-existing insulin lack or resistance, a physiologic stress (eg, an acute illness) can cause further net reduction in the effectiveness of circulating insulin. Concomitant elevations in counter regulatory hormones (eg, glucagon, catecholamines, cortisol, and growth hormone) contribute to impaired glucose use in the peripheral tissues. Hypercortisolemia increases proteolysis, which leads to the production of amino acid precursors for gluconeogenesis, and glucagon induces glycogenolysis. As in DKA, the combination of hepatic glucose production and decreased peripheral glucose use is the main pathogenic etiology for hyperglycemia associated with HHS [2,13,22].

Hyperglycemia leads to glycosuria, hypotonic osmotic diuresis, and dehydration. Glucose is osmotically active and creates an osmotic gradient drawing water from the intracellular to extracellular compartments. As serum concentrations of glucose exceed 180 mg/dL, the kidney's capacity to reabsorb glucose is exceeded [19]. The presence of glucose in the urine impairs the concentrating capacity of the kidney, therefore exacerbating water losses [2]. If fluid intake is adequate, renal excretion of glucose may be sufficient to prevent marked serum hyperglycemia. If the patient is unable to maintain adequate fluid intake (eg, due to acute illness, decreased thirst mechanism, immobility, or other ongoing fluid losses), however, these water losses further decrease kidney perfusion, which markedly exacerbates the hyperglycemia [6]. It is this renal insufficiency in HHS that allows for the extremely high levels of glucose seen with this disorder, much higher than in DKA, resulting in the severe hyperosmolality and intracellular dehydration [34]. The alteration in consciousness seen in HHS directly corresponds to the elevation in effective osmolarity and may be related to intracellular cerebral dehydration, changes in neurotransmitter levels, and microischemia [12].

In the osmotic diuresis, free water is lost in excess of electrolytes, but there is a large loss of sodium, potassium, magnesium, and phosphate in the urine. Losses of electrolytes are more profound that those seen in DKA (Table 1) [13]. Initial measured serum levels of electrolytes may not reflect the actual deficits accurately. The full development of HHS occurs over several days, and the total body water deficit averages 8 to 12 L in HHS, compared with 5 to 7 L in DKA [13]. In its severe form, this prolonged osmotic diuresis results in hypotension and impaired tissue perfusion.

In addition to the degree of fluid loss and dehydration, another key difference between DKA and HHS is the absence of significant ketosis. The reason for this absence of ketosis in HHS is not known, but it is proposed that insulin levels may be adequate to prevent lipolysis and subsequent ketogenesis, yet inadequate to facilitate peripheral glucose uptake and to prevent hepatic

Table 1
Water and electrolyte loss at presentation of hyperosmolar hyperglycemic state and diabetic ketoacidosis [2–4,13]

Electrolyte	HHS*	DKA*
Water (mL/kg)	100–200 (10.5 L)	100 (7 L)
Sodium (mEq/kg)	5–13 (350–910)	7–10 (490–700)
Potassium (mEq/kg)	5–15 (350–1050)	3–5 (210–300)
Chloride (mEq/kg)	3–7 (210–490)	3–5 (210–350)
Phosphate (mmol/kg)	1–2 (70–140)	1–1.5 (70–105)
Magnesium (mEq/kg)	1–2 (70–140)	1–2 (70–140)
Calcium (mEq/kg)	2 (140)	1–2 (70–140)

* Values in parentheses represent total body deficits for a 70 kg patient.

gluconeogenesis [22]. Also, lower levels of counter-regulatory hormones compared with patients with DKA have been found in some studies, and the insulin to glucagon ratio is higher [7]. Finally, hyperosmolality itself may act to decrease lipolysis (the release of free fatty acids) and subsequent ketogenesis [22]. The absence of clinically significant ketoacidosis is a factor in the progression of the pathogenesis of HHS. Lack of physical discomforts associated with ketosis may result in a delay in seeking treatment, and this delay can sustain the osmotic diuresis.

Differential diagnosis

The differential diagnosis of HHS includes any cause of altered level of consciousness, including hypoglycemia, hyponatremia, severe dehydration, uremia, hyperammonemia, drug overdose, and sepsis [20]. Seizures and acute stroke-like syndromes are common presentations. Early measurement of a blood glucose level in any patient with impaired consciousness is imperative. In the unlikely event a level cannot be obtained rapidly, administration of dextrose is indicated to treat possible hypoglycemia, and will only minimally worsen HHS if it is present.

Hyperosmolar hyperglycemic state can be differentiated from DKA by the presentation and laboratory features (Table 2). Mixed syndromes of HHS and DKA can exist. There are essentially no disorders other than uncontrolled diabetes mellitus that produce the marked hyperglycemia seen in HHS [35].

Emergency department evaluation

Laboratory

The initial laboratory evaluation of patients with suspected HHS should consider the frequency of precipitating causes and underlying comorbidities

Table 2
Typical presenting laboratory values associated with hyperosmolar hyperglycemic state compared with diabetic ketoacidosis [2,4,13]

	HHS	DKA
Diagnostic		
Serum glucose (mg/dL)	> 600 (mean: 1166)	> 250 (mean: 475)
Serum osmolality (mOsm/kg)	> 320	< 320
Arterial pH value	> 7.3	< 7.2
Sodium bicarbonate (mEq/L)	> 15	< 15
Serum ketones	Absent or low	Moderate to high
Variable, mean (and SD)		
Serum sodium (mEq/L)	149 (3.2)	134 (1)
Serum potassium (mEq/L)	3.9 (0.2)	4.5 (0.13)
BUN (mg/dL)	61 (10.9)	32 (3.1)
Serum creatinine (mg/dL)	1.4 (0.01)	1.1 (0.01)

associated with HHS. Baseline laboratory assessment includes measurement of serum glucose, serum urea nitrogen (BUN), creatinine, electrolytes, serum ketones, osmolality, urinalysis, complete blood count with differential, and arterial blood glasses if respiratory compromise or acidosis is suspected. Bacterial cultures of urine and blood almost always are indicated. Typical laboratory values in HHS compared with DKA are noted in Table 2.

Glucose

Extreme hyperglycemia defines HHS, and the degree of hyperglycemia is usually proportional to the degree of dehydration and osmolality. Serum glucose levels greater than 600 mg/dL, and often well over 1000 mg/dL, are present. When levels are this high, laboratory determinations, rather than finger-stick bedside measurements, are needed for accurate assessment [16].

Osmolality

The second diagnostic criterion is hyperosmolality. Osmolality is measured directly in the laboratory by determining the freezing point of the serum. This can be approximated by the formula:

$$\text{Osmolarity} = [2 \times \text{Na (mEq/L)}] + \frac{\text{glucose (mg/dL)}}{18} + \frac{\text{BUN (mg/dL)}}{2.8}$$

Because the density of water is 1 kg/L, osmolarity (in osm/L) is roughly equivalent to osmolality (in osm/kg) in water based systems with minimal temperature variation (eg, the human body) and they are often used interchangeably [36]. This calculated value can be compared with the measured value to determine any osmolar gap. This calculation of osmolarity, however, includes urea, which is freely diffusible across cell membranes, is therefore not osmotically active, and is not important in the pathogenesis of HHS. A more useful calculation is the effective osmolarity, which reflects actual tonicity, the osmotic pressure of a solution. The effective osmolarity can be calculated by the formula:

$$\text{Effective osmolarity (mOsm/L)} = 2 \times [(\text{Na}) + (\text{K}^+)] + \text{glucose}/18$$

Measuring the effective osmolarity is important to help guide the optimal choice of fluid for replacement therapy, as elevated BUN and azotemia may mask an actual hypotonicity of the extracellular fluid and can lead to inappropriate administration of hypotonic fluids [6]. The normal serum osmolarity ranges from 275 to 295 mOsm/L. Levels above 320 mOsm/L may involve some alteration in cognitive function, and patients with coma caused by HHS almost always have values of 340 mOsm/L or greater. Rarely, serum osmolarity may be greater than 400 mOsm/L. As reflected in the formula, serum sodium actually contributes more to effective osmolarity than glucose, and most cases of coma are associated with a high serum sodium [28].

Sodium

The measured sodium may be low, normal, or elevated, despite the patient being total body sodium depleted. Because glucose osmotically shifts water into the extracellular space, sodium is diluted, and the measured value is decreased falsely. The measured sodium value should be corrected to a true sodium value that accounts for hyperglycemia by using the formula:

$$\text{Corrected (Na)} = 1.6 \times (\text{glucose} - 100)/100$$

This reflects that the measured serum sodium value is decreased by approximately 1.6 mEq for every 100 mg/dL increase in glucose above 100 [36]. The formula listed is the traditional formula used, although one study has suggested the relationship between glucose and sodium is nonlinear, and that a more accurate correction factor in extreme hyperglycemic states is 2.4 mEq/L for each 100 mg/dL [37]. The dilutional effect of hyperglycemia is counteracted by the glucosuria-induced diuresis, as water is lost more than sodium and potassium. A mild hyponatremia or a normal sodium level usually suggests moderate dehydration. If the serum sodium concentration is high despite severe hyperglycemia, significant water loss has occurred, and extreme volume contraction and dehydration are present [27]. Corrected sodium levels more accurately reflect the state of dehydration and are useful in monitoring treatment [38].

Potassium

Total body potassium depletion is even more profound in HHS than in DKA. The presenting serum potassium concentration, however, is often high because of volume contraction, insulin deficiency, shift of potassium from intracellular to extracellular fluid compartments, and some degree of acidosis. In some instances, this initial serum potassium can be symptomatic [39]. Potassium deficits are common in uncontrolled diabetes and may be especially high in patients who are on diuretics. The presence of normal or low potassium at presentation suggests a profound deficit. Initiation of treatment with volume replacement and insulin will result in a further decrease in the serum potassium concentration. Hypokalemia is a significant risk in the initial treatment phase and should be anticipated.

Other laboratory measurements

Body stores of phosphate and magnesium will be decreased comparable to those of potassium, although serum levels may high or normal. The clinical consequences of magnesium or phosphate deficiency are not as significant as those of potassium in the immediate treatment setting of the ED. Levels tend to normalize during treatment, and there is no evidence that replacement is necessary unless levels are extremely low [4].

Dehydration may cause a rise in the plasma levels of routine chemistries including calcium, protein, amylase, lactate dehydrogenase, transaminases, and creatinine kinase. Underlying disease states associated with these levels need to be excluded, however. Patients present with prerenal azotemia, and the initial BUN to creatinine ratio may exceed 30:1. Leukocytosis is often present secondary to stress, demarginalization, and hemoconcentration [7]. Infection, however, should be ruled out as the cause of any marked elevation in white blood cell count. Hemoglobin and hematocrit concentrations may be elevated falsely because of hemoconcentration, and anemia should be suspected in a patient with a normal hematocrit on examination [20].

A mild high anion gap metabolic acidosis, characterized by an arterial pH above 7.3 and bicarbonate level greater than 15 is common in HHS [22,33]. This acidosis can be multifactorial, contributed to by dehydration, renal failure, starvation, or mild lactic acidosis. Vomiting or the use of thiazide diuretics can cause a metabolic alkalosis that can mask the degree of acidosis [4,12,22]. If acidosis is severe, lactic acidosis caused by hypovolemia and decreased perfusion, underlying infection, or other concurrent severe illness (eg, ischemic bowel) should be considered [4]. Arterial blood gas measurements can help clarify what is sometimes a complicated mixed acid base picture, and indicate other cardiac or pulmonary comorbidities. Although HHS is described as a nonketotic hyperosmolar state, there is often some elevation of serum ketones, including β-hydroxybutyrate, which are related mostly to the starvation ketosis or to dehydration [2,19]. Urinalysis always is indicated and may demonstrate some degree of ketonuria also. Gross proteinuria suggests the presence of underlying renal disease.

Other studies

Other diagnostic studies are obtained routinely in the ED evaluation to look for precipitating or underlying illnesses. The initial chest radiograph may be falsely negative for pneumonitis in light of the state of dehydration, and cardiomegaly in this setting suggests likely cardiomyopathy [19]. An electrocardiogram always is indicated to look for signs of ischemia and infarction, and acute changes related to electrolyte deficiencies. CT of the brain to exclude intracranial pathology is indicated because of the frequent presence of altered cognition. Lumbar puncture and toxicologic studies should be performed if indicated.

Emergency department management

Management in the ED begins with a rapid clinical assessment focused on the elements of history and physical, and with appropriate evaluation and monitoring of respiratory, cardiovascular, and central nervous system function. The diagnosis of the extreme decompensated diabetic state can be made immediately with an early glucose measurement, and a potassium level should follow quickly. The goals of therapy include [7,16]:

- Restoration of hemodynamic stability and correction of hypovolemia
- Maintenance of electrolyte homeostasis
- Gradual correction of hyperglycemia and hyperosmolarity
- Detection and treatment of underlying disease states and precipitating causes
- Avoidance of complications

The most rapid therapy is directed toward hypovolemic shock and life-threatening electrolyte abnormalities.

When faced with such extreme elevations of glucose and abnormalities of osmolarity and sodium as seen in HHS, there is a tendency to think that initial interventions can be gross and inaccurate without consequence. The severity of the disease, however, demands a rational and systematic approach to therapy from the beginning. The initial treatment in the ED can make a difference in the frequency of complications and outcome. Although adherence to protocols and standard treatment algorithms have improved outcomes, therapy must be individualized based on the degree of dehydration and underlying disease states (eg, sepsis, renal failure, and left ventricular dysfunction). Close monitoring in the first hours of treatment is essential. Central venous and urinary catheterization may be required to guide fluid administration. A flow sheet to frequently assess therapy is useful and should be maintained diligently. With prolonged ED stays and EDs serving as holding area for admitted patients, the most critical period for these patients may occur during their ED course. The ED becomes the critical care unit, and patients cannot be forgotten after a few initial interventions. The key is continuing and careful monitoring and therapeutic adjustments.

Fluid therapy

Fluid replacement to expand intravascular volume and restore renal and tissue perfusion is the first priority in managing HHS and is the cornerstone of therapy. Patients invariably are volume depleted, and the approximate fluid deficit can be calculated to help guide therapy. Total body weight is 50% to 60% of usual body weight, and the fluid deficit averages 20% to 25% of total body water, or approximately 12% to 15% of body weight [12]. A range of typical fluid deficits is 8 to 12 L, with the average being 9 L [6,12]. Another way to approximate this deficit is simply 150 mL/kg of body weight or to compare normal recent weight with current weight: every liter of body fluids lost results in 1 kg loss in body weight [6]. The goal is to replace one half of the fluid deficit in the first 12 hours and the remainder in the next 12 to 24 hours [2,12,16,22]. There is general agreement that initial replacement should be with isotonic crystalloid (eg, 0.9% sodium chloride). Sodium chloride will restore intravascular volume effectively but is still hypotonic to the patient's serum osmolality [12]. If the patient is hypotensive and in shock, immediate fluid resuscitation with 0.9% sodium chloride is indicated, and 1 to 2 L are given rapidly until the blood pressure increases, and urine output is established. For most adult patients who are not hypotensive, 0.9% sodium chloride is administered at rates of 15 to 20 mL/kg per hour (average of 1 to 1.5 L) during the first hour [2].

The type of fluid and rate of administration after this should be individualized and adjusted depending upon on vital signs, serum electrolyte levels, and urinary output. In general, once circulating volumes have been restored, replacement will be slower, and the solution changed to 0.45% sodium chloride to avoid further osmotic loads. The ADA guidelines recommend looking to the corrected serum sodium. If it is normal or elevated, 0.45% sodium chloride is infused at 4 to 14 mL/kg per hour (approx 300 to 1200 mL) depending on hydration state, and if low, 0.9% sodium chloride is continued at the same rate [2]. Another approach would be to look at the effective osmolarity. Some authors suggest that 0.9% sodium chloride be used if the serum osmolarity is less than 320 to 330 mOsm/L and 0.45% sodium chloride if it is above this level [6]. Sodium chloride will continue to expand the intravascular volume and slows the decrease in osmolality, but it can be associated with a persistent hypernatremia and runs greater risk of fluid overload. Hypotonic fluids (eg, 0.45% sodium chloride) are more effective in replacing free water loss and prevent hypernatremia, but they may be associated with a more rapid decrease in extracellular osmolarity and sodium [12]. To avoid the risk of cerebral edema, especially in younger patients, the goal is not to exceed a change in serum osmolality greater than 3 mOsm/kg per hour [2]. Early in treatment, a decrease in the plasma glucose level also serves as an index of the adequacy rehydration and restoration of renal perfusion. Failure of the plasma glucose to decrease by 75 to 100 mg/dL per hour usually implies impairment of renal function or inadequate volume administration [6]. Potassium is added to fluids early on, and glucose-containing fluids are begun when the glucose level reaches 300 mg/dL [2]. Carefully monitored, rapid restoration of plasma volume in adult patients with HHS usually is tolerated well. An average fluid administration would be 3 to 4 L in the first 4 hours of therapy.

Underlying disease states (eg, left ventricular dysfunction or renal disease) may modify a patient's ability to handle large volumes of fluid and therefore determine the rate of fluid replacement [27]. Patients with chronic renal insufficiency are especially challenging, and knowledge of a patient's previous renal function can be helpful. In these patients, the glucose can exceed over 1000 mg/dL or even 1500 mg/dL, but because of renal insufficiency, the patient may not establish an osmotic diuresis and may effectively present with hyponatremia and hypochloremia because of the extracellular fluid shift induced by the elevated glucose. The rise in plasma osmolality is limited, as is the likelihood therefore of neurologic symptoms. Overhydration in this subgroup of patients quickly can result in CHF and pulmonary edema. In long-established renal failure or with anuria, the role of fluid therapy in the treatment of HHS is limited, and treatment consists primarily of providing insulin to decrease glucose levels, shift fluid back into the intracellular space, and decrease potassium levels. Patients with underlying renal disease, cardiac disease, or other complicating states are more likely to require invasive monitoring to guide fluid therapy [12].

In pediatric patients (younger than 20 years), fluid replacement objectives are similar to adults. Because of the risk of cerebral edema associated with fluid resuscitation in pediatric patients, however, the rate of administration of 0.9% sodium chloride should be less than that in adults, and should not exceed 50 mL/kg over the first 4 hours of therapy. Continued fluid therapy is calculated to replace the fluid deficit over 48 hours in pediatric patients, compared with 24 hours in adults [2].

Potassium and other electrolytes

Although the potassium level may be initially normal or even high, all patients with HHS are potassium depleted. Losses average 5 to 6 mEq/kg, range as high as 10 to 15 mEq/kg, and are often greater than those seen in DKA [16,27]. After hypovolemic shock, acute hypokalemia is the most serious immediate risk to patients with HHS, and monitoring and replacement of potassium are critical. Treatment of HHS with rehydration and insulin usually results in a rapid decline in the serum concentration of potassium, particularly during the first few hours of therapy. Other factors contributing to this decline include correction of any acidosis and continued potassium loss because of osmotic diuresis [13,40]. Knowledge of the serum potassium level at the beginning of treatment is essential. Patients whose potassium is low initially in the presence of HHS are at the greatest risk of complications including cardiac dysrhythmias, cardiac arrest, and respiratory muscle weakness. If the initial serum potassium level is less than 3.3 mEq/L, potassium replacement should begin immediately with initial fluid therapy at a rate of up to 40 mEq/L per hour until levels are above 3.3 mEq/L. Otherwise, potassium replacement should be initiated as soon urinary output is assured and levels reach 5 mEq/L or below. Routinely, 20 mEq/L potassium chloride can be added to each 1 L of intravenous fluid with the goal being to maintain a serum concentration of potassium within the normal range of 4 to 5 mEq/L [2,12,16]. Initially, the serum concentration of potassium should be measured every 1 to 2 hours, because the most rapid change occurs during the first 5 hours of treatment. Electrocardiogram monitoring is recommended in patients presenting with hypokalemia and receiving replacement therapy. Because insulin facilitates potassium re-entry in to the intracellular compartment, insulin therapy should be delayed until the potassium level is at least 3.3 mEq/L.

Some authorities recommend administering one-third of potassium replacement as potassium phosphate to avoid excess chloride administration and to prevent hypophosphatemia [2]. The rationale for this recommendation has been questioned [4]. Despite the presence of hypophosphatemia, most controlled trials, focused on DKA management, have not demonstrated benefit of phosphate replacement [12]. Although phosphate levels should be measured and treatment initiated when levels are below 1 mg/dL, routine administration of phosphate in the ED setting is not indicated. More gradual replacement, to avoid the complications of hypocalcemia or in the face of renal failure, may be physiologically appropriate in selected patients and can be pursued during inpatient treatment. Likewise, despite total body depletion, replacement of magnesium need only be initiated in the ED when the magnesium level is below normal [29,41]. A total dose of 2 to 3 g of 10% solution can be added to intravenous fluid if renal failure is not present. Because potassium and magnesium regulations are related closely, correction of hypokalemia may be contingent on magnesium replacement [41].

Insulin

Insulin plays a secondary role in the ED management of HHS, and fluid therapy always should precede insulin administration. The osmotic pressure that glucose exerts within the vascular space contributes to maintenance of circulating volume in these severely dehydrated patients. Insulin drives glucose, potassium, and water into cells, and administration of insulin alone could lead to circulatory collapse, shock, and even thromboembolism if fluid has not been replaced first [12,19,27]. Insulin therapy in the ED may not be required at all with appropriate fluid therapy [20]. Once hemodynamic stability is achieved and the kidneys are well perfused, low-dose insulin therapy may be initiated. Also, as noted previously, insulin administration should await measurement of serum potassium and should be delayed if the serum potassium is less than 3.3 mEq/L.

Although glucose initially can drop as much as 80 to 200 mg/dL per hour because of adequate fluid therapy alone, insulin likely will be required [16]. The recommended dose of insulin in HHS is 0.1 U/kg per hour of regular insulin by continuous intravenous infusion with or without an initial bolus of 0.15 U/kg [2]. Steady-state insulin levels can be achieved within 25 minutes of an insulin infusion. No proven benefit of a bolus has been demonstrated, and it specifically is not recommended in pediatric patients [2]. Insulin should be infused separate from other fluids, and the infusion should not be interrupted or suspended once begun [19]. Serum glucose levels should be determined every hour and followed by adjustment of the insulin infusion. In the presence of adequate hydration, this dose of insulin usually decreases plasma glucose concentration at a rate of 50 to 75 dL per hour [2]. The goal is to decrease glucose by no more than 100 mg/dL per hour, and the target is to lower it only to 300 mg/dL [19]. Once the serum concentration of glucose reaches 300 mg/dL or less, dextrose 5% water should be added to the intravenous fluids, and the insulin infusion rate can be decreased by half to 0.05 U/kg per hour [2]. Conversely, if the glucose level does not improve after an hour of insulin infusion, the infusion rate can be doubled until a response is noted; however, the adequacy of fluid therapy should be questioned. Although insulin resistance is present, patients usually respond well to exogenously administered insulin, and less insulin may be required in HHS than in DKA, where insulin also is required to reverse the ketoacidosis.

Underlying illness

Detection and treatment of any underlying predisposing illness is a crucial part of the management of HHS. Antibiotics should be administered early, after appropriate cultures, in patients in whom infection is known or suspected as a precipitant to HHS. Treatment for seizures should avoid phenytoin, which inhibits the release of endogenous insulin and has been associated with HHS [12,20]. A high index of suspicion should be maintained for underlying pancreatitis, GI bleeding, renal failure, and thromboembolic events, especially acute myocardial infarction.

Complications

Complications can occur secondary to the pathophysiology of HHS itself or as a result of treatment. The most common lethal problems of initial treatment include failure to manage the airway and inadequate fluid resuscitation. Hypoglycemia as a consequence of insulin infusion is seen less often than with DKA, and would not be expected during the ED time course. Hypokalemia can occur related to therapy as described previously. Some treatment-related complications of HHS are not typically apparent during the ED course, but ED management could impact their incidence. Serious complications of HHS include thromboembolic events, cerebral edema, adult respiratory distress syndrome, and rhabdomyolysis.

Severe dehydration and elevated serum osmolality in HHS can result in hypotension, low cardiac output, and hyperviscosity of the blood. This and other factors, such as various prothrombotic elements of the diabetic state and frequent presence of underlying atherosclerosis, may predispose the patient to complications such cerebral infarct, myocardial infarction, pulmonary embolism, mesenteric vessel thrombosis, and disseminated intravascular coagulation [13,19]. Such vascular complications may be prevented with aggressive fluid therapy at the onset of treatment to correct the hyperosmolarity and restore perfusion [22]. Because large-vessel thromboembolic events are a cause of late mortality, use of low-dose heparin for prophylaxis is recommended, but full heparinization with either low molecular weight or unfractionated heparin is reserved for clinical evidence of thrombosis [42].

Cerebral edema is a devastating complication that is extremely rare in adults with HHS despite the typically rapid fluid resuscitation. Children with HHS, however, should be assumed to be at similar risk for developing cerebral edema as those with DKA [14]. In the study by Glaser et al, those children who had more severe dehydration at presentation with higher BUN concentrations were at increased risk for cerebral edema [43]. Neurologic deterioration may not occur for an average of 7 hours after initiation of therapy. ED treatment could impact the incidence of this complication, and, in younger patients particularly, gradual correction of the sodium and water deficits and avoidance of rapid decline in plasma glucose concentration are important. The guidelines for slower rehydration should be adhered to meticulously for patients up to 20 years of age [2].

Rhabdomyolysis detected by increasing levels of creatinine kinase is a recognized complication of adult patients with HHS. Related complications occurring at the initial diagnosis of type 2 diabetes mellitus in teenaged children have been reported. Hollander et al described a case series of six adolescent males presenting with HHS complicated by a malignant hyperthermia-like picture with fever, rhabdomyolysis, and severe cardiovascular instability. Four of the six patients died, and all had increased temperature after administration of insulin. Although the etiology of the state is unclear, the authors suggested empiric treatment with dantrolene in this setting [21]. Morales and Rosenbloom reported on seven African-American youth with unrecognized type 2 diabetes mellitus who died from HHS complicated by delayed diagnosis and treatment. One of these patients died from cerebral edema, and one had fever and rhabdomyolysis [14].

Disposition

All patients diagnosed with HHS require hospitalization. Because of the close monitoring and dynamic therapy necessary in these patients, most will require admission to an intensive care setting. Some patients with less severe degrees of metabolic derangement and alteration in consciousness may be considered for step down units if response to initial therapy in the ED is adequate [27]. Careful monitoring of vital signs, fluid balance, and frequent clinical re-evaluation usually obviates the need for invasive monitoring and its associated infection risk [12,28].

Summary

This article has discussed the ED presentation, evaluation, and treatment of HHS. Aggressive volume replacement to restore renal perfusion is the first priority and cornerstone of therapy, with attention on electrolyte balance, especially treatment of hypokalemia. Calculation of the effective osmolarity and corrected sodium values can help guide treatment, and fluid replacement should be more judicious in younger patients. Identification and treatment of any precipitating illness are essential. HHS is usually the result of decompensated type 2 diabetes, and prevention centers on early diagnosis and identification of patients at risk, education of patients and caregivers on the early signs of uncontrolled hyperglycemia, and ensuring proper hydration and consistent monitoring. Finally, maintaining a high index of suspicion for type 2 diabetes mellitus in selected children and especially adolescents, will help prevent presentations of HHS in this age group.

Acknowledgments

The author is grateful for the assistance of Jennifer Zimmer-Young, PharmD, in the preparation of this manuscript.

References

[1] Wachtel TJ. The diabetic hyperosmolar state. Clin Geriatr Med 1990;6(4):797–806.
[2] American Diabetes Association. Hyperglycemic crises in diabetes. Diabetes Care 2004; 27(Suppl 1):S94–102.
[3] English P, Williams G. Hyperglycaemic crisis and lactic acidosis in diabetes mellitus. Postgrad Med 2004;80:253–61.
[4] Ennis ED, Kreisberg RA. Diabetic ketoacidosis and the hyperglycemic hyperosmolar syndrome. In: LeRoith D, Taylor SI, Olefsky JM, editors. Diabetes mellitus: a fundamental and clinical text. 2nd edition. Philadelphia: Lippincott Williams and Wilkins; 2000. p. 326–47.
[5] Wachtel TJ, Tetu-Mouradjian LM, Goldman DL, et al. Hyperosmolarity and acidosis in diabetes mellitus: a three-year experience in Rhode Island. J Gen Intern Med 1991;6: 495–502.
[6] Matz R. Management of hyperosmolar hyperglycemic syndrome. Am Fam Physician 1999; 60:1468–76.
[7] Umpierrez GE, Khajavi M, Kitabchi AE. Review: diabetic ketoacidosis and hyperglycemic hyperosmolar nonketotic syndrome. Am J Med Sci 1996;311(5):225–33.
[8] Engelgau MM, Geiss LS, Saaddine JB, et al. The evolving diabetes burden in the United States. Ann Intern Med 2004;140(11):945–50.
[9] American Diabetes Association. Type 2 diabetes in children and adolescents. Diabetes Care 2000;23(3):381–9.
[10] Perkin RM. The epidemic of pediatric obesity: clinical implications for the ED physician. Pediatric Emergency Medicine Reports 2004;9(6):65–80.
[11] Umpierrez GE, Kelly JP, Navarrete JE, et al. Hyperglycemic crisis in urban blacks. Arch Intern Med 1997;157(6):669–75.
[12] Trence DL, Hirsch IB. Hyperglycemic crises in diabetes mellitus type 2. Endocrinol Metab Clin North Am 2001;30(4):817–31.
[13] Chiasson J, Aris-Jilwan N, Belanger R, et al. Diagnosis and treatment of diabetic ketoacidosis and the hyperglycemic hyperosmolar state. Can Med Assoc J 2003;168(7): 859–66.
[14] Morales AE, Rosenbloom AL. Death caused by hyperglycemic hyperosmolar state at the onset of type 2 diabetes. J Pediatr 2004;144:270–3.
[15] Wachtel TJ, Silliman RA, Lamberton P. Predisposing factors for the diabetic hyperosmolar state. Arch Intern Med 1987;147:499–501.
[16] Delaney MF, Zisman A, Kettyle WM. Diabetic ketoacidosis and hyperglycemic hyperosmolar nonketotic syndrome. Endocrinol Metab Clin North Am 2000;29(4):683–705.

[17] MacIsaac RJ, Lee LY, McNeil KJ, et al. Influence of age on the presentation and outcome of acidotic and hyperosmolar diabetic emergencies. Intern Med J 2002;32:379–85.

[18] Pinies JA, Cairo G, Gaztambide S, et al. Course and prognosis of 132 patients with diabetic nonketotic hyperosmolar state. Diabetes Metab 1994;20:43–8.

[19] Gonzalez-Compoy JM. Hyperosmolar coma. Available at: http://www.emedicine.com/med/topic1091.htm. Accessed June 2, 2004.

[20] Pope D, Zun LS. Hyperosmolar hyperglycemic nonketotic coma. In: Harwood-Nuss A, editor. The clinical practice of emergency medicine, 3rd edition. Philadelphia: Lippincott Williams &Wilkins; 2001. p. 820–3.

[21] Hollander AS, Olney RC, Blackett PR, et al. Fatal malignant hyperthermia-like syndrome with rhabdomyolysis complicating the presentation of diabetes mellitus in adolescent males. Pediatrics 2003;111:1447–52.

[22] Magee MF, Bhatt BA. Management of decompensated diabetes: diabetic ketoacidosis and hyperglycemic hyperosmolar syndrome. Crit Care Clin 2001;17(1):75–106.

[23] Roefaro J, Mukherjee SM. Olanzapine-induced hyperglycemic nonketonic coma. Ann Pharmacother 2001;35:300–2.

[24] Meatherall R, Younes J. Fatality from olanzapine induced hyperglycemia. J Forensic Sci 2002;47(4):893–6.

[25] Abraham MR, Khardori R. Hyperglycemic hyperosmolar nonketotic syndrome as initial presentation of type 2 diabetes in a young cocaine abuser. Diabetes Care 1999;22(8):1380–1.

[26] Umpiarrez G, Freire AX. Abdominal pain in patients with hyperglycemic crises. J Crit Care 2002;17(1):63–7.

[27] Graffeo CS. Hyperosmolar hyperglycemic state. In: Tintanelli JE, editor. Emergency medicine: a comprehensive study guide. New York: Mc Graw Hill; 2004. p. 1307–11.

[28] Larber D. Nonketotic hypertonicity in diabetes mellitus. Med Clin North Am 1995;79(1):39–51.

[29] Gonzalez-Compoy JM, Robertson RP. Diabetic ketoacidosis and hyperosmolar nonketotic state: gaining control over extreme hyperglycemic complications. Postgrad Med 1996;99(6):143–52.

[30] Huff JS. Stroke mimics and chameleons. Emerg Med Clin North Am 2002;20:583–95.

[31] Thurman RJ, Jauch EC. Acute ischemic stroke: emergent evaluation and management. Emerg Med Clin North Am 2002;20:609–30.

[32] Bruno A, Levine SR, Frankel MR, et al. Admission glucose level and clinical outcomes in the NINDS rt-PA Stroke Trial. Neurology 2002;59(5):669–74.

[33] Yared Z, Chiasson JL. Ketoacidosis and the hyperosmolar hyperglycemic state in adult diabetic patients: diagnosis and treatment. Minerva Med 2003;94(6):409–18.

[34] Quinn L. Diabetes emergencies in the patient with type 2 diabetes. Nurs Clin North Am 2001;36(2):341–60.

[35] Rose BD, Robertson RP. Clinical features and diagnosis of diabetic ketoacidosis and non ketotic hyperglycemia. Available at: www.uptodate.com. Accessed May 8, 2004.

[36] Londer M, Hammer D, Kelen GD. Fluid and electrolyte problems. In: Tintanelli JE, editor. Emergency medicine: a comprehensive study guide. New York: McGraw Hill; 2004. p. 167–79.

[37] Hiler TA, Abbott D, Barrett EJ. Hyponatremia: evaluating the correction factor for hyperglycemia. Am J Med 1999;106:399–403.

[38] Liamis G, Gianoutsos C, Elisaf MS. Hyperosmolar nonketotic syndrome with hypernatremia: how can we monitor treatment? Diabetes Metab 2000;26:403–5.

[39] Ting JYS. Hyperosmolar diabetic nonketotic coma, hyperkalaemia and an unusual near death experience. Eur J Emerg Med 2001;8:57–63.

[40] Kitabchi AE, Umpierrez GE, Murphy MB, et al. Management of hyperglycemic crises in patients with diabetes. Diabetes Care 2001;24(1):131–53.

[41] Jones TL. From diabetic ketoacidosis to hyperglycemic hyperosmolar nonketotic syndrome: the spectrum of uncontrolled hyperglycemia in diabetes mellitus. Crit Care Nurs Clin North Am 1994;6(4):703–21.

[42] Kian K, Eiger G. Anticoagulant therapy in hyperosmolar nonketotic diabetic coma. Diabet Med 2003;28:603.

[43] Glaser N, Barnett P, McCaslin I, et al. Risk factors for cerebral edema in children with diabetic ketoacidosis. N Eng J Med 2001;344(4):264–9.

ELSEVIER
SAUNDERS

EMERGENCY
MEDICINE
CLINICS OF
NORTH AMERICA

Emerg Med Clin N Am 23 (2005) 649–667

Hypothyroidism: Mimicker of Common Complaints

Matthew C. Tews, DO[a], Sid M. Shah, MD, FACEP[b],*,
Ved V. Gossain, MD, FACP, FACEP[c]

[a]College of Osteopathic Medicine, Emergency Medicine Residency Program,
Michigan State University–Lansing, P.O. Box 30480, Lansing, MI 48909, USA
[b]Michigan State University, Attending Physician Emergency Medicine,
Ingham Regional Medical, Center 401 W. Greenlawn Avenue, Lansing, MI 48910, USA
[c]Division of Endocrinology, Department of Medicine, Michigan State University,
Lansing, MI 48909, USA

Patients with hypothyroidism may present with vague symptoms such as fatigue, arthralgias, myalgias, muscle cramps, headaches, and "not feeling well." These are also among the more common complaints encountered by the emergency physicians. The disease spectrum of hypothyroidism ranges from an asymptomatic, subclinical condition to the rare, life-threatening myxedema coma, and thus can be a challenging diagnosis to make. A progressive and chronic disease, hypothyroidism results from diminished thyroid hormone production. It slows metabolic functions in every organ system in the body. Commonly, clinical presentation of hypothyroidism can be confused with effects of aging in the elderly, musculoskeletal or a psychiatric illness such as depression in the younger patients.

Spontaneously occurring hypothyroidism is relatively common, with prevalence between 1% to 2%, and is 10 times more common in women than in men [1]. The probability of developing spontaneous hypothyroidism increases with age, with women having a mean age at diagnosis of around 60 years [2]. A recent survey showed that 9.5% out of nearly 26,000 visitors to a statewide health fair in Colorado had elevated circulating thyroid stimulating hormone (TSH) levels, indicating underlying hypothyroidism [3]. One large study performed in England found the prevalence of hypothyroidism to be around 18/1000 women and less than 1/1000 men in the general population studied [4]. The study also revealed a higher

* Corresponding author.
  E-mail address: sidshah@comcast.net (S.M. Shah).

0733-8627/05/$ - see front matter © 2005 Elsevier Inc. All rights reserved.
doi:10.1016/j.emc.2005.03.013   *emed.theclinics.com*

prevalence of subclinical hypothyroidism, defined as an asymptomatic elevation of TSH, found in roughly 8% of women and 3% of men. In a 20-year follow-up to this original study, the authors found the mean incidence from all causes of hypothyroidism to be 4.1/1000 of women and 0.6/1000 of men in survivors [5].

Thyroid disorders pose a particular challenge to emergency physicians because a significant number of patients with thyroid dysfunction are unaware of their condition. A well-known endocrinologist estimates that almost half the people with thyroid dysfunction are not properly diagnosed [6]. Because of this, the American Thyroid Association has recommended measuring serum TSH concentrations in adults starting at age 35 and continuing every 5 years, or more often in those at risk for thyroid dysfunction [7].

Pathophysiology

The production and release of thyroid hormone is the result of a delicate balance of the hypothalamic–pituitary–thyroid axis, which is controlled by a negative feedback loop involving circulating free thyroxine (T4) and triiodothyronine (T3), and TSH release from the thyroid gland. This delicate balance can be altered by causes such as the destruction or removal of the thyroid gland, alterations in the synthesis, release, and conversion of thyroid hormone (secondary to disease or medications), and diseases of the pituitary gland.

The substrate for the synthesis of thyroid hormones is the circulating iodides. The thyroid gland is able to "trap" iodide from the blood stream by an energy requiring mechanism. The trapped iodide is oxidized by the enzyme Peroxidase. The next step in the synthesis of triiodothyronine (T3) and tetraiodothyronine (T4) is iodination of tyrosine to monoiodotyrosine (MIT) and diiodotyrosine (DIT). Coupling of two DIT molecules results in the formation of T4. Some T3 is also formed within the thyroid gland by condensation of one molecule of MIT and DIT. The formed T4 and T3 are stored in the thyroid gland in combination with thyroglobulin. Release of T4 and T3 then occurs by proteolysis and is regulated by TSH.

After its release from the thyroid gland, T4 is bound almost exclusively to proteins in the blood including thyroid-binding globulin (TBG), trans-thyretin (prealbumin), and albumin for transportation to target tissues [8]. Over 99% of T4 is bound to these proteins, leaving <1% free in circulation. It is this small amount of free hormone that is responsible for the negative feedback inhibition on the anterior pituitary and hypothalamus controlling the release of TSH. Even small changes in free hormone levels are reflected in exaggerated changes in TSH secretion; making serum TSH a sensitive marker of thyroid function [9].

Although most of the thyroid hormone released from the thyroid gland is in the form of T4, only about 20% of T3 is released from thyroid, while the other 80% of T3 is formed by deiodination of T4 in peripheral tissues such as the pituitary, liver, kidneys, and hypothalamus [9]. It is T3, however, that has greater biologic activity than T4 at the cellular level.

Etiology

Hypothyroidism is broadly classified either as primary or central hypothyroidism. Ninety-nine percent of cases are primary hypothyroidism, typically resulting from destruction of the gland from either iatrogenic or autoimmune causes [10]. Depending on the cause, patients with hypothyroidism can present with or without a goiter. Central hypothyroidism is divided into pituitary (secondary) or hypothalamic (tertiary) causes, depending on the underlying etiology. Central causes of hypothyroidism make up a very small percentage of hypothyroid cases, with prevalence in the general population of about 0.005% [2]. Congenital hypothyroidism has a prevalence of about 1 in 4000 newborns worldwide. Eighty-five percent of cases of congenital hypothyroidism are due to thyroid dysgenesis, and the remainder are due to central causes [11].

Table 1 lists the causes of hypothyroidism, and the most common causes are discussed here.

Causes of primary hypothyroidism

The most common form of hypothyroidism worldwide is iodine deficiency typically associated with endemic goiter [12]. In iodine-replete

Table 1
Causes of hypothyroidism

Primary hypothyroidism
Chronic autoimmune thyroiditis
Reversible autoimmune thyroiditis (silent and postpartum)
Radioiodine ablation
Surgery
Irradiation
Infiltrative and infectious diseases
Congenital thyroid dysgenesis
Iodine excess or deficiency
Drugs
Central hypothyroidism
Tumors
Trauma
Vascular
Infectious
Infiltrative
Congenital
Drugs

Data from Wiersinga WM. Hypothyroidism and myxedema coma. In: DeGroot LJ, Jameson JL, editors. Endocrinology. 4th edition, volume 2. Philadelphia: W.B. Saunders Company; 2001. p. 1493.

regions, such as the United States, chronic autoimmune disease involving the thyroid gland forms the majority of cases of hypothyroidism.

Autoimmune thyroiditis

Hashimoto's thyroiditis is the most common form of thyroiditis, making this the number one cause of primary hypothyroidism in the developed countries with adequate iodine intake. Hashimoto's thyroiditis is characterized by chronic lymphocytic infiltration and destruction of the thyroid gland over time. It is associated with the presence of antithyroid antibodies. Antithyroid peroxidase (TPO) antibodies are present in more than 90% of cases of chronic autoimmune thyroiditis [13,14]. Hashimoto's thyroiditis is also associated with other autoimmune diseases, and specific association with certain histocompatibility antigens (HLA DR3 and HLA DR5) has also been described [14].

Postpartum thyroiditis is a variant of autoimmune thyroiditis with an incidence of 6.0% to 8.8% in the postpartum period. It typically presents as transient hyperthyroidism, usually between 6 weeks to 6 months postpartum [15]. This period is typically followed by a "hypothyroid phase," which resolves spontaneously in the majority of the cases approximately 1 year postpartum. However, permanent hypothyroidism can develop in up to 23%. It may recur in subsequent pregnancies.

Subacute thyroiditis, thought to be due to an autoimmune viral infection, results in an enlarged, painful, and tender thyroid gland. Patients initially present with hyperthyroidism due to release of preformed hormone, after which there is a brief period of hypothyroidism. The patient typically recovers in a few weeks; although recurrences may occur [16].

Iatrogenic causes

Iatrogenic causes of hypothyroidism are common. Surgical procedures, such as total thyroidectomy, may quickly result in hypothyroidism within 1 month after surgery, while hypothyroidism after subtotal resection for Grave's disease may take up to 10 years to develop [2]. The use of radioiodine (I^{131}) as destructive treatment for thyrotoxicosis frequently causes hypothyroidism. Radioiodine therapy and surgery have an incidence of overt hypothyroidism that is greatest within the first year after treatment [12].

Medications

Often overlooked in the emergency department (ED), medications are a well-known cause of hypothyroidism. Those with underlying autoimmune thyroiditis are more sensitive to the effect of commonly prescribed medications such as lithium, amiodarone, and cytokine therapy [9] Table 2 lists the effects of some medications on thyroid function.

Lithium, along with amiodarone and iodine, causes a decrease in thyroid hormone synthesis and secretion [9]. Lithium is known to cause overt and

Table 2
Medications associated with hypothyroidism

Decreased TSH secretion
  Dopamine
  Glucocorticoids
  Octreotide
Decreased thyroid hormone secretion
  Lithium
  Iodide
  Amiodarone
Decreased T4 absorption
  Colestipol
  Cholestyramine
  Aluminum hydroxide
  Ferrous sulfate
  Sucralfate
Increased thyroid hormone metabolism
  Phenobarbital
  Rifampin
  Phenytoin
  Carbamazepine

Abbreviation: TSH, thyroid stimulating hormone.
Data from Surks MI, Sievert R. Drugs and thyroid function. N Eng J Med 1995; 333(25):1688–94.

subclinical hypothyroidism in up to 20% of patients on long-term treatment [9], and has been shown to precipitate myxedema coma when lithium levels are in the toxic range [17].

Amiodarone, a drug commonly used for atrial and ventricular arrhythmias, is rich in iodine, which makes up about 37% of its molecular weight [18]. It has been shown to cause both hypothyroidism and hyperthyroidism. Amiodarone-induced thyroid dysfunction has an overall incidence of 14% to 18%, and is more common in iodine-sufficient areas. It is more frequently found in women and those with the presence of anti thyroid antibodies, indicating underlying autoimmune thyroid disease. Those who develop hypothyroidism are treated with thyroxine (T4) replacement during amiodarone therapy [18].

Iodine-induced hypothyroidism is from excess iodine, including that obtained from iodine-containing contrast agents for imaging procedures, and can lead to decreased yield of T4 and T3 by inhibiting iodine organification, known as the "Wolff-Chaikoff" effect. Patients with normal thyroid glands typically "escape" from this inhibitory effect, but some patients, especially those with Hashimoto's Thyroiditis or those previously treated with I^{131}, may not and will subsequently become hypothyroid [18].

Anticonvulsants such as phenytoin, carbamazepine, and phenobarbital increase the metabolism of T4 and T3, which can lead to hypothyroidism in those with preexisting thyroid disease [9]. Rifampin, although not an anticonvulsant agent, falls in category of agents that increase metabolism of T4 and T3.

Other medications such as colestipol, cholestyramine, aluminum hydroxide, ferrous sulfate, and sucralfate are known to decrease T4 absorption, thereby inducing hypothyroidism [9].

Central hypothyroidism is caused by trauma, irradiation, neoplasm, and infiltrative diseases of the pituitary such as amyloidosis or sarcoidosis. Pituitary tumors account for over 50% of these cases [19]. Sheehan's syndrome (postpartum pituitary necrosis), is also a cause of panhypopituitarism in the adult, but is rare in developed countries.

Congenital hypothyroidism worldwide is most commonly caused by endemic iodine deficiency. In areas where iodine intake is sufficient, thyroid dysgenesis, or developmental abnormality, is the most common cause [20]. In mothers who have thyroid antibodies, transplacental transmission of maternal thyrotropin receptor blocking antibody can cause transient hypothyroidism in the newborn in 5% of cases [11]. Inborn errors of metabolism make up approximately 10% of cases of congenital disease.

Emergency department presentation

Hypothyroid state involves almost every organ system in the body due to a lowered metabolic state. As a result, the clinical features of hypothyroidism are often subtle, and the diagnosis elusive. Hypothyroidism is indeed a great mimicker of many common complaints encountered in the ED. Common examples are (1) a patient with congestive heart failure complaining of "tingling" (paresthesias), weakness, and weight gain, who is found to be hyponatremic; (2) an elderly "demented" nursing home patient with "behavioral changes;" (3) a young "anemic" woman with frequent episodes of heavy menstrual bleeding, (4) a patient with long-standing well-controlled hypertension who presents repeatedly with episodes of "hypotension" even with reduced dosages of antihypertensive medications; (5) an elderly patient with frequent ED visits for abdominal cramps, constipation, and fecal impaction; (6) a young woman on antidepressant medication seen frequently in the outpatient clinic; now presents with vague complaints of "not feeling well," "loss of energy," weight gain, hoarseness of voice. In such cases, a high index of clinical suspicion allows the emergency physician to test for thyroid dysfunction.

Clinical features

Pertinent history

Many of the common complaints are nonspecific such as: lethargy, fatigue, weight gain, cold intolerance, constipation, dry skin, paresthesias, memory problems, depression, and others. It is not uncommon for a psychiatric condition such as depression to mimic clinical features of hypothyroidism [21]. A state of hypothyroidism has been reported as a common cause of reversible dementia in the elderly, but may not be as common as originally reported [22], see Table 3 for the signs and symptoms of Hypothyroidism.

The American Thyroid Association has published guidelines for detecting thyroid dysfunction [7]. These include a personal history of previous thyroid dysfunction, goiter, surgery, or radioablative therapy on the thyroid gland, diabetes mellitus, vitiligo, pernicious anemia, and the use of medications such as lithium or iodine containing agents. A family history of thyroid disease, diabetes, pernicious anemia, and primary adrenal insufficiency should be elicited.

Table 3
Signs and symptoms of hypothyroidism

Symptoms:
    Fatigue
    Lethargy
    Headache
    Weight gain
    Cold intolerance
    Somnolence
    Decreased appetite
    Dry skin
    Hoarseness of voice
    Constipation
    Menstrual irregularities
    Myalgias
    Paresthesias
    Depression
Signs:
    Nonpitting edema (myxedema)
    Cool, pale skin
    Coarse, dry skin
    Brittle nails
    Bleeding tendencies
    Alopecia
    Macroglossia
    Bradycardia
    Constipation
    Muscle hypertrophy
    Slowed speech
    Dementia
    Ataxia
    Slowed reflexes (with delayed relaxation phase)
    Psychosis
    Diminished libido
    Memory defects

Data from Larsen PR, Davies TF. Hypothyroidism and thyroiditis. In: Larsen PR, Kronenberg HM, Melmed S, Polonsky KS, editors. Williams textbook of endocrinology. 10th edition. Philadelphia: Saunders, 2003;423–55.

Physical examination

General appearance and skin characteristics are the first clues to the diagnosis, particularly in an advanced case of hypothyroidism. The classic presentation of primary hypothyroidism involves nonpitting edema in the face, typically around the eyes (periorbital edema), but also in the hands and pretibial region. This nonpitting edema, termed myxedema, is the result of diminished metabolism of glycosaminoglycans that accumulate in interstitial tissues. In addition to being edematous, the skin feels rough and dry due to decreased secretions of the sebaceous and sweat glands. Skin also feels cool to the touch from decreased cutaneous blood flow. The nails and hair are thin and brittle, and alopecia is present in 50% of patients [2]. The voice can become hoarse, and the tongue can become swollen (macroglossia). The presence of a goiter is most common in areas of iodine deficiency, but sporadic goiters are found in nonendemic areas.

The cardiovascular examination reveals a diastolic elevation in blood pressure due to an elevated systemic vascular resistance. Cardiac contractility and pulse rate are reduced; however, these overall reductions typically result in a cardiac output sufficient to meet the lower oxygen and metabolic needs of the body [23,24]. Intravascular volume is depleted, but rarely enough to cause hypotension unless the patient is critically ill. The heart may be dilated from an infiltrative cardiomyopathy. Pericardial effusion is reported in 3% to 6% of hypothyroid patients, and may take years to develop [25]. Progression to cardiac tamponade is rare.

Pleural effusions can result in diminished breath sounds. The presence of rales and rhonchi on auscultation of the lung fields may be present. Effusions can occur in the absence of congestive heart failure, and can be caused in part by an overall increase in capillary permeability [23].

Decreased peristaltic activity throughout the gastrointestinal tract leads to constipation, which is the most common gastrointestinal complaint associated with hypothyroidism [21]. Abdominal pain and distention can mimic an intestinal obstruction, leading to unnecessary surgery [26]. This occurs when glycoproteins infiltrate the lining of the bowel leading to denervation [27]. Ascites, although rarely from hypothyroidism alone, is produced by the same mechanism as pericardial and pleural effusions [10]. Urinary retention can result from bladder atony, and a distended bladder may be palpated [28].

Behavioral changes include slowed speech or thought process, as well as short-term memory loss, which is common in the elderly. Depression, agitation, hallucinations, and delusions can mask thyroid disease. Now rare, "myxedema madness" is a term used to describe psychosis resulting from hypothyroidism [21,29].

Muscle atrophy, muscular weakness, as well as muscle stiffness and myoclonus can be present. The "pseudomyotonic reflex," with slowing of the relaxation phase of a deep tendon reflex, is considered a classic finding of hypothyroidism, but can be seen with other conditions [30]. An ataxic gait, intention tremor, poor coordination, and evidence of carpel tunnel syndrome or other extremity paresthesias may be present on neurologic examination.

In hypothyroid women of reproductive age, there is an increased incidence of menorrhagia, which resolves with thyroid hormone replacement [31]. Those who become pregnant have an increased risk of premature labor and spontaneous abortion as well as an increased risk of spontaneous abortion [20]. Pregnancy-induced hypertension is also a common finding.

Alterations in the hematologic system can present as easy bruising or prolonged bleeding after tooth extraction due to lower concentration of factors VIII and von Willebrand factor, decreased adhesiveness of platelets, and prolonged bleeding time [2].

Infants with congenital hypothyroidism have different presenting symptoms than adults, and may not present with any symptoms early on. As the disease progresses, hypothermia, poor feeding, bradycardia, jaundice, and an enlarged posterior fontanelle may result [32]. Children and adolescents may present with complaints of delayed growth, seen on clinical examination and on radiographic studies. Hip pain in the adolescent may be the result of a slipped capital femoral epiphysis, which has been reported in conjunction with hypothyroidism [33]. Untreated cretinism can result in underdevelopment of the central nervous system resulting in mental retardation. Because of the serious side effects of untreated congenital hypothyroidism, an initial screening exam measuring T4 by heel prick is performed on all newborns in the North America, followed by a TSH level if the T4 is below the 10th percentile [11].

Laboratory evaluation

Thyroid stimulating hormone

In the past, thyroid function testing included measurement of either a total serum T4, which measures both bound and free hormone, or a free thyroxine estimate (FT4E) using the FT4 index. Total T4 and FT4E are not the most useful indicators of thyroid status, in part because of the effects of variations in serum binding protein levels, but also because T3 is the primary active thyroid hormone and because the relationship between T3 and T4 are not always predictable [34]. On the other hand, use of the clinical TSH measurement for thyroid function in the past was limited by the inability of most immunoassays to differentiate the lower limit of normal from abnormally low levels. The ultrasensitive TSH immunoassay, which uses monoclonal antibodies, is now the best initial screening test of thyroid dysfunction. With the availability of third and fourth-generation ultrasensitive assays, TSH measurement can be done quickly (approximately 20 minutes at our laboratory), and can be more accurate in defining subtle changes in significantly elevated or depressed TSH values [34,35]. This availability of a rapid and accurate screening test for thyroid dysfunction has major implications for certain groups of patients suspected of suffering from thyroid dysfunction presenting to the ED.

Elevated thyroid stimulating hormone

A patient with an elevated TSH and a low free T4 has primary hypothyroidism. The combination of an elevated TSH (TSH value is usually less than 20 mU/L) and normal T4 and T3 is described as subclinical hypothyroidism. It is usually caused by autoimmune thyroid dysfunction that has not yet progressed to severe thyroid failure [36]. This may be associated with positive anti-TPO antibodies, and the patient remains asymptomatic. Less common causes of an elevated TSH and a normal T4 or T3 include an inadequate dose or malabsorption of thyroxine due to other medications or small bowel disease. Apart from medications, the recovery phase of a nonthyroidal illness can cause an elevated TSH as the body attempts to compensate for previously depressed thyroid hormone synthesis. An elevated TSH (usually of short duration: 2 to 3 weeks) is found in patients with acute psychiatric illnesses such as schizophrenia, affective psychosis, and amphetamine abuse [36].

In a patient who has both an elevated TSH and T4, the diagnosis is not related to hypothyroidism, but may be the result of a TSH mediated hyperthyroidism possibly from a TSH secreting pituitary adenoma [36].

Those who have been on thyroid hormone replacement for less than 6 weeks can present with a persistent TSH elevation due to insufficient time for their current dose of hormone to bring their TSH into normal range [37].

Normal thyroid stimulating hormone

A normal TSH usually, but not always, indicates absence of thyroid dysfunction. Central hypothyroidism from pituitary dysfunction can exist with a low T4 and with "normal" levels of TSH, because the pituitary is unable to increase TSH secretion in response to low thyroid hormone levels, but such "normal" levels of TSH are inappropriate for the corresponding T4 levels [36]. A normal TSH and a low T4 may be consistent with a nonthyroidal illness, and can be difficult to differentiate from hypothyroidism clinically. However, a search for a secondary cause of hypothyroidism is necessary in the absence of nonthyroidal illness associated with a "normal" TSH and a low T4.

Low thyroid stimulating hormone

A depressed TSH can be associated with secondary hypothyroidism resulting from an overall reduced TSH production. It can be low due to hyperthyroidism or overtreatment of a patient on thyroxine therapy. In a critically ill patient, use of medications such as dopamine and cortico-steroids can suppress TSH levels [9].

Management

The usual recommended therapy for clinical hypothyroidism is oral T4 replacement with approximately 1.6 µg/kg/d. In the elderly with preexisting coronary artery disease, the initial dose should be 25 micrograms per day and increased slowly to avoid precipitating myocardial infarction from aggressive therapy [38]. After beginning treatment, monitoring of TSH levels at about 6 to 8 weeks is appropriate because it takes about 6 weeks to reach a steady-state drug level, and results before 6 weeks may be misleading [37]. Treatment for subclinical thyroid disease is controversial; therefore, it is prudent to coordinate care with the patient's primary physician before beginning therapy [39]. Risks of overtreatment include atrial fibrillation and the development of an iatrogenic thyrotoxicosis.

Myxedema coma

Myxedema coma is a term used to describe severe manifestations of hypothyroidism. A true medical emergency, it typically occurs in patients with longstanding, untreated, or undiagnosed hypothyroidism. The true incidence of myxedema coma in patients presenting to the ED is not known. The term "myxedema" was originally introduced in 1878 by Ord, and has been used interchangeably with the term hypothyroidism to describe the nonpitting puffy appearance of the skin and soft tissue associated with adult hypothyroidism [23,40]. However, a myxedematous appearance is un-common in most cases of myxedema coma [41,42]. Likewise, the term "coma" does not correctly describe myxedema coma, because not every patient with severe hypothyroidism is comatose. Myxedema coma is better understood to be a state of profound decompensated hypothyroidism usually triggered by a stressor such as infection [42]. Common triggers to myxedema coma include pneumonia and urinary tract infections, surgery, myocardial infarction, congestive heart failure, stroke, hypothermia, and certain medications (see Table 4). A careful review of the patient's prescribed medications may reveal the "trigger agent" such as a sedative, narcotic, or anticonvulsant medication.

Historically, myxedema coma has been associated with a mortality rate as high as 80% [43]. However, more recent studies have reported mortality rate to be closer to 15% to 20%, possibly due to earlier recognition and more aggressive management [44]. One series reported over 90% of cases of coma occurring during the winter months [45]. This wintertime prevalence is likely due to a diminished ability to sense temperature changes with advanced age [46].

Table 4
Precipitating factors for myxedema coma

Infections
Pneumonia
Sepsis
Urinary infections
Influenza
Surgery
Burns
Trauma
Hypothermia
Drugs
Sedatives (narcotics, tranquilizers, barbiturates)
Cardiac medications (amiodarone, beta blockers)
Lithium
Phenytoin
Rifampin
Stroke
Gastrointestinal bleeding
Congestive heart failure

Data from Rhodes Wall C. Myxedema Coma: diagnosis and treatment. Am Fam Phys 2000;62(11):2486.

Clinical findings

Multiple organ systems are involved in myxedema coma, resulting in signs such as altered mental status, hypothermia, bradycardia, hypotension, hypoglycemia, and hypoxia (hypercarbia). Examples of clinical presentations of myxedema coma include: an elderly hypothermic patient who does not "warm up" with usual measures; a patient with profound bradycardia who does not respond to atropine; or a patient on thyroid replacement therapy with acute myocardial infarct who is in "shock" and does not respond to vasopressors. Not all these findings are present in every case, although myxedema coma is unlikely in absence of altered mental status.

For the patient with an altered mental status assumed to be in myxedema coma, the physical examination proceeds in tandem with the primary and the secondary surveys. Attention to the airway, breathing, and circulation are the chief concerns. The initial examination may reveal facial puffiness with periorbital edema, as well as macroglossia and swelling of the pharynx. The neck is examined for an enlarged thyroid or a thyroidectomy scar, or patient may show evidence of hypoventilation. Hypoventilation in myxedema coma is due to a decreased ventilatory response to hypoxia or due to respiratory muscle weakness [47]. The cardiovascular examination may reveal diastolic hypertension, but systemic hypotension may be present due to sepsis or due to other causes of reduced cardiac output. Other contributors to systemic hypotension include: poor cardiac contractility, a decreased intravascular volume, and bradycardia and pericardial effusions. A secondary evaluation reveals many of the typical signs of hypothyroidism including pale, cool skin, dry brittle hair, hypothermia, distant heart sounds, nonpitting or pitting edema of the extremities, and a delayed relaxation of deep tendon reflexes.

Differential diagnosis

Numerous clinical conditions can present similar to myxedema coma. If the patient is comatose, other causes of coma must be considered.

The edematous patient with cardiopulmonary dysfunction can mimic myxedema coma. The presence of cardiomegaly, pleural effusions, low ejection fraction, hypotension, and peripheral pitting edema are all features of cardiac failure in the absence of thyroid dysfunction. However, cardiac failure is a known precipitant of myxedema coma, and both conditions frequently co exist.

Seizures occur in up to 25% of patients with myxedema coma, which often result from electrolyte imbalance such as hyponatremia and hypoglycemia [48]. The use of phenytoin (a medication known to precipitate or worsen a severe hypothyroid state) is avoided when treating seizures in a hypothyroid patient with suspected myxedema coma.

Hypothermia is common in the elderly, even in the absence of thyroid dysfunction secondary to a decline in basal metabolic rate occurring with advancing age [46]. The elderly frequently have comorbid conditions that predispose them to hypothermia such as stroke or malnutrition. The change in temperature that triggers a profound hypothyroid state and a rapid decline in clinical condition does not have to be extreme. However, a core body temperature of less than 35.5°C (95.9°F) is found in around 80% severely hypothyroid comatose patients, and the patient may present without shivering [23].

Thyroid function tests obtained in some critically ill patients may be confused with those that are seen in patients with myxedema coma. Patients with euthyroid sick syndrome, also known as *nonthyroidal illness syndrome*, typically reveal a low T3 and a low or normal T4 and TSH levels. This is likely due to decreased secretion of TSH from the pituitary and reduced peripheral conversion of T4 to T3. Reverse T3 (rT3) is formed when the conversion of T4 to T3 is impaired, and an abnormal level of rT3 may be an indication of a nonthyroidal illness [24,49]. Thyroid function tests return to normal after the resolution of the illness. If low T4 and T3 levels are found along with an elevated TSH (> 25–30 µU/mL) then primary hypothyroidism is the diagnosis [50].

Ancillary laboratory testing

A peripheral smear (complete blood count) demonstrates leukopenia with a mild right shift. The white count may not respond to infection in a typical fashion with a leukocytosis and left shift; however, evidence of elevated "bands" raises suspicion for sepsis [42]. The platelet count is likely to be normal despite abnormal platelet adhesiveness. The hemoglobin typically demonstrates a normochromic normocytic anemia from decreased red cell production and erythropoietin synthesis. Hypochromic microcytic anemia from iron deficiency associated with blood loss is found in women with menorrhagia. A macrocytic anemia can be present secondary to decreased B12 or folate uptake, commonly due to pernicious anemia in patients with autoimmune disease [51].

Hyponatremia is a common electrolyte abnormality in the severe hypothyroid state. This typically results from decreased free water clearance from an increased release of anti diuretic hormone and a decreased renal blood flow from low blood volume or diminished cardiac output [42]. Hypoglycemia results from decreased gluconeogenesis and reduced insulin clearance. Low serum glucose may be a sign of adrenal insufficiency, which is present in 5% to 10% of patients with myxedema coma [23]. A serum creatinine may be elevated, but potassium is generally unchanged. Serum calcium is commonly decreased.

Creatinine phosphokinase (CPK) is often elevated, and can confound the diagnosis of acute myocardial infarction. However, the CPK fraction typically reveals a muscular origin due to increased muscle membrane permeability in myxedema coma [23]. Elevated CPK-MB fractions in myxedema in the absence of acute myocardial injury have been reported [52].

Elevation of serum transaminases, cholesterol levels, and lactate dehydrogenase are common. Arterial blood gas analysis reveals respiratory acidosis with hypoxemia and hypercapnia, which are secondary to a decreased ventilatory drive [53].

A chest radiograph may reveal cardiomegaly and pleural effusions. The lung fields may reveal an infiltrate suggestive of pneumonia, which could be the precipitating factor in the development of myxedema coma. Pericardial effusion is common, with an incidence between 30% to 78% in myxedema coma [23]. Echocardiography can reveal septal hypertrophy and hypertrophic subaortic stenosis in addition to the pericardial effusion.

Electrocardiographic findings include sinus bradycardia, decreased voltage with electrical alternans if a pericardial effusion is present, and nonspecific ST and T wave abnormalities. The ST and T changes on ECG associated with an elevated CPK can confound the diagnosis of acute myocardial injury. To confuse matters more, acute myocardial infarction and myxedema coma frequently coexist with acute myocardial infarct acting as the trigger for the development of myxedema coma [42]. Other ECG abnormalities include the prolongation of the QT interval and conduction abnormalities of varying degrees [23].

A lumbar puncture may be indicated to rule out meningitis or subarachnoid hemorrhage. An increased opening pressure and an elevated protein level in the cerebral spinal fluid are nonspecific findings associated with myxedema coma [30].

A serum cortisol is drawn to rule out concomitant adrenal insufficiency before definitive treatment with thyroid hormone is instituted [28]. Blood and urine cultures are drawn when sepsis is considered in the differential diagnosis.

Management of myxedema coma

Prompt attention to the integrity of the airway is critical, and cardiovascular stabilization follows. Mechanical ventilation may be necessary because of a diminished respiratory drive in response to hypercapnia and hypoxia resulting in a worsening respiratory acidosis. With replacement of thyroid hormone, the central respiratory effort gradually improves over 7 to 14 days. Weaning these patients from the ventilator is especially challenging, and can be achieved after optimal thyroid hormone replacement [53].

Intravascular volume depletion is common, and fluid resuscitation is commonly required even in the absence of associated hypotension. Exacerbation of underlying congestive heart failure and hyponatremia must weigh against the benefits of fluid resuscitation.

Thyroid hormone replacement is the definitive therapy of myxedema coma and the availability of rapid TSH measurement is most helpful in quickly making a diagnosis. However, once the diagnosis of myxedema coma is strongly suspected on clinical grounds, definitive thyroid re-placement therapy is not delayed, and thyroid replacement therapy is started without waiting for laboratory confirmation. A blood sample for free T4 and TSH should be obtained before administration of thyroid hormone. The use of thyroid hormone is associated with the risk of precipitating acute myocardial infarction in elderly patients with preexisting heart disease [42]. These complications must be weighed against the high mortality rate of untreated myxedema coma, and the benefit of treatment in such a clinical scenario outweighs the risk of potential complications. Inadvertent use of thyroid hormone in a euthyroid patient does not increase the risk of complications or morbidity [54].

Thyroid hormone preparations include thyroxine (T4), triiodothyro-nine (T3), or a combination of both T3 and T4. There are no ran-domized clinical trials comparing the efficacy of using these different agents in the treatment of a severe hypothyroid state. Therefore, the use of intravenous (IV) thyroxine (T4) has remained the standard of care in myxedema coma, and is frequently cited as the treatment of choice [23,42–44]. The most common recommendations include 200 to 500 µg of T4 IV to initially raise the peripheral pool of thyroxine. This allows a slow conversion of T4 to T3 in the periphery, thereby re-ducing the possible adverse cardiac effects that may occur with a large dose of T3, especially in those with preexisting heart disease [28,42,49].

Doses of 50 to 100 μg are then given each day until the patient is able to take the medication orally [28]. The use of larger amounts of T4 (>500 μg/d) is associated with higher mortality, and therefore not recommended [44].

Proponents of T3 administration cite the increased biologic activity, quicker onset of action, as well as bypassing the impaired peripheral conversion of T4 to T3 as the reasons for the use of T3 [45,55]. A dosing regimen of 10 to 20 μg intravenously, followed by 10 μg dosed every 4 hours for the first 24 hours and then 10 μg every 6 hours for another 24 to 48 hours until oral intake is possible [56]. Precipitation of cardiac arrhythmias due to an acute rise in serum T3 levels is a concern [28], and high doses of T3 by itself is associated with increased mortality [49]. However, several case reports have cited improved patient outcomes with lower doses of oral T3 [55,57].

Combination therapy can be used providing a loading dose of 200 to 300 μg of T4 IV followed by 100 μg after 24 hours, then 50 μg/d thereafter. An initial dose of 10 μg IV of T3 is started at the same time and is followed by 10 μg every 8 to 12 hours until the patient improves and can take oral T4 [56].

The addition of glucocorticoids to thyroid hormone treatment regimen is recommended to prevent adrenal crisis. Administration of T4 and T3 may cause relative adrenal insufficiency, or if present, adrenal insufficiency may worsen once thyroid hormone replacement is started, due to increased metabolism of cortisol, which is why hydrocortisone is used along with initial thyroid replacement therapy [23]. Stress dose hydrocortisone should be given as 100 μg every 8 hours. A random serum cortisol level should be drawn before initiation of cortisol or thyroid hormone replacement. A high level indicates an adequate stress response and the hydrocortisone can be tapered. A low value will need further investigation. A rapid ACTH stimulation test can be performed in place of the random cortisol level [28].

Hypothermia is treated initially with passive rewarming, such as regular blankets and a warm room temperature. The use of heated blankets or warmed IV fluids lead to a rapid rewarming and peripheral vasodilation, which can cause (in theory) hypotension and vascular collapse. The restoration of normal body temperature and thermoregulation is restored with thyroid hormone administration [28].

Hyponatremia can be treated with fluid restriction and thyroid hormone replacement. If the hyponatremia is more severe (serum Na <120 mEq/L) or associated with seizures, cautious use of 3% normal saline is recommended. The use of hypotonic fluids should be avoided because there is already a problem with free water clearance.

Underlying infections (reported in up to 35% of patients with myxedema coma) are frequently the triggers for myxedema coma, and are aggressively treated [41].

Prognostic indicators

Factors associated with a poor outcome in myxedema coma include advanced age, a low serum level of T3, a body temperature <93°F, and hypothermia that does not respond within 3 days of therapy. Those with bradycardia less than 44 beats per minute, sepsis, myocardial infarction, and hypotension also have a poor outcome [41]. Yamamoto and others [44] also observed that advanced age, cardiac complications, and high-dose thyroid hormone replacement (>500 μg/d) were associated with a fatal outcome within 1 month of treatment. Pulmonary complications did not seem to be a factor associated with mortality.

Disposition

All patients in myxedema coma are admitted to the intensive care unit. Hospitalization is recommended for those with profound hypothyroidism who are clinically stable in the ED, to search for the underlying triggering event. Those who have mild symptoms can be sent home if clinically stable for close follow-up with their primary care physicians. Asymptomatic alterations in TSH levels can be evaluated further as an outpatient.

Summary

Hypothyroidism is a common condition presenting with many common complaints. This can pose a challenge to emergency physicians in diagnosing the underlying etiology of such vague complaints. Fortunately, testing for thyroid disease is now quicker and more sensitive than in the past with the newer generation TSH assays. This may prove especially helpful in the diagnosis of critically ill patients who are suspected of being in myxedema coma, a serious condition that arises when the body is in a decompensated hypothyroid state from a precipitating event. Even with the speed of the serum TSH assay, early treatment of suspected myxedema coma with thyroid hormone replacement (before TSH results) is necessary to avoid higher patient mortality. To do this, the emergency physician must maintain a high degree of clinical suspicion for thyroid disease in the ED.

References

[1] Vanderpump MPJ, Tunbridge WMG. Epidemiology and prevention of clinical and subclinical hypothyroidism. Thyroid 2002;12(10):839–47.
[2] Wiersinga WM. Hypothyroidism and myxedema coma. In: DeGroot LJ, Jameson JL, editors. Endocrinology. 4th edition, volume 2. Philadelphia: W.B. Saunders; 2001. p. 1491–506.
[3] Canaris GJ, Manowitz NR, Mayor G, et al. The Colorado thyroid disease prevalence study. Arch Intern Med 2000;160:526–34.
[4] Tunbridge WMG, Evered DL, Hall R, et al. The spectrum of thyroid disease in the community: The Whickham Survey. Clin Endocrinol 1977;7:481–93.

[5] Vanderpump MPJ, Tunbridge WMG, French JM, et al. The incidence of thyroid disorders in the community: a twenty-year follow-up of the Whickham Survey. Clin Endocrinol 1995; 43:55–68.

[6] Landers SJ. Overlooked, underdiagnosed? Am Med News 2004;47(9):25–6.

[7] Ladenson PW, Singer PA, Ain KB, et al. American Thyroid Association guidelines for detection of thyroid dysfunction. Arch Intern Med 2000;160(11):1573–6.

[8] Stockigt JR. Thyroid hormone binding and metabolism. In: DeGroot LJ, Jameson JL, editors. Endocrinology. 4th edition, volume 2. Philadelphia: W.B. Saunders; 2001. p. 1314–26.

[9] Surks MI, Sievert R. Drugs and thyroid function. N Engl J Med 1995;333(25):1688–94.

[10] Larsen PR, Davies TF. Hyopthyroidism and thyroiditis. In: Williams textbook of endocrinology. 10th edition. Philadelphia: W.B. Saunders; p. 423–56.

[11] LaFranchi S. Congenital hypothyroidism: etiologies, diagnosis, and management. Thyroid 1999;9:735–40.

[12] Vanderpump M, Tunbridge WMG. The epidemiology of thyroid disease. In: Braverman LE, Utiger RD, editors. Werner and Ingbar's the thyroid: a fundamental and clinical text. 8th edition. Philadelphia: Lippincott Williams and Wilkins; 2000. p. 467–73.

[13] Mariotti S, Caturegli P, Piccolo P, et al. Antithyroid peroxidase autoantibodies in thyroid diseases. J Clin Endocrinol Metab 1990;71:661–9.

[14] Pearce EN, Farwell AP, Braverman LE. Current concepts: thyroiditis. N Engl J Med 2003; 348(26):2646–55.

[15] Stagnaro-Green A. Recognizing, understanding and treating postpartum thyroiditis. Endocrinol Metab Clin North Am 2000;29(2):417–30.

[16] Emerson CH, Farwell AP. Sporadic silent thyroiditis, postpartum thyroiditis, and subacute thyroiditis. In: Braverman LE, Utiger RD, editors. Werner and Ingbar's the thyroid: a fundamental and clinical text. 8th edition. Philadelphia: Lippincott Williams and Wilkins; 2000. p. 578–81.

[17] Santiago R, Rashkin MC. Lithium toxicity and myxedema coma in an elderly woman. J Emerg Med 1990;8:63–6.

[18] Martino E, Bartalena L, Bogazzi F, et al. The effects of amiodarone on the thyroid. Endocrinol Rev 2001;22(2):240–54.

[19] Samuels MH, Ridgway EC. Central hypothyroidism. Endocrinol Metabol Clin North Am 1992;21:903–19.

[20] Smallridge R. Hypothyroidism and pregnancy. Endocrinologist 2002;12(5):454–64.

[21] Westphal SA. Unusual presentation of hypothyroidism. Am J Med Sci 1997;314(5):333–7.

[22] Dugbartey AT. Neurocognitive aspects of hypothyroidism. Arch Intern Med 1998;158: 1413–8.

[23] Olson CG. Myxedema coma in the elderly. J Am Board Fam Pract 1995;8(5):376–82.

[24] Klein I, Ojamaa K. Thyroid hormone and the cardiovascular system. N Engl J Med 2001; 344(7):501–9.

[25] Gupta R, Munyak J, Haydock T, et al. Hypothyroidism presenting as acute cardiac tamponade with viral peicarditis. Am J Emerg Med 1999;17:176–8.

[26] Bergeron E, Mitchell A, Heyen F, Dube S. Acute Colonic Surgery and Unrecognized Hypothyroidism. A warning: report of six cases. Dis Colon Rectum 1997;40:859–61.

[27] Salerno N, Grey N. Myxedema psudoobstruction. Am J Roentgenol 1978;130:175–6.

[28] Ringel MD. Management of hypothyroidism and hyperthyroidism in the intensive care unit. Crit Care Clin 2001;17(1):59–74.

[29] Talbot-Stern JK, Green T, Royle TJ. Psychiatric manifestations of systemic illness. Emerg Med Clin North Am 2000;18(2):199–209.

[30] Swanson JW, Kelly JJ Jr, McConahey WM. Neurological aspects of thyroid dysfunction. Mayo Clin Proc 1981;56:504–12.

[31] Brenner PF. Differential diagnosis of abnormal uterine bleeding. Am J Obstet Gynecol 1996; 175(3):175–9.

[32] Foley TP Jr. Congenital hypothyroidism. In: Braverman LE, Utiger RD, editors. The thyroid: a fundamental and clinical text. 8th edition. Philadelphia: Lippincott Williams and Wilkins; 2000. p. 977–82.

[33] Hirano T, Stamelos S, Harris V, et al. Association of primary hypothyroidism and slipped capital femoral epiphysis. J Pediatr 1978;93(2):262–4.

[34] Whitley RJ. Thyroid function. In: Burtis CA, Ashwood ER, editors. Tietz textbook of clinical chemistry. 3rd edition. Philadelphia: W.B. Saunders; 1999. p. 1504–8.

[35] Supit EJ, Peiris AN. Interpretation of laboratory thyroid function tests for the primary care physician. South Med J 2002;95(5):481–5.

[36] Dayan CM. Interpretation of thyroid function tests. Lancet 2001;357:619–24.

[37] Smith SA. Commonly asked questions about thyroid function. Mayo Clin Proc 1995;70: 573–7.

[38] Locker GJ, Kotzmann H, Frey B, et al. Factitious hyperthyroidism causing acute myocardial infarction. Thyroid 1995;5(6):465–7.

[39] Surks MI, Ertiz D, Daniels GH, et al. Subclinical thyroid disease: scientific review and guidelines for diagnosis and management. JAMA 2004;291(2):228–38.

[40] Ord WM. On myxedema, a term proposed to be applied to an essential condition in the "cretinoid" affection occasionally observed in middle aged women. Med Chir Trans 1878;61: 57–78.

[41] Jordan RM. Myxedema coma. Med Clin North Am 1995;79:185–92.

[42] Nicoloff JT, LoPresti JS. Myxedema coma: a form of decompensated hypothyroidism. Endocrinol Metab Clin North Am 1993;22(2):279–90.

[43] Holvey DN, Goodner CJ, Nicoloff TJ, et al. Treatment of myedema coma with intravenous thyroxine. Arch Intern Med 1964;113:89–96.

[44] Yamamoto T, Fukuyama J, Fujiyoshi A. Factors associated with mortality of myxedema coma: report of eight cases and literature survey. Thyroid 1999;9(12):1167–74.

[45] Forester CF. Coma in myxedema. Arch Intern Med 1963;111:734–43.

[46] Ballester JM, Harchelroad FP. Hypothemia: an easy-to-miss, dangerous disorder in winter weather. Geriatrics 1999;54(2):51–7.

[47] Zwillich CW, Pierson DJ, Hofeldt FD, et al. Ventilation control in myxedema and hypothyroidism. N Engl J Med 1975;292(13):662–5.

[48] Stathatos N, Wartofsky L. Thyroid emergency: are you prepared? Emerg Med 2003;2(22): 22–30.

[49] Hylander B, Rosenquist U. Treatment of myxoedema coma—factors associated with fatal outcome. Acta Endocrinol (Copenh) 1985;108:65–71.

[50] Umpierrez GE. Euthyroid sick syndrome. South Med J 2002;95(5):506–13.

[51] Klein I, Levey GS. Unusual manifestations of hypothyroidism. Arch Intern Med 1984;144: 123–8.

[52] Nee PA, Scane AC, Lavelle PH, et al. Hypothermic myxedema coma erroneously diagnosed as myocardial infarction because of increased creatine kinase MB. Clin Chem 1987;33(6): 1083–4.

[53] Behnia M, Clay AS, Farber MO. Management of myxedema respiratory failure: review of ventilatory and weaning principles. Am J Med Sci 2000;320(6):368–72.

[54] Brent GA, Hershman JM. Thyroxine therapy in patients with severe nonthyroidal illness and low serum thyroxine concentration. Ann Intern Med 1986;63(1):1–8.

[55] Pereira VG, Haron ES, Lima-Neto N, et al. Management of myxedema coma: report on three successfully treated cases with nasogastric or intravenous administration of triiodothyronine. J Endocrinol Invest 1982;5:331–4.

[56] Wartofsky L. Myxedema coma. In: Braverman LE, Utiger RD, editors. Werner and Ingbar's the thyroid: a fundamental and clinical text. 8th edition. Philadelphia: Lippincott Williams and Wilkins; 2000. p. 843–7.

[57] McCulloch W, Price P, Wass JAH. Effects of low dose oral triiodothyronine in myxoedema coma. Intensive Care Med 1985;11:256–62.

ELSEVIER
SAUNDERS

EMERGENCY
MEDICINE
CLINICS OF
NORTH AMERICA

Emerg Med Clin N Am 23 (2005) 669–685

Hyperthyroidism

Nathanael J. McKeown, DO[a], Matthew C. Tews, DO[a],
Ved V. Gossain, MD, FACP, FACEP[b],
Sid M. Shah, MD, FACEP[c],*

[a]College of Osteopathic Medicine, Emergency Medicine Residency Program,
Michigan State University, PO Box 30480, Lansing, MI 48909, USA
[b]Division of Endocrinology, Department of Medicine, B234 Clinical Center,
138 Service Road, Michigan State University, Lansing, MI 48824, USA
[c]Michigan State University, Emergency Medicine, Ingham Regional Medical Center,
401 West Greenlawn, Lansing, MI 48910, USA

Hyperthyroidism is a hypermetabolic state that results from excess synthesis and release of thyroid hormone from the thyroid gland. Thyrotoxicosis is a general term referring to all causes of excess thyroid hormone in the body, including exogenous intake of thyroid hormone preparations. Although the terms hyperthyroidism and thyrotoxicosis are by definition not the same, they often are used interchangeably [1].

The clinical spectrum of hyperthyroidism varies from asymptomatic, subclinical hyperthyroidism to the life-threatening thyroid storm. Subclinical hyperthyroidism is diagnosed in asymptomatic patients on the basis of abnormal laboratory tests (low thyrotropin [TSH] but normal free T4 and free T3), and is probably more common than generally believed. Overt clinical hyperthyroidism presents with typical signs and symptoms. Thyroid storm is the severe life-threatening form of hyperthyroidism. It usually is brought about by a precipitating event in patients with undiagnosed or undertreated hyperthyroidism.

Epidemiology and pathophysiology

The overall incidence of subclinical and overt hyperthyroidism has been estimated to be 0.05 to 0.1% in the general population [2]. It occurs at all ages, but it is more common in women than in men. In a recent US study

---

* Corresponding author.
E-mail address: sidshah@comcast.net (S.M. Shah).

0733-8627/05/$ - see front matter © 2005 Elsevier Inc. All rights reserved.
doi:10.1016/j.emc.2005.03.002

(National Health and Nutrition Examination Survey III), the prevalence of hyperthyroidism was found to be 1.2% (0.5% clinical and 0.7% subclinical) in a sample of randomly selected people [3]. Of those who have hyperthyroidism, only 1% to 2% will progress to thyroid storm [4]. Overall, Graves' disease is the most common cause of spontaneously occurring thyrotoxicosis, except in the elderly, where toxic nodular goiter is more common than Graves' disease [5].

Thyroid function is controlled by a negative feedback loop that is regulated by circulating TSH and thyroid hormones (T4 and T3). Thyroid gland mainly produces T4 and a smaller amount of T3. Most T3 (80%) is formed in the periphery by conversion of T4 to T3 [6]. T3 is approximately three to four times more biologically active compared with T4. Excess T3 triggers a sequence of molecular events that cause the tissue responses seen in hyperthyroidism such as excessive energy and heat production and deleterious effects on the central nervous system and cardiac function.

Etiologies

The most common cause of hyperthyroidism in the developed countries, Graves' disease is an autoimmune disease in which antibodies against TSH receptors develop. The result is unopposed stimulation of the thyroid gland causing increased synthesis and release of thyroid hormone and enlargement of the thyroid gland. Laboratory abnormalities include high serum thyroid hormone levels and a high radioiodine uptake by the thyroid gland. Graves' disease is more common in areas of high iodine intake, such as the United States, and generally presents between 30 to 40 years of age [6,7]. There is also a genetic component leading to an increased risk of developing the disease in those with a family history of hyperthyroidism or in those with an autoimmune disease such as type 1 diabetes mellitus [6]. Other triggers include stressful events, sex steroids, smoking, or dietary iodine intake [1].

Graves' disease can affect the neonate of a mother who has active Graves' disease or a history of Graves' disease. This is caused by transplacental passage of thyroid-stimulating immunoglobulin (TSI) that is present in maternal serum [8]. The fetus is at increased risk of neonatal hyperthyroidism, especially if the antibody titer is elevated in the third trimester. This hyperthyroid state, however, typically resolves as the maternal TSI is removed from the neonate after birth. If the mother has been on antithyroid medications for Grave's disease, the hyperthyroidism can be masked until the drug is cleared from the neonatal system over the period of days. Developmental and growth retardation may occur if thyroid abnormalities are not discovered and treated in a timely fashion after birth. Mandatory screening for T4 by heel stick at birth is now common in the United States.

Although Graves' disease is by far the most common cause of hyperthyroidism now, toxic multinodular goiter is the second leading cause of hyperthyroidism worldwide [9]. This is caused by excess release of thyroid hormone from multiple autonomously functioning nodules in the thyroid gland. It is more common in the elderly, and in areas of iodine deficiency. It develops slowly over a period of years and typically has milder symptoms than Graves' disease.

Toxic (adenoma) nodular goiter is a solitary nodule in the thyroid gland that has increased production of thyroid hormone [1]. It is more common in areas of iodine deficiency and in women, with an increasing frequency associated with age. It presents as a unilateral area of hyperfunctioning thyroid tissue that suppresses serum TSH. On I^{123} radioiodine scan, it is evident as a hot nodule.

Iodine-induced hyperthyroidism is another less common cause of thyrotoxicosis. It is often present in areas with endemic goiters and iodine deficiency, but it can be present in iodine replete and nonendemic goiter areas [7]. Hyperthyroidism results from one or more areas of autonomously functioning areas in the thyroid gland following administration of iodides or iodine-containing preparations for diagnostic tests.

In the past, a frequent cause of hyperthyroidism was iatrogenic, a surge of thyroid hormone caused by manipulation of the gland during thyroidectomy. This event now is prevented by pretreatment with agents such as inorganic iodide, or β-blockers before thyroid surgery [10].

Hashimoto's thyroiditis, the most common type of thyroiditis, is caused by an autoimmune etiology. It is characterized by chronic lymphocytic infiltration of the thyroid gland and the presence of high titers of antithyroid antibodies, most often thyroid peroxidase antibodies in up to 90% of patients. Twenty percent to 50% of patients have a high concentration of antithyroglobulin antibodies [11]. It is the most frequent cause of hypothyroidism and goiter in iodine-replete areas [7]. Most patients present with a painless goiter and are usually euthyroid. Rarely, patients may present with hyperthyroidism (Hashi toxicosis), but eventually hypothyroidism develops in most of these patients.

Subacute thyroiditis, also known as de Quervain's thyroiditis, is a painful inflammation of the thyroid that usually is preceded by a viral upper respiratory infection [11]. A common presentation includes malaise, pharyngitis, and fatigue, followed by fever and neck pain and swelling and symptoms of thyrotoxicosis up to 50% of the time. Inflammation causes leakage of stored hormone into the circulation, causing hyperthyroidism. The resulting hyperthyroidism is usually transient, resolving when the inflammation subsides and the hormone stores are depleted. This may be followed by a hypothyroid phase. Eventually, most of the patients make a complete recovery, although occasionally hypothyroidism may be permanent.

Postpartum thyroiditis, occasionally referred to as silent thyroiditis, is a variant of autoimmune thyroiditis. It presents with clinical features similar to subacute thyroiditis except that there is no pain or tenderness of the thyroid, hence the term silent. This transient form of hyperthyroidism develops between 6 weeks to 6 months postpartum with an incidence of about 5% to 10% of all women [12]. This is followed by a hypothyroid state with a return to baseline after about 1 year, although some women may develop permanent hypothyroidism. There is usually a small, nontender goiter, and symptoms are usually mild, the result of either the hyperthyroid or hypothyroid state. There is approximately a 70% chance of recurrence in subsequent pregnancies in those who had postpartum thyroiditis with their first pregnancy [12].

Sporadic thyroiditis is a condition similar in clinical course to postpartum thyroiditis, but it is not associated with pregnancy [11]. Up to 20% of these patients eventually develop lasting hypothyroidism.

Suppurative thyroiditis is an infection of the thyroid gland typically caused by a bacterial infection, and less commonly by fungal, mycobacterial, or parasitic infections [11]. Although rare, it is more common in those with pre-existing thyroid disease and in immunocompromised patients. Clinical features include a painful thyroid gland (anterior neck pain with erythema), fever, dysphagia, and dysphonia.

Amiodarone-induced thyroiditis is associated with either symptomatic or asymptomatic hyperthyroidism. It occurs in about 10% of patients in iodine-deficient areas, and less commonly in iodine-replete areas [7]. The mechanism of thyroid dysfunction from the use of amiodarone is caused either by the release of the iodine from the drug itself or by the development of destructive thyroiditis. Individuals with underlying autoimmunity are at increased risk for developing hyperthyroidism if they are taking amiodarone. Nodular and multinodular goiters, which are more common in the elderly, are a predisposing factor for amiodarone-induced thyroiditis [7].

Clinical features

Thyroid hormone affects nearly every organ system in the body. Patients with elevated thyroid hormone present in a hypermetabolic state with signs of increased β-adrenergic activity. Severity of the symptoms and signs of thyrotoxicosis are related to the duration of the disease, the magnitude of thyroid hormone excess, and age [13]. Although the diagnosis is frequently straightforward in patients with overt features of hyperthyroidism, a high degree of clinical suspicion has to be exercised in those with subtle clinical features of hyperthyroidism.

History

Constitutional

Many nonspecific complaints are common, particularly when hyperthyroidism is not yet advanced or when it occurs in the elderly. Complaints such as fatigue, nervousness, or anxiety can lead one to consider a psychiatric disorder. Excessive weight loss can prompt an evaluation for occult malignancy. On average, patients weigh 15% below their usual body weight [14]. Heat intolerance and an increase in perspiration are also common. Thyroid hormone increases basal metabolic rate and stimulates lipogenesis and lipolysis [14].

Cardiac

Thyroid hormone influences cardiac function by its direct effects on the myocardium and the systemic vasculature. Palpitations, irregular heart beats, shortness of breath on exertion, and orthopnea are among the more frequent complaints in the emergency department (ED). A reduced exercise tolerance is common [15]. Anginal symptoms are triggered in patients with cardiovascular disease. Chest pain similar in character to angina, presenting in absence of known cardiovascular disease, is thought to be caused by increased myocardial oxygen demand or coronary artery spasm.

Pulmonary

Dyspnea at rest and on exertion is common. The cause of dyspnea in a hyperthyroid state is multifactorial: weakness of respiratory muscles, high output cardiac failure causing an engorgement of pulmonary vasculature, increased ventilatory drive to breathe, increased airway resistance, diminished lung compliance, and tracheal compression caused by enlarged thyroid. In an ED setting, the combination of dyspnea, tachypnea, and tachycardia can confound the diagnosis and lead one to suspect pulmonary embolus.

Gastrointestinal

Gastrointestinal symptoms are common and nonspecific. Difficulty swallowing, secondary to compression of the esophagus [13] from a swollen thyroid is not as common as in the past. There is also a decrease in force of propulsion of pharyngeal muscles and in closure of upper esophageal sphincter, which also contribute to dysphagia [16]. Other complaints include frequent bowel movements and a rapid intestinal transit time secondary to increased motor contractions [13]. Nausea and vomiting can occur frequently.

Reproductive

Changes in menstrual cycle including anovulation, oligomenorrhea, menometrorrhagia, and amenorrhea are common. Infertility is very common in thyrotoxicosis. Postmenopausal women with thyrotoxicosis and especially subclinical thyrotoxicosis have greatly accelerated development of osteoporosis [17]. Males present with signs of increased estrogen activity

such as gynecomastia, spider angiomas, and decrease in libido. Gynecomastia, a very common complaint, is reported to be present in 83% of men
with thyrotoxicosis [18].

Neuromuscular

Over half of patients with thyrotoxicosis have myopathy—easy fatigabil-
ity and generalized weakness [19]. Muscular weakness most often involves
proximal muscle groups of the shoulder and muscle girdles. Weakness in
their shoulders presents as difficulty combing hair. Other examples of
proximal muscle group weakness include difficulty climbing stairs and
standing up from a squatting position or rising to standing position after
sitting in a deep chair.

Psychiatric

Patients and family members also may mention problems in cognitive
function and behavior, including memory loss and poor attention span [13].
Complaints of feeling jittery, restless, and the inability to sit still are
common. Family members report an increased emotional lability. Episodic
anxiety is a common complaint noted by the patient and others. Patients
may complain of insomnia, vivid dreams, and even nightmares [20]. In other
situations, the only presenting complaint may be altered mental status
prompting an evaluation for thyrotoxicosis. This may be more common in
the elderly [21].

Physical examination

Integument

The skin feels warm, smooth, and velvety, similar to an infant. Scalp hair
can be fine but brittle. Diffuse alopecia can occur. There may be localized or
generalized hyperpigmentation thought to be caused by increased release of
pituitary adrenocorticotropic hormone compensating for increased cortisol
degradation [20]. Localized dermopathy, termed pretibial myxedema, which
is a mucopolysaccharide infiltration of the dermis most commonly located
over pretibial region, is noted in advanced cases. The skin becomes raised
and discolored, and the lesions are painless, firm, and nonpitting [17]. Nail
changes are seen rarely. Plummer's sign refers to separation of the nail from
the nail bed.

Orbitopathy

A characteristic stare and exophthalmos, which is a measurable proptosis
from enlargement of the extraocular muscles, typifies the classic presentation of Graves' disease. Mild proptosis caused by elevation of the

levator palpebrae superioris due to sympathetic hyperactivity can be seen in patients with thyrotoxicosis from any cause. Depending on the degree of proptosis, there is associated lid lag, infrequent blinking, chemosis, and vasodilation of the conjunctiva and edema of the lids [22]. The proptosis and extraocular muscle fibrosis may cause diplopia. Inability to close the eyelids may lead to corneal ulceration and in extreme cases visual obscuration or even vision loss [23].

Thyroid gland

Almost all patients with hyperthyroidism have some palpable abnormality in their thyroid gland. Patients with Graves' disease reveal a diffusely enlarged thyroid gland, whereas a single nodule or a multi-nodular goiter may be palpable in others. Patients with thyroiditis also reveal a diffusely enlarged gland, which may be tender on palpation. A bruit resulting from increased blood flow to the gland over the thyroid gland is virtually pathognomonic for thyrotoxicosis [13].

Cardiovascular

Most patients (over 90%) have a resting tachycardia [15]. A widened pulse pressure results in a bounding pulse. Mean blood pressure may be normal or slightly increased. Carotid upstroke is rapid and brisk. Heart sounds are crisp. Soft to moderately loud systolic flow murmurs are a result of increased blood flow over the aortic outflow tract. Approximately 10% of patients have atrial arrhythmias including atrial fibrillation or flutter [15]. The occurrence of atrial fibrillation is more common in the elderly and may precipitate congestive heart failure (CHF). A search for underlying cause of CHF is being undertaken.

Pulmonary

The increase in basal metabolic rate leads to an increase in oxygen requirements and consequently an increase in carbon dioxide production. The respiratory system accommodates by increasing the respiratory rate. In a patient with underlying lung disease, an exacerbation of underlying disease is precipitated when such additional demands are placed. A reduction in vital capacity and decreased lung compliance can occur. Several case reports have described worsening airway reactivity in patients with asthma, which improved only after treatment of thyrotoxicosis was begun [24]. Other studies, however, contradict this assertion and maintain that a consistent relationship between asthma and thyrotoxicosis does not exist [25,26].

Musculoskeletal

A state of chronic hyperthyroidism is associated with decreased muscle volume and as a result decreased muscular strength. Proximal muscle groups including pelvic girdle and shoulder muscles are affected more commonly. Muscular atrophy is noted in longstanding thyrotoxicosis, especially in the thenar and hypothenar muscles [13]. Profound muscular weakness may affect respirations as a result of involvement of the diaphragm [1]. Case reports of hypokalemic periodic paralysis have been reported in conjunction with thyrotoxicosis. More common in Asian men, hypokalemic periodic paralysis also is encountered in others [27]. Onset of symptoms is typically sudden and involves muscle stiffness and cramps. The best treatment is a rapid reduction in thyroid hormone production. Hypokalemia is treated with potassium replacement therapy.

Neurological

Patients appear nervous and fidgety. A resting tremor occurs frequently. This can be severe enough for some patients to seek urgent medical attention. Characteristically, it is a fine rapid tremor that is present at rest and with movement. It is exaggerated with the arms outstretched and fingers spread apart. The tremor also can affect the feet, tongue, and even lip or facial muscles [28]. Hyperactivity and rapid-fire speech can be observed. Brisk reflexes with a rapid relaxation phase are common in thyrotoxicosis.

Hyperthyroidism in the elderly

The usual hyperkinetic and ocular signs and symptoms may not be evident in the elderly, making the clinical diagnosis even more challenging. The older person is much more likely to present with the involvement of a single system such as atrial fibrillation and CHF. Many nonspecific, subtle signs may be attributed to other illnesses or to the aging process [29]. A goiter may not be palpable in as many as 70% of patients [30]. Elderly patients present with apathetic facies, small goiter, presence of depression, lethargy, absence of eye changes, muscular weakness, and excessive weight loss. These patients are said to have apathetic hyperthyroidism. The diagnosis of hyperthyroidism is considered in the elderly when investigating a new-onset atrial fibrillation, weight loss, myopathy, or worsening of cardiovascular disease, especially if it appears to be resistant to the usual cardiotonic drugs. Because the signs and symptoms of hyperthyroidism may be too subtle for clinical diagnosis, some endocrinologists suggest a periodic screening for T4 levels in the elderly [30].

Thyrotoxicosis in pregnancy

Graves' disease complicates one in about 500 pregnancies [31]. It is a major cause of fetal morbidity and mortality. Complications include miscarriage, premature labor, low birth weight, and eclampsia [32]. Clinical features of thyrotoxicosis in pregnancy may be indistinguishable from normal physiological changes of pregnancy. Euthyroid pregnant females frequently have increased skin warmth and heat intolerance. An increase in cardiac output with a systolic flow murmur, mild tachycardia, and widened pulse pressure can occur in normal pregnancy. Weight loss is common in thyrotoxicosis; however this may be obscured by the normal weight gain in pregnancy. The presence of a goiter, sinus tachycardia above 100 beats per minute that does not slow with Valsalva maneuver, weight loss and onycholysis (separation or loosening of a fingernail or toenail from its nail bed) are rarely seen in pregnancy, but the presence of these features may indicate thyrotoxicosis [31]. Total T4 levels are increased because of an increase in thyroxine binding globulin in pregnancy, but free T4 and TSH levels are normal in euthyroid pregnant patients.

Thyrotoxicosis in the neonate

Although rare, thyrotoxicosis in the neonate accounts for 1% of cases of thyrotoxicosis in childhood [20]. Most cases are caused be Graves' diseases, usually with the mother having a history of the same. Clinical features include a low birth weight and premature delivery but with accelerated skeletal maturation. Microcephaly, enlargement of cerebral ventricles, frontal bossing, or triangular facies may be present. Weight gain is poor despite adequate or even increased caloric intake. Most of theses infants have prominent eyes and small diffuse goiter. Other features include: tachycardia and bounding pulses, cardiomegaly, CHF, jaundice, hepatos-plenomegaly, and sometimes thrombocytopenia [20]. Diagnosis is confirmed with TSH and free T4 levels. Treatment options include the use of both methimazole (MMI) and propylthiouracil (PTU). Propranolol can be given to severely ill infants who have extreme tachycardia and increased hyperactivity in doses of 2 mg/kg per day [20].

Thyroid storm

Thyroid storm is a severe life-threatening form of thyrotoxicosis, almost always brought about by a precipitating (trigger) event. There is often a history of untreated or partially treated thyrotoxicosis [1]. Untreated thyroid storm is fatal, and even with treatment, mortality ranges from 20% to 50% [33]. The clinical features of thyrotoxicosis are accentuated in thyroid storm.

Excessive diaphoresis and severe hyperpyrexia (with body temperatures even as high as 106°F) can occur [34]. Cardiovascular findings are common. Sinus tachycardia is the most common cardiac dysrhythmia, with the heart rate often over 140 beats per minute [29,30]. Atrial fibrillation and other tachyarrhythmias occur often. CHF may ensue, particularly in the elderly, although younger patients with no history of heart disease can develop CHF. Altered mental status indicative of metabolic encephalopathy may help distinguish thyroid storm from simple thyrotoxicosis. The mental status changes include agitation, emotional lability, chorea, delirium, convulsions, or even coma [30]. Volume depletion caused by vomiting or diarrhea with subsequent vascular collapse can occur. Acute abdomen pain can mimic bowel obstruction [20].

In the past, the most common trigger for thyroid storm was thyroid surgery in patients with uncontrolled hyperthyroidism. Now, with early recognition and pretreatment before surgery, this is rare. Infection (or sepsis) is now the most common precipitant of thyroid storm [20].

The differentiation between thyrotoxicosis and thyroid storm is not made easily based on laboratory values alone. Serum T4 and TSH values can be similar and are abnormal in patients with thyroid storm just as in un-complicated thyrotoxicosis [33]. The diagnosis of thyroid storm is a clinical one, aided by abnormal thyroid hormone levels.

Hyperglycemia secondary to glycogenolysis and catecholamine-mediated inhibition of insulin release is a common finding in thyroid storm. Other abnormal findings include leukocytosis with left shift, even in absence of infection, while other hematologic values are usually normal. Serum electrolytes are usually normal except mild hyperglycemia and a high serum calcium secondary to hormone-stimulated bone resorption. Serum lactate dehydrogenase, aspartate aminotransferase, alanine aminotransferase, and total bilirubin may be elevated, indicating some degree of liver dysfunction. Serum cortisol levels are high because of stress, and normal levels should be interpreted as an indication of some degree of adrenal insufficiency [20].

Laboratory diagnosis

The laboratory diagnosis of thyrotoxicosis is relatively straightforward. In the ED, TSH and free T4 levels are the most commonly obtained thyroid function tests. Third-generation chemiluminescent TSH assays can detect small changes in thyroid hormone levels. Serum free T4 values can be measured in two ways: directly by equilibrium dialysis techniques or indirectly by calculation of free-thyroxine index [35]. In thyrotoxicosis, the TSH is suppressed except where hyperthyroidism is pituitary-dependent. An elevated serum T4 is seen in approximately 95% of patients [36]. An increased serum free T3 and a normal T4 occurs in less than 5% of patients with hyperthyroidism (T3-toxicosis) [13]. Total T4, although a test commonly obtained, can be difficult to interpret because of alterations caused by thyroid binding proteins. Therefore, it is not a useful screening test. Several drugs including iodine, interleukins, and interferons can confound the diagnosis of thyrotoxicosis through their effects on the binding proteins [35]. With the easy availability of reliable free T4 assays, the need for estimation of total T4 has been eliminated and should not be used routinely for diagnosing thyroid disorders.

Other ancillary tests are considered depending on the clinical situation. Serum thyroglobulin levels have some utility in distinguishing Graves' disease from factitious thyrotoxicosis. It is elevated in Graves' disease and decreased in factitious disorder [35].

Treatment

Therapy for thyrotoxicosis depends identifying the underlying cause. The three main treatment strategies include: antithyroid drugs, radioactive iodine, and thyroid surgery. The choice frequently depends on clinician familiarity, usage, and preference of the patient. In developed countries, the thionamides, PTU and MMI are the two most commonly used antithyroid medications. These medications block the synthesis of T4 by inhibiting organification of tyrosine residues [37]. PTU also blocks peripheral conversion of T4 to T3. Compliance is better with MMI with its once-daily dosage. MMI dosage is 10 to 30 mg per day; for PTU, the dosage is 200 to 400 mg per day. Thyroid function tests are repeated every 4 to 6 weeks for the first 4 to 6 months [1]. On average, 30% to 40% of patients treated with antithyroid drugs go into remission lasting 10 years or more [38]. Common adverse effects of the drugs are abnormal sense of taste, pruritus, urticaria, fever, and arthralgias. Serious complications include cholestatic jaundice, thrombocytopenia, lupus-like syndrome, hepatitis, and agranulocytosis [39]. Patients are advised to seek medical attention if they develop a sore throat, fever, or malaise.

Radioactive iodine is the most common treatment for adults with Graves' disease [40]. Thyroid function returns to normal in approximately 2 to 6 months, and hypothyroidism occurs within 4 to 12 months as a natural complication of the radioiodine; as a consequence, lifelong therapy with L-thyroxine is routine. The relationship of I_{131} therapy and Graves' ophthalmopathy is controversial. An exacerbation of ophthalmopathy, especially in smokers, has been reported. This, however, may be prevented by administration of glucocorticoid agents given along with the radioiodine therapy. The glucocorticoid therapy is tapered slowly over a period of 2 to 3 months [41]. The use of radioiodine is efficacious in those with toxic nodules and toxic multi-nodular goiter.

Surgery is the most invasive and most costly option. Patients are rendered euthyroid before surgery can be performed safely. The treatment is rapid and effective, especially in patients with large goiters. It also may cause permanent hypothyroidism. In experienced hands, surgical complications are rare and include recurrent laryngeal nerve damage and permanent hypoparathyroidism. Transient hypocalcemia is seen in up to 25% of post-thyroidectomy patients [42], and this can be treated with oral calcium supplements and vitamin D supplementation if ionized calcium levels are less than 1.12 mmol/L. If the patient is symptomatic or has ionized calcium of less then 1.0 mmol/L, intravenous calcium is the therapy of choice [43].

Treatment for thyroiditis

Treatment for subacute thyroiditis is initially aspirin or other non-steroidal agents. Glucocorticoid therapy sometimes is needed and may be given as prednisone in doses of 40 to 60 mg once daily for a week, followed by gradual tapering over 4 weeks. Relief of pain usually starts after 1 to 2 days of therapy. β-blocking agents also are used. The thyrotoxicosis generally resolves spontaneously, and no further treatment is needed [41,44].

Treatment of thyrotoxicosis in pregnancy

Antithyroid medications and β-blocking agents are the mainstay of treatment. The use of radioactive iodine is contraindicated, and thyroid surgery rarely is recommended. Surgery, however, can be performed safely in the second trimester if patients prefer surgical treatment as the definitive treatment for their hyperthyroidism. Both MMI and PTU can be used, and both these agents have similar frequency of neonatal hypothyroidism [45]. MMI rarely has been associated with scalp defects and more serious congenital malformations; hence it is used much less often [39]. Both MMI and PTU are secreted in breast milk. Because PTU is more protein-bound, it is secreted in breast milk to a lesser extent. PTU is the drug of choice for breast-feeding mothers, although MMI can be used [31].

β-blocking agents can be used for the symptomatic treatment of palpitations in pregnancy. Because these agents cross the placenta and can exert some adverse effects on the fetus, such as intrauterine growth retardation, prolonged labor, neonatal bradycardia, hypotension, hypogly-cemia, and prolonged hyperbilirubinemia, they are used on a case-by-case basis based on the risk-to-benefit analysis [46].

Treatment for thyroid storm

The clinical management of thyroid storm is directed at four areas: (1) therapy to control the overactive thyroid gland, (2) therapy to block the peripheral effects of thyroid hormone, (3) supportive care, and (4) iden-tification and treatment of the precipitating event.

Therapy to control the overactive thyroid gland

The two main medications for preventing new hormone synthesis, PTU and MMI, are not available in parenteral forms and are given orally or through an orogastric tube. These agents also can be given by rectal administration [47,48]. PTU inhibits peripheral conversion of T4 to T3. In thyroid storm, the initial oral loading dose of PTU is between 600 to 1000 mg, and then 200 to 250 mg administered every 4 hours. MMI can be given initially as a 20 mg dose repeated every 4 hours [33,49].

Although PTU and MMI are very effective at preventing new synthesis, they have little effect on release of preformed hormone. Both iodine preparations and lithium are effective in blocking the release of preformed hormone from the thyroid gland. Iodine preparations have been studied more extensively. The iodine preparation is given at least 1 hour after the first dose of PTU or MMI, because iodides potentially can increase the intrathyroidal hormone stores by providing more substrate for further hormone production. The iodine preparations include iopanoic acid, Lugol's iodine, and saturated solution of potassium iodide (SSKI). The usual dose of iopanoic acid is 1 g every 8 hours for the first 24 hours, then 500 mg twice daily. The dosage of Lugol's iodide or SSKI is 4 to 8 drops every 6 to 8 hours [49]. When iodides are used along with thionamide agents, serum T4 levels are reduced rapidly and approach normal levels in 4 to 5 days [50]. The use of iodides may preclude the use radioiodine for several months.

Patients with an iodine-induced anaphylaxis may be treated with lithium carbonate to block further release of hormone. The dosage of lithium is 300 mg every 6 hours orally or by nasogastric tube, and then adjusted to maintain serum lithium levels of approximately 1 mEq/L [33].

Therapy to block peripheral effects of the thyroid hormones

The goal of blocking peripheral effects is to antagonize the sympathetic hyperstimulation that results from thyrotoxicosis. This includes blocking the peripheral conversion of T4 to T3 and reducing or removing thyroid hormone from the circulation. Both iopanoic acid and PTU have some effect on inhibition of the peripheral conversion of T4 to T3. β-blockers and high-dose glucocorticoid medications also contribute to a smaller effect.

β-Blockers are used to control the sympathetic effects such as tachycardia and tremors. Propranolol has been used most extensively secondary to its familiarity and to its inhibition of peripheral conversion to T4 to T3. For thyroid storm the dosage is 60 to 80 mg orally every 4 hours. The onset of action of oral propranolol is within 1 hour of administration. In selected cases, an intravenous loading dose of propranolol can be given (0.5 to 1 mg) every 15 minutes as needed until the oral therapy becomes effective. Esmolol also can be used (0.25 to 0.5 µg/kg loading dose, then infusion of 0.05 to 0.1 µg/kg per minute); however, close cardiac monitoring is needed [51,52]. Contraindications for the use of β-blocking agents include patients with moderate to severe CHF or those with a history of asthma or bronchospasm. In those individuals, either guanethidine 30 to 40 mg orally every

6 hours or reserpine 2.5 to 5 mg intramuscularly every 4 hours may be given [50,53]. The use of these medications is contraindicated in hypotension.

In cases where clinical improvement is not discernible despite aggressive conventional therapy, the use of other methods for removal of the thyroid hormones such as hemodialysis, peritoneal dialysis, plasmapheresis, charcoal hemoperfusion, exchange transfusion, and plasma exchange should be considered [54–56].

Supportive care

Fever is treated with antipyretics and cooling measures. The use of salicylates is avoided, because salicylates potentially can exacerbate the thyrotoxicosis by decreasing thyroid protein binding, thereby increasing free T4 and T3. Cooling measures include ice packs, cooling blankets, and cool mist. Shivering is avoided. Dehydration is common, and fluid requirements of 3 to 5 L/day may be needed. Intravenous fluids should contain 5% to 10% dextrose in addition to electrolytes to replace depleted glycogen stores. The elderly and those with CHF should be monitored closely to avoid fluid overload.

Treatment of the precipitating cause

An aggressive search for an underlying precipitating cause of thyroid storm is being undertaken. Searching for a source of infection is especially challenging, because both fever and white blood cell counts are elevated in thyroid storm and in underlying infection. Blood, urine, and sputum cultures are obtained in a febrile thyrotoxic patient. Empiric use of antibiotics is not recommended [33]. In a few challenging cases, an identifiable cause of thyroid storm may not be found.

Disposition

All patients with suspected thyroid storm require admission to an intensive care unit. Symptomatic thyrotoxic patients may require hospitalization. Patients with mild or moderate hyperthyroidism can be evaluated for signs of thyrotoxicosis in the ED, and most of these patients can be referred for further outpatient evaluation and continuity of care.

Summary

Hyperthyroidism is a common form of thyroid disease that mimics many of the common complaints in the ED. Most of these complaints refer to the overt or sometimes undiagnosed state of hypermetabolism caused by excess thyroid hormones. The diagnosis of hyperthyroidism is often challenging because of many physical and even psychiatric complaints. The most common worldwide cause of thyrotoxicosis is Graves' disease. Thyroid storm is considered in patients presenting with profound hyperpyrexia, tachycardia, altered mental status, and an underlying history of thyroid disease. The diagnosis of thyroid storm is primarily a clinical one aided by selected laboratory tests. Appropriate clinical suspicion and rapidly available laboratory tests measuring sensitive TSH and free T4 levels make the diagnosis of hyperthyroidism and thyroid storm possible in the ED setting. Radioactive iodine is the most common treatment for hyperthyroidism in a stable patient; however. the use of other therapeutic modalities can be considered. In the acutely ill patient who is suspected to have thyroid storm, therapy should begin immediately. First-line treatment typically includes the use of PTU, inorganic iodides, and β-blocking agents along with supportive care.

References

[1] Cooper DS. Hyperthyroidism. Lancet 2003;362:459–68.
[2] Glauser J, Strange GR. Hypothyroidism and hyperthyroidism in the elderly. Emerg Med Rep 2002;1(2):1–12.
[3] Hollowell JG, Staehling NW, Flanders WD, et al. Serum TSH, T3 and thyroid antibodies in the United States population (1988–1994): National Health and Nutrition Examination Survey (NHANES III). J Clin Endocrinol Metab 2002;87:489–99.
[4] Wogan JM. Selected endocrine disorders. In: Marx JA, Hockberger RS, Walls RM, editors. Rosen's emergency medicine: concepts and clinical practice. 5th edition. St. Louis (MO): Mosby; 2002. p. 1770.
[5] Diez JJ. Hyperthyroidism in patients older than 55 years: an analysis of the etiology and management. Gerontology 2003;49:316–23.
[6] Streetman DD, Khanderia U. Diagnosis and treatment of Graves' disease. Ann Pharmacother 2003;37:1100–9.
[7] Roti E, Uberti E. Iodine excess and hyperthyroidism. Thyroid 2001;11(5):493–500.
[8] Zimmerman D, Lteif AN. Thyrotoxicosis in children. Endocrinol Metab Clin North Am 1998;27(1):113–4.
[9] Seigel RD, Lee SL. Toxic nodular goiter: toxic adenoma and toxic multi-nodular goiter. Endocrinol Metab Clin North Am 1998;27:151–68.
[10] Baeza J, Aguayo M, Barria M, et al. Rapid preoperative preparation in hyperthyroidism. Clin Endocrinol 1991;35:439–42.
[11] Pearce EN, Farwell AP, Braverman LE. Thyroiditis. N Engl J Med 2003;348:2646–55.
[12] Stagnaro-Green A. Recognizing, understanding, and treating postpartum thyroiditis. Endocrinol Metab Clin North Am 2000;29:417–30.
[13] Dabon-Almirante CLM, Surks MI. Clinical and laboratory diagnosis of thyrotoxicosis. Endocrin Metabol Clin 1998;27:25–35.
[14] Motomura K, Brent GA. Mechanisms of thyroid hormone action: Implications for the clinical manifestation of thyrotoxicosis. Endocrin Metab Clin 1998;27:1–23.
[15] Klein I, Ojamaa K. Thyrotoxicosis and the heart. Endocrin Metabol Clin 1998;27:51–62.
[16] Marks P, Anderson J, Vincent R. Thyrotoxic myopathy presenting as dysphagia. Postgrad Med J 1980;55:669.
[17] Mazzaferri EL. Recognizing thyrotoxicosis. Hosp Pract 1999;34(5):43–58.
[18] Carlson HE. Current concepts—gynecomastia. N Engl J Med 1980;303:795.
[19] Kudrjavcev T. Neurologic complications of thyroid dysfunction. Adv Neurol 1978;19:619–36.

[20] Braverman LE, Utiger RD. Werner and Ingbar's the thyroid: a fundamental and clinical text. 7th edition. Philadelphia: Lipponcott-Raven; 1996.

[21] American College of Emergency Physicians. Clinical policy for the initial approach to patients presenting with altered mental status. Ann Emerg Med 1999;33:251–81.

[22] Bahn R, Heufelder A. Pathogenesis of Graves' ophthalmopathy. N Engl J Med 1993;329: 1468–75.

[23] Ginsberg J. Diagnosis and management of Graves' disease. CMAJ 2003;168:575–85.

[24] Settipane GA, Schoenfeld E, Hamolsky MW. Asthma and hyperthyroidism. J Allergy Clin Immunol 1972;49:348.

[25] Roberts JA, McLellan AR, Alexander WD. Effect of hyperthyroidism on bronchial reactivity in nonasthmatic patients. Thorax 1989;445:603.

[26] Hollingsworth HM, Pratter MR, Dubois JM, et al. Effect of tri-iodothyronine-induced thyrotoxicosis on airway hyper-responsiveness. J Appl Physiol 1991;71:438.

[27] Ober KP. Thyrotoxic periodic paralysis in the United States: report of 7 cases and review of the literature. Mayo Clin Proc 1966;41:785.

[28] Shaw PJ. Neurological abnormalities associated with thyroid disease. Handbook of Clinical Neurology 1998;70:81.

[29] Lahey FH. The crisis of exopthamlic goiter. N Engl J Med 1928;199:255–7.

[30] Lamberg BA. The medical thyroid crisis. Acta Med Scand 1959;164:479–96.

[31] Masiukiewicz US, Burrow GN. Hyperthyroidism in pregnancy: diagnosis and treatment. Clin Endocrinol 1999;9:647–52.

[32] Davis LE, Lucas MJ, Hankins GDV, et al. Thyrotoxicosis complicating pregnancy. American J Obstet Gynecol 1989;160:63–70.

[33] Burch HB, Wartofsky L. Life-threatening thyrotoxicosis. Endocrinol Metab Clin North Am 1993;22:263–77.

[34] Howton JC. Thyroid storm presenting as coma. Ann Emerg Med 1988;17:343–5.

[35] Dayan CM. Interpretation of thyroid function tests. Lancet 2001;357:619–24.

[36] Ladenson PW, Singer PA, Ain KB, et al. American Thyroid Association guidelines for detection of thyroid dysfunction. Arch Intern Med 2000;160:1573–5.

[37] Cooper DS. Antithyroid drugs for the treatment of hyperthyroidism caused by Graves' disease. Endocrinol Metab Clin North Am 1998;27:225–47.

[38] Weetman AP. Graves' disease. N Engl J Med 2000;343:1236–48.

[39] Fisher JN. Management of thyrotoxicosis. South Med J 2002;95:493–505.

[40] Solomon B, Glinoer D, Lagasse R, et al. Current trends in the management of Graves' disease. J Clin Endocrinol Metab 1990;70:1518–24.

[41] Bartalena L, Pinchera A, Marcocci C. Management of Graves' ophthalmopathy: reality and perspectives. Endocr Rev 2000;21:168–99.

[42] Bourrel C, Uzzan B, Tison P, et al. Transient hypocalcemia after thyroidectomy. Ann Otol Rhinol Laryngol 1993;102:496–501.

[43] Prendiville S, Burman KD, Wartofsky L, et al. Evaluation and treatment of post-thyroidectomy hypocalcemia. Endocrinologist 1998;8:34–40.

[44] Singer PA. Thyroiditis—Acute, subacute and chronic. Med Clin NA 1991;75:61–7.

[45] Momotani N, Noh JY, Ishikawa N, et al. Effects of propylthiouracil and methimazole on fetal thyroid status in mothers with Graves' hyperthyroidism. J Clin Endo Metab 1997; 82(11):3633–6.

[46] Gladstone GR, Hordof A, Gersony WM. Propranolol administration during pregnancy: effects on the fetus. J Pediatr 1975;121:242–5.

[47] Nareem N, Miner DJ, Amatruda JM. Methimazole: an alternative route of administration. J Clin Endocrinol Metab 1982;54:180–1.

[48] Walter RM, Bartle WR. Rectal administration of propylthiouracil in the treatment of Graves' disease. Am J Med 1990;88:69–70.

[49] Ringel MD. Management of hypothyroidism and hyperthyroidism in the intensive care unit. Crit Care Clin 2001;17:59–74.

[50] Tietgens ST, Leinung MC. Thyroid storm. Med Clin North Am 1995;79:169–84.

[51] Brunette DD, Rothong C. Emergency department management of thyrotoxic crisis with esmolol. Am J Emerg Med 1991;9:232–4.

[52] Isley WL, Dahl S, Gibbs H. Use of esmolol in managing a thyrotoxic patient needing emergency surgery. Am J Med 1990;89:122–3.

[53] Waldstein SS, Slodki SJ, Kaganiec GL, et al. A clinical study of thyroid storm. Ann Intern Med 1960;52:626–42.

[54] Candrina R, Distegano O, Spandrio S, et al. Treatment of thyrotoxic storm by charcoal plasma perfusion. J Endocrinol Invest 1989;12:133–4.

[55] Ashkar FS, Katims RB, Smoak WM III, et al. Thyroid storm treatment with blood exchange and plasmapheresis. JAMA 1970;214:1275–9.

[56] Tajiri J, Katsuya H, Kiyokawa T, et al. Successful treatment of thyrotoxic crisis with plasma exchange. Crit Care Med 1984;12:536–7.

ELSEVIER
SAUNDERS

EMERGENCY
MEDICINE
CLINICS OF
NORTH AMERICA

Emerg Med Clin N Am 23 (2005) 687–702

Recognition and Management of Adrenal Emergencies

Susan P. Torrey, MD[a,b]

[a]Tufts University School of Medicine, 136 Harrison Avenue Boston, MA 02111, USA
[b]Department of Emergency Medicine, Baystate Medical Center,
759 Chestnut Street, Springfield, MA 01199, USA

Case 1.   A 52-year-old woman presents to the emergency department (ED) with the chief complaint of palpitations, sweating, and chest tightness. This has been a recurrent problem for the patient over the prior 6 months. She has been treated with benzodiazepines by her primary care provider. Although the symptoms are improving on presentation to the ED, she says she felt like she was going to die. PMH is otherwise negative. She does not smoke and denies drug or regular alcohol use. Exam in the ED includes: vital signs: 188/104, 108, 20, 98.8°F, oxygen saturation 98%; lungs: clear without wheeze or rales; cardiac: regular without murmur; abdomen: soft, nontender; neurologic: nonfocal exam. Is this simply another presentation of an anxiety attack in the ED?

Pheochromocytomas

Pheochromocytomas are notorious but rare catecholamine-secreting tumors of neuroectodermal origin. There are several clinical issues of importance to emergency physicians, ranging from the potential for presentation as a hypertensive emergency to the recognition of more subtle symptoms masquerading as yet another anxiety attack. Although pheochromocytoma will be diagnosed or treated infrequently in the emergency ED, it is an important entity to consider in the differential diagnosis of several presentations.

Pheochromocytomas can occur anywhere along the sympathetic chain, although 85% to 90% are discovered within the adrenal gland. In adults, at least 10% are extra-adrenal; 10% are bilateral, and 10% are malignant, with

E-mail address: susan.torrey@bhs.org

a propensity to metastasize to bone, liver, and lung [1]. In children, there is approximately a 20% incidence of extra-adrenal location, bilateral occurrence, and malignancy [2].

Pheochromocytomas occur sporadically, or, in approximately 10% of cases, in association with familial disorders, like multiple endocrine neoplasia type IIA (MEN-IIA), von Hippel-Lindau disease or neurofibromatosis. Multiple endocrine neoplasia type IIA is characterized by the familial association of medullary thyroid cancer, pheochromocytoma, and parathyroid hyperplasia. Patients with von Hippel-Lindau disease develop early-onset bilateral kidney tumors and cysts, pheochromocytomas, cerebellar and spinal hemangioblastomas, retinal angiomas, and pancreatic cysts and tumors. Von Hippel-Lindau disease and MEN IIA have a similar prevalence—approximately 1 in 30,000 [3]. Hereditary pheochromocytomas are typically intra-abdominal and bilateral. Patients with hereditary tumors present at a younger age than those with sporadic disease.

Emergency department presentation

The classic signs and symptoms of pheochromocytomas are caused by the excretion of catecholamines, including norepinephrine and epinephrine, into the circulation. Typical symptoms include hypertension (sustained or paroxysmal), with episodes of headache, palpitations, pallor, and sweating [4,5]. Catecholamine excess also may produce anxiety and a sense of impending doom. In addition to frequently being misdiagnosed as an anxiety condition, in many middle-aged women, these symptoms are assumed to be perimenopausal symptoms, delaying the diagnosis for years [6]. A recent case review found hypertension in 82% of patients, headaches in 58%, palpitations in 48%, and sweating in 37% of patients [6]. Although excessive sweating, palpitations, and a history of headaches in a hypertensive patient should suggest the possibility of pheochromocytoma, the absence of these three symptoms in a hypertensive patient has been shown to effectively exclude pheochromocytoma in most cases [1]. Sustained hypertension is seen in approximately 50% of patients, paroxysmal hypertension in 30%, and normal blood pressure in less than 20% of patients [4].

Cardiovascular presentations of pheochromocytoma include dilated cardiomyopathy from sustained catecholamine excess, myocarditis with inflammatory infiltrates, and acute ischemic disease including ST-elevation myocardial infarction (MI) [4,7]. Classic electrocardiographic signs of pheochromocytoma include sinus tachycardia, left ventricular hypertrophy, and diffuse T wave inversion. Reported changes noted during hypertensive paroxysms included marked prolongation of the QT interval and deep and symmetrically inverted T waves in the anterior leads [7].

Pheochromocytomas occasionally can present as a hypertensive crisis following some precipitating event, typically surgery, trauma, or during pregnancy [8,9]. This scenario often is associated with acute hemorrhage into the pheochromocytoma, a particularly vascular tumor, with abrupt and excessive release of catecholamines. The patient will present with flank pain, significant hypertension, and vomiting. With a differential diagnosis that more commonly includes renal colic or even rupture of an abdominal aortic aneurysm, hemorrhage into an occult pheochromocytoma usually will be discovered as an unexpected finding on abdominal CT scan.

The most severe, and fortunately rare, presentation of a pheochromocytoma is multiple organ system failure, a condition that has been called pheochromocytoma multi-system crisis [10]. This unusual presentation consists of multi-organ impairment, a temperature often greater than 40°C, encephalopathy, and vascular liability (hypertension or hypotension). The symptoms tend to progress despite appropriate medical management. Successful treatment demands prompt diagnosis, vigorous medical treatment, and emergency tumor removal if the patient's condition continues to deteriorate.

Emergency department evaluation

Recommendations for screening for pheochromocytoma include patients with (1) episodic symptoms of headache, palpitations and diaphoresis (with or without hypertension); (2) a family history of pheochromocytoma or multiple endocrine neoplasia syndrome; (3) incidental adrenal or abdominal masses; (4) unexplained paroxysms of tachycardia, hypertension during intubation, unexplained paroxysms at induction of anesthesia, parturition, or prolonged, unexplained hypotension after surgery; and (5) spells or attacks occurring during exertion, twisting of the torso, straining, or coitus [5].

Diagnosis of pheochromocytomas includes biochemical tests for screening and appropriate imaging studies for localization of the tumor. The combination of urinary metanephrines and vanillylmandelic acid (VMA) has a diagnostic sensitivity of 98% for detecting pheochromocytoma [6]. More recently, the measurement of plasma metanephrines has shown sensitivity approaching 100%, and a normal value has a negative predictive value of 100% [11]. The main difficulty with simple reliance on measurement of plasma metanephrines is its lack of specificity, with a false-positive rate of 15%. More plainly stated, even if the prevalence of pheochromocytoma was estimated to be as high as one in every 200 screened patients, this test would result in 30 patients with false-positive tests for every one patient diagnosed with a pheochromocytoma [12]. The increased sensitivity of a diagnostic test is always at the expense of specificity; however, a knowledgeable clinician can use the negative predictive value of the plasma metanephrine test to exclude pheochromocytoma from consideration, understanding that a positive result will require further screening with 24-hour urine collection for catecholamines and VMA.

In addition to the problems inherent with the specificity and sensitivity of measurements of catecholamines, certain clinical situations may increase plasma and urinary catecholamine metabolites to levels often seen with pheochromocytomas. These situations include: (1) acute clonidine withdrawal, (2) acute alcohol withdrawal, (3) vasodilator therapy with hydralazine, (4) acute myocardial ischemia, (5) acute cerebrovascular accident, (6) cocaine abuse, and (7) severe congestive heart failure (CHF) [5].

Once the diagnosis of a pheochromocytoma is confirmed biochemically, the tumor will need to be localized. CT and MRI have excellent sensitivity (98% and 100%, respectively), while both have lower specificity (approximately 70% for each) [6,13]. Either test is generally adequate for identifying a pheochromocytoma suggested by biochemical testing. An additional imaging technique that can be helpful if no definite tumor is identified with CT or MRI is the Meta-iodo-Benzyl-Guanidine (MIBG) scan, with specificity for pheochromocytoma of 100%.

Emergency department management

In preparation for surgery, essentially all pheochromocytomas are managed with catecholamine blockade. Typically, phenoxybenzamine, an α-blocker, is initiated first. In many patients, this is combined with metytosine, which directly inhibits the synthesis of catecholamines. Thus, both the production and the actions of catecholamines are reduced. Surgery is the definitive treatment for pheochromocytoma, and with good imaging techniques for tumor localization, preoperative catecholamine blockade, and improved anesthesia, the need for an extensive thoracoabdominal incision has been replaced with more locally targeted approaches, including a current trend toward laparoscopic adrenalectomy. Laparoscopic resection of benign pheochromocytomas has been shown to be safe and effective, with resultant short hospital stays [14].

Treatment of hypertension associated with pheochromocytoma depends in part on the clinical situation. Although phenoxybenzamine frequently is used preoperatively, it produces significant orthostatic hypotension and reflex tachycardia that can limit its use in outpatient therapy. Selective postsynaptic α-1 adrenergic receptor antagonists (prazosin, terazosin, doxazosin) have been used to circumvent some of the disadvantages of phenoxybenzamine. This class of drugs does not produce reflex tachycardia and has a shorter duration of action, permitting more rapid adjustment of dosage. Labetalol, an α- and β-adrenergic blocker, has been reported to be effective for controlling hypertension and other manifestations of pheochromocytoma, although there are a few reported cases of it precipitating hypertensive crisis. In general, β-blockers should be avoided in patients with pheochromocytoma who are not already adequately α-blocked, as unopposed alpha effects are extremely dangerous. Calcium channel blockers have been successful in controlling blood pressure and are tolerated well, particularly in patients with occasional episodes of paroxysmal hypertension. Calcium channel blockers also prevent catecholamine-induced coronary vasospasm. A hypertensive crisis associated with pheochromocytoma may present with signs and symptoms suggestive of either an acute MI or CHF. In this situation, sodium nitroprusside should be used to control blood pressure. β-adrenergic blockade is added as need to control tachycardia. Esmolol provides rapid-onset and short-duration β-blockade.

Adrenal gland physiology

Cortisol is the major corticosteroid hormone synthesized by the adrenal cortex, and it is required for normal function of all cells in the body. Cortisol is required for carbohydrate, protein, and lipid metabolism; immune function; synthesis and action of catecholamines; wound healing; vascular tone and permeability; and numerous other vital functions. The production of cortisol by the adrenal cortex is stimulated by corticotropin (ACTH) produced by the anterior pituitary gland, which in turn is released in response to corticotropin-releasing hormone (CRH) from the hypothalamus. Each step in this cascade is controlled by elaborate feedback mechanisms; adequate cortisol levels limit the production of ACTH and CRH. In addition, proinflammatory cytokines, including interleukins and tumor necrosis factor, stimulate ACTH production, thus augmenting the production of cortisol under stress conditions [15].

Case 2. A 40-year-old woman presents to the ED with a complaint of severe generalized weakness and orthostatic dizziness associated with nausea, vomiting, and diarrhea for several days. Initial examination reveals VS: 90/40, 120, 20, 100.4°, 98% oxygen saturation; abdomen: soft, nontender. Laboratory results include white blood cell (WBC) count of 8200, Hct 38.0, Na 128, K 5.8, HCO₃ 20, serum urea nitrogen 28, creatinine 1.0. Initial treatment included 2 L of normal saline intravenously and promethazine hydrochloride. Repeat vital signs revealed only slight improvement after fluid resuscitation. Blood pressure 98/54, heart rate 110, and the patient still complained of dizziness when she attempted to ambulate. What further evaluation or treatment should be considered?

Pathophysiology

Adrenal insufficiency is defined as the impaired ability of the adrenal cortex to produce cortisol in response to normal physiologic demands. Primary adrenal insufficiency occurs when there is destruction of adrenal tissue resulting in diminished excretion of cortisol. Secondary adrenal insufficiency occurs with diminished ACTH stimulation, either because of chronic suppression of the adrenal–pituitary axis by exogenous steroids or compromise of the pituitary–hypothalamic system. Both primary and secondary adrenal insufficiency can be defined further as chronic or acute. Table 1 lists the important causes of adrenal insufficiency based on this definition scheme [16].

Primary adrenal insufficiency, or Addison's disease, is caused most commonly by autoimmune adrenalitis, which may be isolated (40%) or part of an autoimmune polyendocrine syndrome (60%) [17]. Addison's disease typically presents after a chronic and insidious course with symptoms that are often vague and nonspecific. Patients complain of fatigue and generalized weakness and may appear clinically depressed. Occasionally gastrointestinal (GI) symptoms may predominate, with nausea, vomiting, and diarrhea as primary complaints. In many cases, the diagnosis is made only when the patient presents with an acute crisis during an intercurrent illness [18].

Because of the chronic nature of primary adrenal insufficiency, and deficiency of both glucocorticoid and mineralocorticoid, there are some unique signs and symptoms associated with Addison's disease that are conspicuously absent with secondary causes of adrenal insufficiency (Box 1). Patients with Addison's disease typically have hyperpigmented skin, particularly of sun-exposed areas, axillae, palmar creases, and mucous membranes. The cause of hyperpigmentation in Addison's disease is believed to reflect increased stimulation of melanocyte receptors by ACTH. In addition, the mineralocorticoid deficiency often produces significant salt craving, and evidence in laboratory analysis, including hyperkalemia and hyponatremia [19].

Table 1
Etiologies of adrenal insufficiency

	Primary adrenal insufficiency	Secondary adrenal insufficiency
Chronic	Autoimmune adrenalitis	Pituitary or metastatic tumor
	Tuberculosis	Pituitary surgery
	AIDS	Sarcoidosis
	Metastatic CA (lung, breast)	Chronic steroid use
Acute	Adrenal hemorrhage	Pituitary apoplexy
	(sepsis, warfarin, thrombosis, trauma)	Postpartum pituitary necrosis (Sheehan's syndrome)

Box 1. Clinical characteristics of adrenal insufficiency

Adrenal insufficiency of any cause
Fatigue and weakness, mental depression
Anorexia and weight loss
Nausea, vomiting, diarrhea
Hyponatremia, hypoglycemia, mild normocytic anemia

Primary adrenal insufficiency
Hyperpigmentation
Hyperkalemia
Vitiligo
Autoimmune thyroid disease

Secondary adrenal insufficiency
Pallor
Amenorrhea, diminished libido
Scanty axillary and pubic hair
Headache and visual symptoms

Other causes of primary adrenal insufficiency include infiltrative and infectious processes. Tuberculous adrenalitis was formerly the most common cause of primary adrenal insufficiency, and it remains a frequent cause in developing countries [17]. Most cases of adrenal tuberculosis are found 10 to 15 years after the primary infection, and bilateral adrenal calcifications is the most common radiologic feature [20]. Two other important clinical conditions that impair adrenal gland function include HIV infection and metastatic cancer. Regardless of the process that impairs adrenal function, adequate hormone production is maintained until 80% to 90% of both adrenal glands are destroyed. Thus function typically is maintained despite the surprising frequency of adrenal involvement in many of these processes. Adrenal metastases frequently are encountered during autopsy but uncommonly of clinical importance. One large case review of patients with metastatic disease to the adrenal gland found that only 4% of patients became symptomatic [21].

Adrenal involvement in HIV infection increasingly has been reported in recent years. The adrenal gland is the endocrine organ most commonly involved in patients infected with HIV [22]. Potential etiologies of adrenal insufficiency include direct involvement with HIV, opportunistic infections, neoplasms, and medications used in these disorders. Primary adrenal infections include many of the usual opportunistic infections associated with HIV: cytomegalovirus (CMV), *Mycobacterium avium-intracellulare* (MAI), tuberculosis, cryptococcosis, histoplasmosis, toxoplasmosis, and

Pneumocystosis carinii. In addition, malignancies like Kaposi sarcoma and non-Hodgkin lymphoma can cause adrenal insufficiency in patients with HIV. Medications that interfere with adrenal function include ketoconazole, rifampin, phenytoin, and megestrol acetate. Autopsy studies revealed involvement of the adrenal glands in more than 50% of patients with HIV infection [23]. A study of patients with HIV found risk factors for adrenal insufficiency included prolonged time since diagnosis of HIV infection, CD4 counts less than 50 cells/mm3, and a history of opportunistic infections. Patients with tuberculosis and disseminated cytomegalovirus infection appear to be at particular risk of developing adrenal insufficiency [24,25].

Although clinical manifestations of adrenal dysfunction are uncommon in patients with HIV, subclinical functional abnormalities of hypothalamic-pituitary-adrenal axis are frequent, particularly in critically ill patients. Using stringent criteria for diagnosis of adrenal insufficiency (both stress cortisol and low-dose ACTH stimulation levels less than 18 µg/dL), Marik et al recently found 21% of critically ill patients with HIV had diminished adrenal function. These authors recommended evaluation of adrenal function in seriously ill HIV patients (critical illness, surgery or trauma) and the consideration of hydrocortisone treatment as indicated [22].

Emergency department presentation

Acute adrenal insufficiency may present to the ED as a life-threatening event, requiring astute diagnostic suspicion and aggressive therapeutic interventions. The most common cause of acute adrenal crisis is abrupt withdrawal of chronic steroid use, or the addition of a substantial stress to relative adrenal insufficiency caused by prolonged steroid use or an occult pathologic process impairing adrenal gland function. Acute adrenal insufficiency presents with hypotension unresponsive to fluid resuscitation and pressors. Recognition of this condition requires prompt replacement of corticosteroids (typically 100 mg hydrocortisone intravenously); however, if doubt as to the diagnosis exists, it is helpful to future management of the patient if some diagnostic or provocative testing can be accomplished. At the very least, a random cortisol level should be sent. This level can be interpreted in light of the current stressful physiologic event that should raise the cortisol level. If time allows, an even better approach is to administer 10 mg dexamethasone intravenously, which should not alter the cortisol assay, and carry out a cosyntropin stimulation test.

Several unique presentations of acute adrenal insufficiency are described. These include adrenal hemorrhage or infarction and catastrophic pituitary failure. Massive and bilateral adrenal failure mainly is associated with profound hypotension and multi-organ failure, which in turn accompanies surgery or sepsis. The classic presentation of this entity was described independently by Waterhouse and Friderichsen in the early 1900s and was termed purpura fulmanans to describe the extensive purpura than accompanied meningococcal sepsis [26]. Autopsies revealed extensive hemorrhagic infarction of the adrenal glands. Today, bilateral adrenal infarction is recognized as a cause of adrenal insufficiency with meningococcal sepsis and other overwhelming infections, including *Streptococcus pneumoniae* and β hemolytic *Streptococcus* group A, *Pseudomonas aueriginosa,* and *Escherichia coli* [27–29].

Although adrenal hemorrhage associated with overwhelming infection and shock has a high mortality, even with early institution of corticosteroid replacement, there are several causes of adrenal hemorrhage that allow a short latent period (on the order of hours to a few days) between hemorrhage and acute decompensation from adrenal insufficiency. The mortality from these causes is related directly to the recognition of the adrenal insufficiency and appropriate steroid replacement. These causes of adrenal hemorrhage include those associated with trauma, anticoagulant therapy, metastatic disease to the adrenal glands, heparin-induced thrombocytopenia, and antiphospholipid antibody syndrome [30–32].

Antiphospholipid antibody syndrome is characterized by recurrent venous or arterial thrombosis, and as applicable, a history of spontaneous fetal loss. The disorder is primary, and not associated with another systemic disorder, in up to 70% of patients [33]. In other cases, antiphospholipid antibodies are associated with collagen vascular diseases, especially systemic lupus erythematosus. In a recent case review, adrenal insufficiency was the first clinical manifestation of antiphospholipid antibody syndrome in 36% of cases [33]. These patients presented with abdominal pain (55%), hypotension (54%), fever (40%), nausea and vomiting (31%), weakness and fatigue (31%), and lethargy or altered mental status (19%). The main finding on imaging these patients was adrenal hemorrhage, and histopathology revealed hemorrhagic infarction associated with vessel thrombosis. Hemorrhage is typically bilateral in this situation [30], which helps to explain the high incidence of adrenal insufficiency. Lupus anticoagulant was detected in 97% of patients, and anticardiolipin antibodies were positive in 93% of patients. Baseline cortisol was decreased in 98% of patients who presented with adrenal insufficiency in this cohort, and cosyntropin stimulation testing was positive in 100% of patients [33]. These authors concluded that screening for lupus anticoagulant and anticardiolipin antibodies is appropriate in all cases of adrenal hemorrhage and in adrenal insufficiency of uncertain cause. Conversely, it is also appropriate to screen for adrenal hemorrhage and hypoadrenalism in any patient with known antiphospholipid antibody syndrome who complains of abdominal pain and any of the previously mentioned symptoms [33–35].

Another important cause of acute adrenal insufficiency is pituitary apoplexy, caused by sudden hemorrhage or infarction of the pituitary gland. This entity presents in a typical fashion. Patients present with severe headaches associated with neuro–ophthalmologic signs and symptoms and altered mental status [36–39]. Disruption of the dural covering of the pituitary may allow blood and necrotic material into the subarachnoid space, causing meningeal irritation, nausea, vomiting, fever, and impaired consciousness. Pituitary apoplexy should be considered whenever subarachnoid hemorrhage or meningitis is considered. Expansion of the sellar contents may compress the optic chiasm and optic nerves, resulting in visual field deficits, or impinge on cranial nerves III, IV, and VI, resulting in ophthalmoplegia, diplopia, ptosis, and mydriasis, thus mimicking an expanding anterior cerebral artery aneurysm.

Most cases of pituitary apoplexy involve pre-existing pituitary adenomas that are particularly prone to hemorrhage and necrosis. The rate of hemorrhagic degeneration of these tumors is 10% to 15%. Hemorrhage may be precipitated by pregnancy, anticoagulation, head trauma, and surgery [40]. A recent case report suggests that pituitary apoplexy should be considered in a dialysis patient who presents with headache and sudden hypotension [41]. Postpartum pituitary necrosis (Sheehan's syndrome) occurs after hypotension associated with peripartum bleeding [42,43]. Many patients have panhypopituitarism following the acute event, and most have adrenal insufficiency, including the frequent finding of hyponatremia, which can be a potential clue to this emergency.

CT is the most useful test for diagnosing pituitary apoplexy in the acute setting. MRI is more helpful in detecting hemorrhage in the subacute setting (4 days to 1 month). Neurosurgical decompression by means of a transsphenoidal approach is the definitive therapy for pituitary apoplexy. Indications for surgery include obtundation or rapidly progressive deterioration. Severe visual loss is a relative indication for surgery, because decompression may restore sight completely [39].

Emergency department evaluation

Cortisol production exhibits a diurnal pattern, with cortisol levels highest in the early morning. Interpretation of random cortisol levels is complicated by several factors, including the cross-reactivity of corticosteroid supplements [44,45]. Hydrocortisone, methylprednisolone, and prednisone will be detected by cortisol assays, but dexamethasone will not be measured. These first medications should be avoided within 24 hours of a cortisol assay. Because little of the hormone exists in the free or unbound state, measured serum cortisol is also a function of the concentration of the predominant binding protein, cortisol-binding globulin (CBG). Estrogen stimulates hepatic production of CBG, thereby resulting in higher total serum cortisol levels. Many chronic or sustained diseases cause decreased protein production, diminished total cortisol measurements, but a normal physiologic hormone level. The ability to measure serum-free cortisol levels in the near future, particularly in critically ill patients with hypoproteinemia, will prevent the incorrect diagnosis of adrenal insufficiency and the unnecessary use of glucocorticoid therapy [46]. In current practice, there is one helpful value to bear in mind when interpreting random cortisol levels. A cortisol level less than 18 μg/dL, particularly if measured during a stressful clinical situation, implies deficient cortisol production.

A provocative test, using cosyntropin, a synthetic corticotropin analog, may be of further benefit in diagnosing adrenal insufficiency. The low-dose cosyntropin test (1 μg) is being used increasingly because of a decreased frequency of false-negative results compared with the traditional high-dose (250 μg) cosyntropin test. Cortisol levels are measured before and 30, or preferably, 60 minutes after 1 μg cosyntropin administered intravenously. Adrenal function is considered normal if either the basal or postinjection plasma cortisol level is at least 20 μg/dL.

Corticosteroid therapy

Corticosteroid therapy is common among many patients, including those with chronic pulmonary, rheumatologic, oncologic, or GI diseases, and as an immunosuppressive agent following transplant surgery. In emergency medicine, steroids frequently are prescribed for short courses for acute exacerbations of asthma, chronic obstructive pulmonary disease and dermatologic disorders. Several clinical concerns are associated with therapeutic use of steroids, including decisions about amount and duration of therapy, risks of adverse effects, and possibility of suppression of the adrenal gland resulting in adrenal insufficiency. A review of the literature on these questions finds little recent research. Most of the pertinent data come from studies done over 20 years ago.

Adverse effects encountered with short-term steroid use include many findings common to Cushing syndrome. Corticosteroids inhibit fibroblast growth and collagen synthesis, leading to decreased structural stability of connective tissue. Cutaneous manifestations of steroid use include acne, frequent ecchymoses after minor trauma, thinning of the skin, and striae. With the possible exception of striae, all cutaneous symptoms are reversible upon cessation of the steroid therapy [47]. Steroids may cause an acute or chronic form of myopathy. Both proximal and distal muscle weakness occur acutely, usually associated with a significant elevation of serum creatinine phosphokinase. The chronic form of myopathy generally is limited to proximal muscle weakness, often manifested as difficulty climbing stairs or lifting the arms over the head.

Psychologic adverse effects from steroid use can vary widely, from mood alterations and insomnia, to frank psychosis. Significant emotional and psychologic effects have been described in approximately 5% of patients receiving steroids. These effects are unpredictable and cannot be anticipated on the basis of previous steroid-related problems or previous psychiatric disorders. There is an association between higher steroid doses and an increased likelihood of psychologic effect [47]. Psychotic reactions develop most frequently within the first 5 days of use in patients receiving 40 mg or more of prednisone daily. These often are associated with emotional lability, anxiety, pressured speech, delusions, hypomania, and even visual or auditory hallucinations. Treatment with phenothiazines may be necessary. Withdrawal from corticosteroids also may be associated with psychologic manifestations, including depression, irritability, fatigue, insomnia, and memory problems. These symptoms may persist for 6 to 8 weeks after steroids have been discontinued.

Common laboratory evidence of adverse effects includes glucose intolerance, hypokalemia, and elevation of the peripheral WBC count [47,48]. Hyperglycemia may develop in select patients on steroids, even in those not predisposed to the development of diabetes mellitus. Risk factors for steroid-induced hyperglycemia include the dose of steroid used and patient age, body weight, and family history of diabetes. Hyperglycemia usually resolves with in a few days of reducing or discontinuing steroids. Hypokalemia is a common adverse effect of using hydrocortisone, prednisone, or prednisolone, probably related to the mineralocorticoid effect of these medications. Dexamethasone has no mineralocorticoid effect and thus does not cause hypokalemia. Corticosteroid therapy increases the total peripheral leukocyte count, as neutrophils are shifted from the marginated pool into the circulation. The elevated leukocyte count, which may approach 14,000 to 20,000/mm^3, usually returns to normal within 1 week of discontinuing steroid therapy.

Perhaps the most important detrimental effect of corticosteroid therapy is the potential for significant symptoms when treatment is withdrawn. Symptoms can appear with cessation of steroid therapy or with rapid reduction in dosage. Symptoms may be caused by recurrence of the underlying disease, development of adrenal insufficiency, or rarely, appearance of steroid withdrawal syndrome. The degree of adrenal suppression depends on the glucocorticoid dose, duration of treatment, and dosage intervals. Moderate doses of glucocorticoid (less than 40 mg of prednisone given in the morning for less than 7 days) usually will not cause suppression of the adrenal gland [49]. Alternate day steroid therapy suppresses adrenal responsiveness less than daily doses. This advantage primarily has been used as part of a tapering regimen after long-term steroid use [50]. An alternate approach to withdrawal of long-term steroid therapy requires reducing prednisone to a daily dose of 5 mg or less. Spontaneous recovery of adrenal function is the rule at this steroid dosage [51]. Even if no overt symptoms develop when steroids are withdrawn, it can take up to 9 months for complete recovery of hypothalamic-pituitary-adrenal function. During this time, patients may require supplemental treatment with corticosteroids during the stress of surgery, trauma, or an acute illness [52,53]. Corticotropin stimulation testing will confirm possible insufficient adrenal response to stress.

Some patients develop symptoms during withdrawal of corticosteroid therapy that initially may be interpreted as adrenal insufficiency; however, when tested, they have normal adrenal function. This scenario has been called the steroid withdrawal syndrome, and symptoms include weakness, fatigue, nausea, arthralgias, and dizziness. Patients with steroid withdrawal syndrome respond normally to hypothalamic-pituitary-adrenal axis testing and are not predisposed to adrenal crisis. It is theorized that the steroid withdrawal syndrome may be caused by elevated circulating interleukin 6 or other inflammatory mediators [54]. Corticosteroid therapy must be tapered very slowly to avoid recurrent symptoms. Nonsteroidal anti-inflammatory agents may be helpful in ameliorating some complaints.

Symptoms caused by the withdrawal of steroid therapy are identified infrequently in patients because of the vague and insidious nature of the symptoms that often may be ascribed to somatic or emotional problems. Patients who have been withdrawn from steroids and present with these symptoms need to have HPA function tested [55].

Incidental adrenal (incidentalomas)

With the increasing use of noninvasive abdominal imaging, the discovery of incidental (clinically inapparent) adrenal tumors has increased. Current estimates suggest that an incidental adrenal mass is found in 1% to 4% of abdominal CT scans [56]. This estimate agrees with autopsy studies in which an adrenal mass is found in at least 3% of persons older than 50 years [57]. Most (80%) of these incidental tumors are benign, nonfunctioning, adrenocortical adenomas, but they must be distinguished from pheochromocytomas, adrenal carcinomas, and adrenal metastases [58]. The size of the incidentaloma is predictive of its etiology. Twenty-five percent of tumors greater than 6 cm are adrenal cortical carcinomas, and therefore, most institutions and a recent National Institutes of Health consensus report recommend surgical removal of adrenal masses greater than 6 cm [57]. In addition, patients with known primary cancers that metastasize to the adrenal gland (lung, stomach, liver) need further evaluation of incidentalomas to rule out metastatic disease. Finally, all patients with incidental adrenal tumors, regardless of size, should be screened biochemically for pheochromocytoma with free plasma metanephrine levels, and for hypercortisolism with a dexamethasone suppression test [59,60]. Recent reports suggest that up to 20% of patients with adrenal incidentaloma have some form of subclinical hormone dysfunction [57].

References

[1] Rusnak R. Adrenal and pituitary emergencies. Emerg Med Clin North Am 1989;7(4): 903–25.
[2] Caty M, Coran A, Geagen M, et al. Current diagnosis and treatment of pheochromocytoma in children. Arch Surg 1990;125:978–81.

[3] Pacak K, Linehan W, Eisenhofer G, et al. Recent advances in genetics, diagnosis, localization, and treatment of pheochromocytoma. Ann Intern Med 2001;134(4):315–29.

[4] Dluhy R, Lawrence J, Williams G. Endocrine hypertension. In: Larsen P, Kronenberg H, Melmed S, et al, editors. Williams textbook of endocrinology. 10th edition. Philadelphia: WB Saunders; 2003. p. 552–85.

[5] Bravo E. Pheochromocytoma. Cardiol Rev 2002;10(1):44–50.

[6] Goldstein R, O'Neill J, Holcomb G, et al. Clinical experience over 48 years with pheochromocytoma. Ann Surg 1999;229(6):755–66.

[7] Liao W, Liu C, Chiang C, et al. Cardiovascular manifestations of pheochromocytoma. Am J Emerg Med 2000;18(5):622–5.

[8] May E, Beal A, Beilman G. Traumatic hemorrhage of occult pheochromocytoma: a case report and review of the literature. Am Surg 2000;66(8):720–4.

[9] Kizer J, Koniaris L, Edelman J, et al. Pheochromocytoma crisis, cardiomyopathy, and hemodynamic collapse. Chest 2000;118(4):1221–3.

[10] Newell K, Prinz R, Pickleman J, et al. Pheochromocytoma multisystem crisis. A surgical emergency. Arch Surg 1988;123(8):956–9.

[11] Lenders J, Pacak K, Walther M, et al. Biochemical diagnosis of pheochromocytoma—which test is best? JAMA 2002;287(11):1427–34.

[12] Kudva Y, Sawka A, Young W. The laboratory diagnosis of adrenal pheochromocytoma: the Mayo Clinic experience. J Clin Endocrin Metab 2003;88(10):4533–9.

[13] Ilias I, Pacak K. Current approaches and recommended algorithm for the diagnostic localization of pheochromocytoma. J Clin Endocrin Metab 2004;89(2):479–91.

[14] Jaroszewski D, Tessier D, Schlinkert R, et al. Laparoscopic adrenalectomy for pheochromocytoma. Mayo Clin Proc 2003;78:1501–4.

[15] Stewart P. The adrenal cortex. In: Larsen P, Kronenberg H, Melmed S, et al, editors. Williams textbook of Endocrinology. 10th edition. Philadelphia: WB Saunders; 2003. p. 491–551.

[16] Oelkers W. Adrenal insufficiency. N Engl J Med 1996;335(16):1206–12.

[17] Ten S, New M, MacLaren N. Addison's disease 2001. J Clin Endocrin Metab 2001;86(7): 2909–22.

[18] Arlt W, Allolio B. Adrenal insufficiency. Lancet 2003;361:1883–93.

[19] Kong M, Jeffcoate W. Eighty-six cases of Addison's disease. Clin Endocrin 1994;41: 757–61.

[20] Alevritis E, Sarubbi F, Jordan R, et al. Infectious causes of adrenal insufficiency. South Med J 2003;96(9):888–90.

[21] Lam K, Lo C. Metastatic tumors of the adrenal glands: a 30-year experience in a teaching hospital. Clin Endocrin 2002;56(1):95–101.

[22] Marik P, Kiminyo K, Zaloga G. Adrenal insufficiency in critically ill patients with human immunodeficiency virus. Crit Care Med 2002;30(6):1267–73.

[23] Eledrisi M, Verghese A. Adrenal insufficiency in HIV infection: a review and recommendations. Am J Med Sci 2001;321(2):137–44.

[24] Piedrola G, Casado J, Lopez E, et al. Clinical features of adrenal insufficiency in patients with acquired immunodeficiency syndrome. Clin Endocrin 1996;45:97–101.

[25] Mayo J, Collazos J, Martinez E, et al. Adrenal function in the human immunodeficiency virus-infected patient. Arch Intern Med 2002;162:1096–8.

[26] Varon J, Chen K, Sternbach G. Rupert Waterhouse and Carl Friderichsen: adrenal apoplexy. J Emerg Med 1998;16(4):643–7.

[27] Hamilton D, Harris M, Foweraker J, et al. Waterhouse-Friderichsen syndrome as a result of non-meningococcal infection. J Clin Pathol 2004;57:208–9.

[28] Karakousis P, Page K, Varello M, et al. Waterhouse-Friderichsen syndrome after infection with group A streptococcus. Mayo Clin Proc 2001;76:1167–70.

[29] Giraud T, Dhainaut J, Schremmer B, et al. Adult overwhelming meningococcal purpura. Arch Intern Med 1991;151:310–6.

[30] Vella A, Nippoldt T, Morris J. Adrenal hemorrhage: a 25-year experience at the Mayo Clinic. Mayo Clin Proc 2001;76(2):161–8.

[31] Udobi K, Childs E. Adrenal crisis after traumatic bilateral adrenal hemorrhage. J Trauma 2001;51(3):597–600.

[32] Carey R. The changing clinical spectrum of adrenal insufficiency. Ann Intern Med 1997; 127(12):1103–5.

[33] Espinosa G, Santos E, Cervera R, et al. Adrenal involvement in the antiphospholipid syndrome: clinical and immunologic characteristics of 86 patients. Medicine 2003;82(2): 106–18.

[34] Takebayashi K, Aso Y, Tayama K, et al. Primary antiphospholipid syndrome associated with acute adrenal failure. Am J Med Sci 2003;325(1):41–4.

[35] Satta M, Corsello S, Della Casa S, et al. Adrenal insufficiency as the first clinical manifestation of the primary antiphospholipid antibody syndrome. Clin Endocrin 2000;52: 123–6.

[36] Randeva H, Schoebel J, Byrne J, et al. Classical pituitary apoplexy: clinical features, management and outcome. Clin Endocrin 1999;51:181–8.

[37] Kaiser U. Case records of the Massachusetts General Hospital –15–2001. N Engl J Med 2001;344(20):1536–42.

[38] Vidal E, Cevallos R, Vidal J, et al. Twelve cases of pituitary apoplexy. Arch Intern Med 1992; 152:1893–9.

[39] Lee C, Cho A, Carter W. Emergency department presentation of pituitary apoplexy. Am J Emerg Med 2000;18(3):328–31.

[40] Biousse V, Newman N, Oyesiku N. Precipitating factors in pituitary apoplexy. J Neurol Neurosurg Psychiatry 2001;71:542–5.

[41] De la Torre M, Alcazar R, Aguirre M, et al. The dialysis patient with headache and sudden hypotension: consider pituitary apoplexy. Nephrol Dial Transpl 1998;13(3):787–8.

[42] Perlitz Y, Varkel J, Markovitz J, et al. Acute adrenal insufficiency during pregnancy and puerperium: case report and literature review. Obstet Gynecol Surv 1999;54(11):717–24.

[43] Chandraharan E, Arulkumaran S. Pituitary and adrenal disorders complicating pregnancy. Curr Opin Obstet Gynecol 2003;15:101–6.

[44] Dorin R, Qualls C, Crapo L. Diagnosis of adrenal insufficiency. Ann Intern Med 2003; 139(3):194–204.

[45] Grinspoon S, Biller B. Laboratory assessment of adrenal insufficiency. J Clin Endocrin Metab 1994;79(4):923–31.

[46] Hamrahian A, Oseni T, Arafah B. Measurement of serum free cortisol in critically ill patients. NEJM 2004;350(16):1629–38.

[47] Buchman A. Side effects of corticosteroid therapy. J Clin Gastroenterol 2001;33(4):289–94.

[48] Melby J. Systemic corticosteroid therapy: pharmacology and endocrinologic considerations. Ann Intern Med 1974;81(4):505–12.

[49] Byyny R. Withdrawal from glucocorticoid therapy. N Engl J Med 1976;295(1):30–2.

[50] Ackerman G, Nolan C. Adrenocortical responsiveness after alternate-day corticosteroid therapy. N Engl J Med 1968;278(8):405–9.

[51] LaRochelle G, LaRochelle A, Ratner A, et al. Recovery of the hypothalamic-pituitary-adrenal (HPA) axis in patients with rheumatic diseases receiving low-dose prednisone. Am J Med 1993;95(3):258–64.

[52] Coursin D, Wood K. Corticosteroid supplementation for adrenal insufficiency. JAMA 2002; 287(2):236–40.

[53] Lamberts S, Bruining H, de Jong F. Corticosteroid therapy in severe illness. N Engl J Med 1997;337(18):1285–92.

[54] Krasner A. Glucocorticoid-induced adrenal insufficiency. JAMA 1999;282(7):671–6.

[55] Dixon R, Christy N. On the various forms of corticosteroid withdrawal syndrome. Am J Med 1980;68:224–30.

[56] Cook D, Loriaux L. The incidental adrenal mass. Am J Med 1996;101:88–94.

[57] Grumbach M, Biller B, Braunstein G, et al. Management of the clinically inapparent adrenal mass (incidentaloma). Ann Intern Med 2003;138(5):424–9.

[58] Hanna N, Kenady D. Advances in the management of adrenal tumors. Curr Opin Oncol 2000;11:49–53.

[59] Barzon L, Boscaro M. Diagnosis and management of adrenal incidentalomas. J Urol 2000; 163:398–407.

[60] Thompson G, Young W. Adrenal incidentaloma. Curr Opin Oncol 2003;15(1):84–90.

ELSEVIER
SAUNDERS

EMERGENCY
MEDICINE
CLINICS OF
NORTH AMERICA

Emerg Med Clin N Am 23 (2005) 703–721

Bone and Mineral Metabolism

John Sarko, MD

Department of Emergency Medicine, Maricopa Medical Center,
2601 E. Roosevelt Street, Phoenix, AZ 85008, USA

In addition to providing strength, support for the body, and serving as the attachment for muscles to allow movement to occur, bone is extremely active on a metabolic level and is important in the regulation of several endocrine functions. It is the major source of calcium; it buffers against acidosis, and can adsorb toxins and heavy metals. Calcium, phosphate, and magnesium are minerals vital to the function of all cells. They are tightly regulated by several hormones, and disorders in their metabolism are common. In this article, bone structure and function, and mineral metabolism are reviewed. Conditions leading to bone loss are discussed, as diseases increasing bone density are rare and less likely to be encountered by emergency physicians.

Bone and bone metabolism

Anatomy of bone

Bone comprises approximately 14% of the adult weight. Two types of bone exist: cortical (compact) and cancellous (spongy) [1]. Compact bone comprises 85% of the skeleton, is strong, solid, and very organized. Its basic structural unit is the Haversian system (osteon), a cylindrical entity that runs along the long axis of the bone (see Fig. 1). It is comprised of concentric rings of matrix called lamellae, which contain small holes called lacunae with an osteocyte in each. The center of the Haversian system is an opening called the Haversian canal, which contains blood vessels and nerves. Haversian canals and lacunae are connected to each other by canaliculi that are oriented parallel to the horizontal axis of the bone.

Cancellous (spongy) bone makes up 15% of the skeleton, and most bones contain at least some of each type. The vertebrae are predominately

E-mail address: sarkoj@yahoo.com

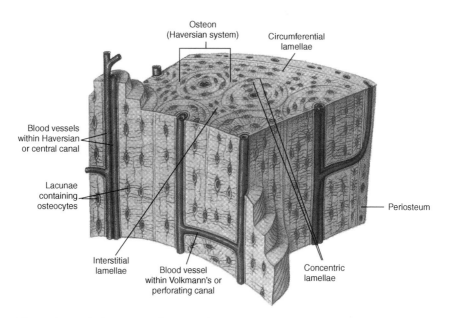

Fig. 1. Anatomical structure of compact bone. (*Adapted from* Thibodeau GA, Patton KT. Anatomy and physiology. 5th edition. St. Louis (MO): Mosby, 2003; with permission.)

cancellous bones, and flat bones such as the skull and iliac also contain a greater percentage of this spongy bone. It lacks the Haversian system, and the lamellae are arranged instead as trabeculae—plates or rods that branch and connect with each other to form a meshwork. The pattern of meshwork is not random but is determined by the stress the bone is subject to.

Physiology of normal bone metabolism

Three main types of cells are involved in bone metabolism: osteoblasts, osteocytes, and osteoclasts. Osteoblasts are derived from mesenchymal precursors and are responsible for bone formation. They secrete collagen and osteoid, which is nonmineralized bone matrix. Once the matrix is formed mineralization begins. This involves the deposition and precipitation of calcium and phosphate that eventually leads to the formation of hydroxyapatite crystals. The result is a very hard, strong Haversian system.

As matrix is laid around the osteoblasts, they become isolated from other cells. Some of them die a programmed death [2], some remain on the surface to form new layers of bone, and some become osteocytes. Osteocytes are found in the lacunae of the Haversian system, and they synthesize and provide nutrients to the matrix. Their blood supply is via capillaries coursing through the canaliculi. Osteoclasts are the cells that resorb bone. They attach to mineralized matrix and initiate resorption by secreting lysozymal enzymes, citric and lactic acid [1,3].

Once formed, bone is continually remodeled. Remodeling is a finely regulated interaction of osteoblasts and osteoclasts. Patterns of stress (mechanical or microdamage) and metabolic demands affect the balance of formation and resorption. Many factors, both local and systemic, influence this balance [3,4]. Locally, cytokines, prostaglandins, growth factors, and colony stimulators can cause or prevent bone loss.

Effects of hormones on normal bone metabolism

Systemic factors regulating bone metabolism are numerous as well. Estrogen is one of the most important hormones regulating normal bone turnover [5]. It acts by decreasing the number of osteoclasts, and its deficiency leads to increased bone resorption and decreased bone mass.

Parathyroid hormone (PTH) and vitamin D play the major roles in storing and mobilizing calcium, which is the major metabolic function of bone. Parathyroid hormone stimulates osteoclasts to release calcium and phosphate from bone, leading to increased resorption [6]. It can also stimulate bone formation. Parathyroid hormone has a greater effect on cortical bone than cancellous bone, resorbing the former to a much greater extent than the latter, and possibly increasing bone formation in cancellous bone [7–9]. This most likely protects bones subject to mechanical loads. The effects of vitamin D are indirect, by altering the absorption of calcium from the gastrointestinal tract. Calcitonin has little, if any, effect on calcium stores.

Other hormones influencing bone metabolism include glucocorticoids, growth hormone, and thyroid hormone. Glucocorticoids increase bone resorption and decrease bone formation, resulting in a net loss of bone, as seen with glucocorticoid-induced osteoporosis. Growth hormone and thyroid hormone increase both resorption and formation.

Emergency department presentation

Patients with abnormalities in bone metabolism severe enough to affect bone strength are at high risk for fractures, and this is usually why they present to the emergency department. The elderly are especially at risk, as they are more often subject to falls. Fractures of the vertebrae and forearm are typical in patients with hyperparathyroidism [10,11], and decreased bone mass, especially due to osteoporosis, can predispose a patient to a fracture of almost any bone [12,13].

Pathophysiology

Many conditions affect bone metabolism. Hyperparathyroidism leads to prolonged resorption and decreased bone density, which can be reversed by surgical correction [8,9]. Chronic renal failure causes chronic hypocalcemia. This leads to a secondary hyperparathyroidism with chronic bone resorption, and is associated with the risk of fractures [14,15]. Chronic renal failure also produces chronic metabolic acidosis, and bone is the second line of defense against this. Protons are absorbed by the matrix, resulting in its dissolution. Osteoclasts are also stimulated and osteoblasts inhibited, leading to an efflux of calcium, carbonate, and phosphate [16–20]. Thus, systemic pH is regulated but at the expense of mineral stores.

Many medications can affect metabolism resulting in bone loss (see Box 1). Anticonvulsants reduce cortical bone by altering osteoblast and osteoclast activity, and by decreasing vitamin D activity [21,22]. The effects are more pronounced with a longer duration of the treatment and when multiple drugs are used. Long-term heparin use and chronic alcoholism are also associated with osteoporosis. Social drinking does not appear to have a negative effect on bone density, and the effects appear to be reversible if alcohol use ceases [23].

Osteoporosis is the most common metabolic disorder of bone, and is due to a reduced amount of estrogen in most cases. Without adequate estrogen, bone loss exceeds its replacement, leading to a structurally weaker bone.

Emergency department management

Treatment of fractures is specific for the type of fracture identified. Reducing the risk of falls may help prevent future fractures. Treatment of osteoporosis is directed at reducing the risk of fracture by increasing bone density and strength. Ensuring an adequate calcium and vitamin D intake, regular weight bearing exercise, moderating alcohol intake, and quitting

---

Box 1. Medications causing bone loss

Anticonvulsants
Heparin
Ethanol
Glucocorticoids
Neuroleptics
Thyroid hormone (postmenopausal women or at
    supraphysiologic doses)
Methotrexate
Aluminum, aluminum hydroxide (antacids)
Lithium
Cyclosporin
Medroxyprogesterone (premenopausal women)
Leuteinizing hormone releasing hormone agonists
    (eg., leuprolide acetate)
Aromatase inhibitors (eg., anastrozole, letrozole)
Cholestyramine

smoking are behavioral treatments used. Drug treatments include bi-sphosphonates to bind hydroxyapatite crystals and to inhibit resorption, calcitonins to inhibit osteoclastic activity, and selective estrogen receptor modulators to inhibit resorption [24].

Disposition

Disposition of the patient depends upon the type of fracture, reason for the fall (if the cause of the fracture), and any other abnormalities found during the examination and evaluation of the patient.

Mineral metabolism

Calcium metabolism

Calcium concentration in the extracellular fluid is regulated by the interplay of factors affecting the gut, kidney, and bone. Abnormalities in calcium metabolism have multiple causes that usually exert their effects on these three organ systems. The resulting abnormal extracellular calcium level has effects on a variety of cell functions.

Normal calcium metabolism

Calcium metabolism is normally balanced, with urinary excretion approximating dietary intake. Of the typical daily intake of 1 g, only approximately 150 mg is absorbed into the blood [6]. Bone stores 99% of the 1 to 1.3 kg of the body's calcium in the form of hydroxyapatite. Less than 1% of bone stores are in bone fluid that can exchange freely with the extracellular fluid.

The major hormones affecting calcium are parathyroid hormone, $1,25(OH)_2$ vitamin D_3 (vitamin D; calcitriol), and calcitonin. Without parathyroid hormone and vitamin D, calcium levels always fall. Parathyroid hormone is secreted by the parathyroid glands and is the key hormone in maintaining serum calcium levels [25]. Parathyroid hormone is secreted in response to a fall in plasma calcium concentration, and its release is inhibited by a rise in this ion. Its action on bone is to stimulate osteoclast activity, leading to resorption of bone and release of calcium and phosphate into the blood. In the kidneys it also stimulates tubular calcium reabsorption, so that less calcium is excreted in the urine. Parathyroid hormone inhibits phosphate reabsorption, and the net effect is to raise plasma calcium concentration and lower phosphate levels. Parathyroid hormone also stimulates the kidney enzyme 1α-hydroxylase to convert the vitamin D precursor into its most active form, calcitriol. As the calcium level returns to normal, the negative feedback loop returns parathyroid hormone levels to normal.

The main effect of vitamin D is to stimulate intestinal absorption of calcium and phosphate by activating an active transport protein in the gut mucosa [26]. Without vitamin D, passive absorption across the gut is not adequate to prevent a net total loss of calcium. Vitamin D also has secondary actions in the kidney, facilitating calcium absorption and enhancing the effect of parathyroid hormone [27]. Vitamin D exerts a negative feedback on the parathyroid gland.

Vitamin D is initially formed in the skin and then hydroxylated twice: first, in the liver, and then in the kidneys to its final form. 25(OH) vitamin D_3 is also an active form. In young people, most vitamin D is derived from sun-activated formation in the skin, with food being a relatively minor source. As people age, this conversion is reduced, and vitamin D supplements are frequently needed to maintain adequate absorption of calcium and prevent bone loss.

Calcitonin is a peptide produced by parafollicular "C" cells of the thyroid gland. Increases in ionized calcium produce an increase in calcitonin levels, and decreases in ionized calcium produce a fall. The exact role and importance of calcitonin in calcium homeostasis is unclear. Calcitonin appears to have a very minor physiologic role on bone outside of skeletal development. It inhibits osteoclastic activity, but appears to play no significant role in normal individuals. No skeletal disease has been found due to calcitonin deficiency, and patients with excess calcitonin production do not suffer from abnormal calcium metabolism [6,28]. Its current uses are for the treatment of postmenopausal osteoporosis, Paget's disease of bone, and hypercalcemia [29].

Hypercalcemia

Emergency departmemt presentation

In general, the body is better at preventing hypocalcemia than hypercalcemia. Hypercalcemia is defined as an ionized calcium >2.7 mEq/L or serum calcium >10.5 mg/dL [25]. Patients are usually asymptomatic until their calcium rises over 12 mg/dL. As calcium is used in every tissue of the body, the effects are widespread, and symptoms can involve many organ systems. Most important are the neurologic and cardiovascular systems. Patients can present with altered level of consciousness or coma, can be confused, irritable, ataxic, depressed, and be hyporeflexic and hypotonic. Hypertension is a common finding. On EKG a shortened QT_c, wide T wave, ST segment depression, and bradycardia can be seen. Nausea, vomiting, constipation, abdominal pain, and pancreatitis are common gastrointestinal findings. Polyuria is common, as the kidneys attempt to excrete the excess calcium being resorbed from bone. As a result, patients are very dehydrated, despite a normal or increased blood pressure. The old mnemonic "stones, bones, moans, and groans" is an uncommon finding, as most patients with increased calcium not due to malignancy are discovered by incidental laboratory testing and have few symptoms, if any.

Pathophysiology

Many diseases alter calcium homeostasis (see Box 2). Hyperparathy-roidism and malignancy are the two most common causes of hyper-calcemia. Parathyroid hormone-related protein is secreted by malignant cells and appears to be responsible for the hypercalcemia. It acts by stimulating osteoclastic resorption and renal tubular reabsorption of calcium [30,31]. If hypercalcemia of malignancy is not suspected, the primary disorder is most likely hyperparathyroidism. It is important to exclude vitamin D, vitamin A, and thiazide use, and immobilization

---

Box 2. Causes of abnormal calcium metabolism

Hypercalcemia
  Malignancy
  Hyperparathyroidism
  Hyperthyroidism
  Adrenal insufficiency
  Acromegaly
  Granulomatous disease
  Immobilization
  Paget's disease
  Phosphate depletion syndrome
  Drugs (especially thiazides and lithium)
Hypocalcemia
  Vitamin D deficiency
  Malabsorption syndrome
  Drugs
    Loop diuretics
    Phosphates
    Phenytoin
    Phenobarbital
    Aminoglycosides
    Heparin
  Hypoparathyroidism and pseudohypoparathyroidism
  Chronic renal insufficiency
  Alcoholism
  Sepsis
  Pancreatitis
  Massive blood transfusions
  Rhabdomyolysis
  Hypomagnesemia
  Surgery

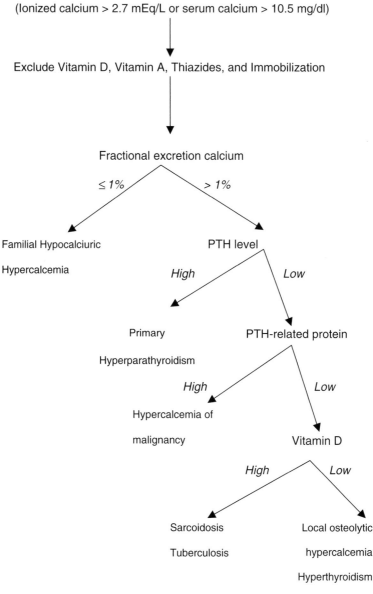

Fig. 2. Evaluation of hypocalcemia.

(see Fig. 2). Measuring phosphate at the same time will help to differentiate between vitamin D and parathyroid hormone abnormalities [25].
It is also important to correct the calcium for hypoalbuminemia, if
present, as this affects the ionized calcium. In patients with an abnormal

calcium (<4 g/dL), the corrected total calcium is: measured calcium $+ 0.8$ (4-albumin).

Emergency department management

Treatment of hypercalcemia begins with replenishing intravascular volume, as patients are dehydrated (see Table 1). Once patients are no longer volume depleted, renal excretion of calcium is undertaken, using a loop diuretic such as furosemide. Hypokalemia and hypomagnesemia occur commonly, and these must be corrected. Finally, calcium mobilization from bone is decreased. Several drugs are available for this purpose. Bisphosphonates such as etidronate and pamidronate are useful for temporarily lowering serum calcium [32,33]. Mithramycin or calcitonin are also effective. Consideration should be given to the use of glucocorticoids. One study found that serum ionized calcium was lower in a group of patients with hypercalcemia of malignancy treated with prednisolone (25 mg orally three times a day for 8 days), hydration, and furosemide than in

Table 1
Treatment of severe hypercalcemia

Treatment	Dose
Hydration	
Normal saline	1–2 liters IV or more if needed
Enhance renal excretion	
Loop diuretic (eg, furosemide)	20–60 mg IV
Decrease calcium mobilization	
from bone	
Etidronate	7.5 mg/kg IV over 4 h for 3–7 days
Pamidronate	Moderate hypercalcemia: 60 mg IV infusion over 4 h initial
	Severe hypercalcemia: 90 mg IV infusion over 24 h initial
Reduce bone turnover	
Gallium nitrate	Severe hypercalcemia: 200 mg/m^2/d IV for 5 d in 1 L of NS or D$_5$W
	Mild hypercalcemia: 100 mg/m^2/d IV for 5 d in 1 L of NS or D$_5$W
Multiple actions	
Calcitonin	4 IU/kg IM/SC 12 h
Inhibit cytokine release	
Hydrocortisone	200–300 mg IV for 3 days
Unknown mechanism	
Mithramycin	25 μ/kg IV over 4–6 h; repeat q24–48 h prn for 3–4 days;
(aka plicamycin)	dose may be repeated at 1-week (or more) intervals prn until satisfactory response is obtained
Calcimimetic agent	
Cinacalcet (Used	30 mg po qd initially
for secondary	
hyperparathyroidism	
or hypercalcemia with	
parathyroid carcinoma)	

a group treated with hydration and furosemide alone [34]. Gallium nitrate is effective, but is associated with renal toxicity, so its use is limited [35]. Phosphates are no longer used.

Disposition

Patients with severe hypercalcemia, or who are symptomatic, should be admitted. An incidental discovery of hypercalcemia can be further evaluated on an outpatient basis.

Hypocalcemia

Emergency department presentation

Hypocalcemia is defined as an ionized calcium <2.0 mEq/L or serum calcium <8.5 mg/dL when corrected for the serum albumin level [25]. Symptoms of hypocalcemia depend in large part upon the rapidity of the decrease. Neurologic findings include tetany, paresthesias of the perioral area and fingers, and Chvostek or Trousseau signs. Chvostek sign is a twitch of the upper lip when the cheek over the facial nerve is tapped. Trousseau's sign is seen when carpopedal spasm develops after a blood pressure cuff is inflated to a pressure greater than the systolic blood pressure for 3 minutes. Seizures, confusion, and extrapyramidal signs can be seen as well. Heart failure is possible, as myocardial contractility is diminished. The QT_c interval can be prolonged, with a normal T wave width. Muscular weakness and cramps can occur.

Pathophysiology

Hypocalcemia is defined as an ionized calcium <2.0 mEq/L or serum calcium <8.5 mg/dL when corrected for the serum albumin level [25]. Mechanisms include lack of parathyroid hormone, lack of vitamin D, or end-organ resistance to parathyroid hormone. The causes of hypocalcemia are many (see Box 2). Phosphate measurements can help in the diagnosis. A high phosphate level with normal renal function suggests hypoparathyroidism, while a low phosphate suggests a lack of vitamin D. A high parathyroid hormone suggests end-organ resistance or lack of vitamin D [25].

Emergency department management

The treatment is calcium replacement and correction of the underlying cause. Intravenous (IV) calcium should be reserved for symptomatic or severe hypocalcemia (ionized calcium <1.3 mEq/L). Oral calcium is available in many preparations: carbonate, citrate, lactate, glubionate, and ascorbate. Calcium carbonate is the cheapest, but requires an acidic gut environment for absorption. Generally, 1 to 3 g of elemental calcium are needed each day, in doses of 500 mg or less. When needed, IV calcium gluconate (10–30 mL of 10% solution) or calcium chloride (10 mL of 10% solution) can be given over 10 to 20 minutes. If this does not alleviate the symptoms, a continuous infusion of 100 mg/h can be given to adults for several hours, provided calcium levels are measured closely [36]. Magnesium and potassium must also be replaced if low.

Disposition

It may not be possible to correct severe hypocalcemia during a short stay in an emergency department, and patients may need admission to a monitored bed for continued replacement. Many will need admission because of the underlying disease causing the electrolyte abnormality. Incidentally discovered, asymptomatic hypocalcemia can be corrected in the emergency department and further treated on an outpatient basis.

Phosphate metabolism

Inorganic phosphate is essential for many cellular functions, such as DNA and RNA synthesis, glycolysis and gluconeogenesis, protein phosphorylation, and skeletal mineralization. Most phosphate is found in bone as hydroxyapatite (85%), with about 1% in the extracellular fluid. The remainder resides in the intracellular space. Therefore, serum levels may not accurately reflect total body stores. Dietary phosphate is generally 800 to 1600 mg/d, and is absorbed in all segments of the small bowel, predominately in the jejunum [37]. Most absorption is passive, but an active transport process exists that is also vitamin D_3 dependent. The majority of absorbed phosphate is then renally excreted. It is filtered through the glomerulus, and then 80% or more is reabsorbed in the proximal and distal tubules. Renal phosphate reabsorption is influenced by several hormones and by diet. Phosphate restriction, calcitriol, thyroid hormone, growth hormone, and insulin-like growth factor-1, all stimulate reabsorption. Parathyroid hormone, calcitonin, atrial natriuretic factor, glucocorticoids, and PTH-related hormone inhibit this process.

Plasma phosphate concentration is maintained in a narrow range that varies according to age (2.8–4.5 mg/dL in adults). It is important to be aware of this when interpreting phosphate levels, because hypophosphatemia in children can be missed if adult values are used. Levels are highest in infants and then decline gradually until adulthood. Phosphate levels also vary with time of day, peaking in the early morning and reaching a nadir 4 to 6 hours later. Calcium and phosphate levels are inversely proportional to each other, and the calcium-phosphate product, obtained by multiplying the two levels, is normally 30 to 40.

Hyperphosphatemia

Emergency department presentation

The manifestations of hyperphosphatemia are related to its effect on serum calcium. Tetany may occur when the phosphate level increases rapidly (due to hypocalcemia). A rise in the calcium–phosphate product to >70 causes calcium to precipitate in soft tissues, leading to hypocalcemia. This is most often seen in patients with chronic renal failure who take vitamin D supplements.

Pathophysiology

Hyperphosphatemia is most often due to reduced renal phosphate excretion, seen most commonly with acute or chronic renal failure (see Box 3). A reduction in the filtered load of phosphate is responsible for this. Hyperphosphatemia induces PTH release by an unknown mechanism.

An increased endogenous load of phosphate is seen in patients with tumor lysis syndrome, rhabdomyolysis, bowel infarction, hemolysis, and malignant hyperthermia. Metabolic acidosis also shifts phosphate to the extracellular fluid.

An increased exogenous phosphate load is seen in cases of vitamin D overdose or with the administration of high quantities of phosphate—IV phosphate infusions, or phosphate containing enemas, for example. The ability of the kidneys to excrete this phosphate is exceeded.

Emergency department management

Reducing intestinal phosphate absorption is the most effective treatment. Decreasing protein intake and using phosphate-binding salts (eg, aluminum hydroxide or aluminum carbonate) are beneficial. Intravenous infusions and phosphate supplements should be stopped. Dialysis is rarely needed.

Disposition

As with hypophosphatemia, patients who are hyperphosphatemic may have other abnormalities that need to be evaluated and treated on an inpatient basis.

Hypophosphatemia

ED presentation

Symptomatic hypophosphatemia usually develops when phosphate falls below 1 mg/dL. Emergency physicians will encounter this disorder in patients with alcohol withdrawal and recovery from DKA or alcoholic ketoacidosis. Hyperventilation is a frequent precipitating cause. Myopathy, dysphagia, ileus, and rhabdomyolysis may occur in severe cases. Respiratory failure due to muscle weakness may occur, and can make weaning a patient from a ventilator difficult. Hemolysis and thrombocytopenia can occur and metabolic encephalopathy may also develop.

Box 3. Causes of phosphate abnormalities

Hypophosphatemia
  Respiratory alkalosis
  Recovery from diabetic ketoacidosis (DKA)
  Sepsis
  Hyperparathyroidism
  Abnormal Vitamin D metabolism
  Kidney transplantation
  Volume expansion
  Alcohol abuse
  Acidosis
  Antacid overuse
  Dietary restriction
  Chronic diarrhea
Hyperphosphatemia
  Intravenous infusion
  Oral intake
  Excess Vitamin D
  Phosphate containing enemas
  Tumor lysis syndrome
  Rhabdomyolysis
  Malignant hyperthermia
  Hemolysis
  Renal failure
  Hypoparathyroidism
  Bisphosphonate therapy
  Magnesium deficiency
  Multiple myeloma (pseudohyperphosphatemia)
  Hypertriglyceridemia (pseudohyperphosphatemia)

Pathophysiology

Dietary phosphate deficiency is rare in Western countries because most Westerners have a high phosphate diet. Hypophosphatemia has a number of causes (see Box 3), and is defined as a plasma phosphate level below 2.3 mg/dL. It is seen in 0.25% to 2% of hospitalized patients.

Pathophysiologic mechanisms include intracellular redistribution, urinary losses, and decreased intestinal reabsorption. Combinations of mechanisms exist, but an intracellular shift of the ion is the most common cause. Respiratory alkalosis, recovery from DKA, and increased insulin release during glucose administration are the most common causes of hypophosphatemia due to intracellular shifts that emergency physicians encounter. These conditions stimulate glycolysis, which consume phosphate, leading to the shift [38].

The most common cause of hypophosphatemia due to urinary losses is seen in hypoparathyroidism. Patients usually have a moderate hypophosphatemia and an associated hypercalcemia. A resistance to PTH develops, which limits the phosphate wasting. Volume expansion and alcohol abuse are also common causes. Chronic antacid use can occasionally reduce intestinal absorption to the point where phosphate deficiency and hypophosphatemia develops.

Emergency department management

Replacement of phosphate is generally easy. Oral replacement is preferred, except when patients are symptomatic or the level is less than 1 mg/dL. One thousand milligrams per day orally is adequate for most patients. Cow's milk contains 1 mg/mL of phosphate, or phosphate replacement can also be given as potassium or sodium phosphate (2 g/d). Intravenous phosphate replacement (2.5 mg/kg body weight over 6 hours) should be given carefully to patients with severe or symptomatic hypophosphatemia as it can cause hypocalcemia. When given IV, phosphate levels should be measured after each infusion.

Disposition

Most patients with hypophosphatemia have other abnormalities in electrolytes or disease processes that may necessitate admission. Symptomatic or severely hypophosphatemic patients should be treated as inpatients. Mild hypophosphatemia can be treated with milk or phosphate supplements on an outpatient basis.

Magnesium metabolism

Magnesium is primarily an intracellular cation. The body contains approximately 0.33 mg/kg of magnesium, with 0.66 stored in bone, and about 0.33 found in cardiac muscle, skeletal muscle, and the liver. Less than 1% is found in the extracellular fluid. Magnesium homeostasis is dependent on dietary intake, and there is no known regulatory system to mobilize it from bone or elsewhere. Two hundred to 350 mg are ingested daily, and about one half of this is absorbed, mostly in the jejunum and ileum, by both active and passive mechanisms. The kidneys excrete about 125 mg a day, with serum magnesium levels being the primary determinant of renal reabsorption. Parathyroid hormone, vitamin D, hypocalcemia, metabolic alkalosis, and intravascular volume depletion also increase its reabsorption. Diuretics, metabolic acidosis, hypercalcemia, hypophosphatemia, and intravascular volume overload reduce it. Insulin use, IV solutions with glucose, and amino acid infusions shift magnesium into cells, and ischemia and acidosis lead to its efflux. Normal serum magnesium levels are 1.5 to 2.5 mEq/L.

Hypermagnesemia

ED presentation
Small elevations have no clinical significance, but extreme elevations can cause hypotension, bradycardia, loss of deep tendon reflexes, decreased level of consciousness, respiratory depression, and cardiac arrest.

Pathophysiology
This is an unusual finding in emergency department patients. Patients with renal failure taking magnesium-containing drugs are the ones most likely to present with this abnormality (see Box 4). Rhabdomyolysis is another likely cause.

Emergency department management
As most cases are iatrogenic, magnesium administration should be stopped. Intravenous fluids followed by a loop diuretic may help. Severe symptomatic hypermagnesemia should be treated with calcium chloride (5 mL of 10% calcium chloride) because calcium directly counters the effects of magnesium. Dialysis also removes magnesium, and is used in life-threatening cases.

Disposition
As with other electrolyte disorders, patients may need admission because of coexisting illnesses. Those with severe elevations of magnesium or who are symptomatic should be admitted.

Hypomagnesemia

Emergency department presentation
Most symptoms are nonspecific and usually associated with deficiencies of other ions such as potassium and calcium. Therefore, neuromuscular hyperexcitability can be seen. Chvostek and Trousseau signs are possible. The ECG may show widening of the QRS complex, peaked T waves, and prolongation of the PR interval. Severely hypomagnesemic patients may develop ventricular dysrhythmias and be sensitive to cardiac glycosides.

Pathophysiology
This is a common finding in hospitalized patients—up to 65% of intensive care unit patients [39] and 12% on general wards [40]. Box 4 shows a partial list of causes of magnesium deficiency. Diuretics lead to a mild hypomagnesemia because the associated volume depletion increases

---

Box 4. Causes of abnormal magnesium levels

Hypomagnesemia
  Renal losses
    Drugs
      Diuretics
      Alcohol
      Foscarnet
      Pentamidine
      Aminoglycosides
    Hypercalcemia
    Hypokalemia
    Phosphate depletion
    Volume expanded states
    Hyperparathyroidism
    Hyperthyroidism
    Syndrome of inappropriate antidiuretic hormone (SIADH)
  Gastrointestinal losses
    Malabsorption
    Malnutrition
    Acute pancreatitis
Hypermagnesemia
  Renal failure
  Tumor lysis syndrome
  Rhabdomyolysis
  DKA
  Treatment of preeclampsia
  Hyperparathyroidism
  Adrenal insufficiency

---

proximal tubular reabsorption. In the emergency department, alcoholism and chronic malnutrition are the usual reasons hypomagnesemia is seen.

Emergency department management

Oral magnesium replacement is preferred in patients with mild to moderate deficiency. With up to 6 g magnesium sulfate (50 mEq magnesium) required for replacement when the deficiency is severe, 5 to 10 g of IV magnesium may be given per day at a rate of 1 g/h. Much of the magnesium will be lost in the urine, but the net balance will be positive [41]. In addition, when both hypokalemia and hypomagnesemia coexist, magnesium must be replenished for the potassium deficiency to be corrected [38,41].

Disposition

Magnesium deficiency is frequently diagnosed along with other electrolyte abnormalities. When not severe, it can be treated on an outpatient basis. Symptomatic patients must be treated as inpatients.

Summary

Although not often appreciated, the structure and metabolism of bone is intimately involved the homeostasis of electrolytes that emergency physicians evaluate daily. Assessment of calcium, phosphate, and magnesium in the evaluation of metabolic dysfunction is necessary in symptomatic emergency department patients. Diagnosis and treatment of these mineral abnormalities is essential due to their interrelation with many cellular functions.

References

[1] Crowther CL, Mourad LA. Structure and function of the musculoskeletal system. In: McCance KL, Huether SE, editors. Pathophysiology. The biologic basis for disease in adults and children. 4th edition. St. Louis (MO): Mosby; 2002. p. 1338–43.

[2] Jilka RL, Weinstein RS, Bellido T, et al. Osteoblast programmed cell death (apoptosis): modulation by growth factors and cytokines. J Bone Miner Res 1998;13(5):793–802.

[3] Raisz LG. Physiology and pathophysiology of bone remodeling. Clin Chem 1999;45(8 Pt 2): 1353–8.

[4] Raisz LG. Osteoporosis: current approaches and future prospects in diagnosis, pathogenesis, and management. J Bone Miner Metab 1999;17:79–89.

[5] Harada S, Rodan GA. Control of osteoblast function and regulation of bone mass. Nature 2003;423(6937):349–55.

[6] Mundy GR, Guise TA. Hormonal control of calcium homeostasis. Clin Chem 1999;45 (8 Pt 2):1347–52.

[7] Parisien M, Silverberg SJ, Shane E, et al. The histomorphometry of bone in primary hyperparathyroidism: preservation of cancellous bone structure. J Clin Endocrinol Metab 1990;70(4):930–8.

[8] Abdelhadi M, Nordenstrom J. Bone mineral recovery after parathyroidectomy in patients with primary and renal hyperparathyroidism. J Clin Endocrinol Metab 1998;83(11): 3845–51.

[9] Silverberg SJ, Locker FG, Bilezikian JP. Vertebral osteopenia: a new indication for surgery in primary hyperparathyroidism. J Clin Endocrinol Metab 1996;81(11):4007–12.

[10] Khosla S, Melton LJ 3rd, Wermers RA, et al. Primary hyperparathyroidism and the risk of fracture: a population-based study [see comment]. J Bone Miner Res 1999;14(10):1700–7.

[11] Vestergaard P, Mollerup CL, Frokjaer VG, et al. Cohort study of risk of fracture before and after surgery for primary hyperparathyroidism. BMJ 2000;321(7261):598–602.

[12] Stone KL, Seeley DG, Lui LY, et al. BMD at multiple sites and risk of fracture of multiple types: long-term results from the Study of Osteoporotic Fractures. J Bone Miner Res 2003; 18(11):1947–54.

[13] Seeley DG, Browner WS, Nevitt MC, et al. Which fractures are associated with low appendicular bone mass in elderly women? The Study of Osteoporotic Fractures Research Group. Ann Intern Med 1991;115(11):837–42.

[14] Korkor AB. Reduced binding of [3H]1,25-dihydroxyvitamin D3 in the parathyroid glands of patients with renal failure. N Engl J Med 1987;316(25):1573–7.

[15] Pitts TO, Piraino BH, Mitro R, et al. Hyperparathyroidism and 1,25-dihydroxyvitamin D deficiency in mild, moderate, and severe renal failure. J Clin Endocrinol Metab 1988;67(5): 876–81.

[16] Arnett T. Regulation of bone cell function by acid-base balance. Proc Nutr Soc 2003;62(2): 511–20.

[17] Bushinsky DA, Lechleider RJ. Mechanism of proton-induced bone calcium release: calcium carbonate-dissolution. Am J Physiol 1987;253(5 Pt 2):F998–1005.

[18] Bushinsky DA, Ori Y. Effects of metabolic and respiratory acidosis on bone. Curr Opin Nephrol Hypertens 1993;2(4):588–96.

[19] Bushinsky DA, Wolbach W, Sessler NE, et al. Physicochemical effects of acidosis on bone calcium flux and surface ion composition. J Bone Miner Res 1993;8(1):93–102.

[20] Bushinsky DA, Frick KK. The effects of acid on bone. Curr Opin Nephrol Hypertens 2000; 9(4):369–79.

[21] Pluskiewicz W, Nowakowska J. Bone status after long-term anticonvulsant therapy in epileptic patients: evaluation using quantitative ultrasound of calcaneus and phalanges. Ultrasound Med Biol 1997;23(4):553–8.

[22] Tannirandorn P, Epstein S. Drug-induced bone loss. Osteoporos Int 2000;11(8):637–59.

[23] Peris P, Pares A, Guanabens N, et al. Bone mass improves in alcoholics after 2 years of abstinence. J Bone Miner Res 1994;9(10):1607–12.

[24] Yew KS, DeMieri PJ. Disorders of bone mineral metabolism. Clin Fam Pract 2002;4(3): 525–65.

[25] Fukugawa M, Kurokawa K. Calcium homeostasis and imbalance. Nephron 2002; 92(Suppl 1):41–5.

[26] Heaney RP, Weaver CM. Calcium and vitamin D. Endocrinol Metab Clin North Am 2003; 32(1):181–94 [vii–viii].

[27] Yamamoto M, Kawanobe Y, Takahashi H, et al. Vitamin D deficiency and renal calcium transport in the rat. J Clin Invest 1984;74(2):507–13.

[28] Silverman SL. Calcitonin. Endocrinol Metab Clin North Am 2003;32(1):273–84.

[29] Novartis P. Mialcin. Available at: www.pharma.us.novartis.com/product/pi/pdf/miacalcin_injection.pdf. Accessed May 4, 2004.

[30] Cisneros G, Lara LF, Crock R, et al. Humoral hypercalcemia of malignancy in squamous cell carcinoma of the skin: parathyroid hormone-related protein as a cause. South Med J 2001;94(3):329–31.

[31] Motellon JL, Javort Jimenez F, de Miguel F, et al. Parathyroid hormone-related protein, parathyroid hormone, and vitamin D in hypercalcemia of malignancy. Clin Chim Acta 2000; 290(2):189–97.

[32] Atula ST, Tahtela RK, Nevalainen JI, et al. Clodronate as a single-dose intravenous infusion effectively provides short-term correction of malignant hypercalcemia. Acta Oncol (Madr) 2003;42(7):735–40.

[33] Pecherstorfer M, Steinhauer EU, Rizzoli R, et al. Efficacy and safety of ibandronate in the treatment of hypercalcemia of malignancy: a randomized multicentric comparison to pamidronate. Support Care Cancer 2003;11(8):539–47.

[34] Kristensen B, Ejlertsen B, Holmegaard SN, et al. Prednisolone in the treatment of severe malignant hypercalcaemia in metastatic breast cancer: a randomized study. J Intern Med 1992;232(3):237–45.

[35] Hughes TE, Hansen LA. Gallium nitrate. Ann Pharmacother 1992;26(3):354–62.

[36] Bringhurst FR, Demay MB, Kronenberg HM. Hormones and disorders of mineral metabolism. In: Larsen P, Kronenberg HM, Melmed S, Polonsky KS, editors. Williams textbook of endocrinology. 10th edition. Philadelphia: W.B. Saunders; 2003. p. 1347–8.

[37] DiMeglio LA, White KE, Econs MJ. Disorders of phosphate metabolism. Endocrinol Metab Clin North Am 2000;29(3):591–609.

[38] Weisinger JR, Bellorin-Font E. Magnesium and phosphorus [see comment]. Lancet 1998; 352(9125):391–6.

[39] Ryzen E. Magnesium homeostasis in critically ill patients. Magnes Trace Elem 1989;8: 201–12.

[40] Wong ETRR, Singer FR. A high prevalence of hypomagnesemia in hospitalized patients. Am J Clin Pathol 1983;79:348–52.

[41] Hamill-Ruth RJ, McGory R. Magnesium repletion and its effect on potassium homeostasis in critically ill adults: results of a double-blind, randomized, controlled trial. Crit Care Med 1996;24(1):38–45.

ELSEVIER
SAUNDERS

EMERGENCY
MEDICINE
CLINICS OF
NORTH AMERICA

Emerg Med Clin N Am 23 (2005) 723–747

Disorders of Potassium

Timothy J. Schaefer, MD[a,b,*],
Robert W. Wolford, MD, MMM[c,d]

[a]Section of Emergency Medicine, Department of Surgery, University of Illinois College
of Medicine at Peoria, Peoria, IL 61605, USA
[b]Department of Emergency Medicine, OSF Saint Francis Medical Center,
530 Northeast Glen Oak Avenue, Peoria, IL 61637, USA
[c]Program in Emergency Medicine, Michigan State University College of Human Medicine,
Saginaw Campus, Saginaw MI 48601, USA
[d]Emergency Care Center, Covenant Healthcare, 900 Cooper, Saginaw, MI 48602, USA

Of all the electrolytes, the serum potassium is probably the most tested for, titrated, and treated. A potassium disorder is the most common electrolyte abnormality in hospitalized patients, and this is likely true of emergency department (ED) patients as well [1–3]. Of the two conditions, hypokalemia is more common; affecting a broader range of patients, while hyperkalemia is potentially more serious and occurs almost exclusively in patients with some underlying renal abnormalities [4,5].

Physiology, total body balance, and pathophysiology of potassium

A brief review of the physiology and the body's handling of potassium will help in understanding the pathophysiology, causes, and management of hypo- and hyperkalemia. The total body potassium content is approximately 50 mEq/kg, and is distributed asymmetrically in the body. (Note, for potassium, 1 mEq = 1 mmol = 39.09 mg. The potassium concentration of milliequivalents per liter (mEq/L) and millimoles per liter (mmol/L) are used interchangeably throughout this article.) About 98% is intracellular, and approximately 75% of the intracellular component is in muscle [6,7]. Only 65 to 70 mEq, or 2%, is extracellular and of this extracellular component, about 15 mEq or 0.4% of the total body potassium is measurable in the

* Corresponding author.
E-mail address: tjschaefer@pol.net (T.J. Schaefer).

0733-8627/05/$ - see front matter © 2005 Elsevier Inc. All rights reserved.
doi:10.1016/j.emc.2005.03.016

plasma [6,7]. This tiny fraction of total body potassium is maintained in a fairly narrow serum concentration of 3.5 to 5.0 mmol/L. In comparison, the intracellular potassium concentration is about 150 mmol/L. The intracellular to extracellular ratio (150 mmol/L/4 mmol/L) results in a voltage gradient across the cell membrane and plays a major role in establishing the resting cell membrane potential, particularly in cardiac and neuromuscular cells [4]. It is apparent that changes in the large, intracellular concentration would have little effect on this ratio, but even small changes in the extracellular concentration will have significant effects on this ratio, the transmembrane potential gradient, and thereby the function of neuromuscular and cardiac tissues [4]. The sodium–potassium adenosinetriphosphate (Na-K-ATPase) enzyme pump, located in the cell membrane, maintains the potassium concentration gradient by actively transporting potassium into and sodium out of cells.

All disorders of potassium occur because of abnormal potassium handling in one of three ways: problems with potassium intake (relatively too much or too little), problems with distribution of potassium between the intracellular and extracellular spaces (ie, transcellular shifts and alterations in the normal ratio), or problems with potassium excretion (relatively too much or too little excreted).

Intake disorders

Normally functioning kidneys protect against hyperkalemia by excreting excess ingested potassium and handle large dietary intakes with little problem [3,8]. Although the kidney protects against hyperkalemia, it is unable to stop all urinary potassium losses. An inadequate intake, over a period of time, may lead to hypokalemia [8,9].

Transcellular shifting disorders

Transcellular potassium shifting is affected by a variety of factors including; integrity of the cell membrane, Na-K-ATPase activity, and the internal state of the body, that is, potassium concentration, acid-base status, and serum tonicity. For example, rhabdomyolysis may cause a massive leak of potassium to the extracellular space because approximately 70% to 75% of the total body potassium is stored in muscle cells [7]. Insulin or beta 2-adrenergic catecholamines increase the Na-K-ATPase activity and drives potassium intracellularly leading to decreased serum potassium levels, whereas patients with impaired insulin production (eg, diabetes mellitus), are predisposed to the development of hyperkalemia [4]. Finally, the internal state of the body may affect transcellular shifting. In acidosis, the high extracellular hydrogen ion concentration results in hydrogen ion movement into and potassium movement out of cells to maintain electroneutrality [4]. Conversely, alkalemia and hypertonicity (eg, hyperglycemia) will result in the movement of potassium into cells.

Excretion disorders

Last, potassium excretion may be relatively too much or too little, which is primarily related to kidney function. The kidney accounts for 90% of potassium excretion with the remainder primarily from the gastrointestinal tract and generally negligible amounts in sweat [3,5]. About 85% to 90% of filtered potassium is reabsorbed before the distal cortical collecting tubules. It is the remaining 10% to15% that is either excreted or reabsorped [3,10]. Normally functioning kidneys, with adequate perfusion, can compensate for a wide range of potassium intake by increasing or decreasing potassium urinary output. The kidneys are able to lower urinary potassium concentration to as little as 5 mEq/L but cannot stop excretion completely [4].

The amount of potassium renally excreted is primarily influenced by three factors: the plasma potassium concentration, plasma aldosterone, and the delivery of sodium and water to the distal collecting tubules [3,11,12]. Increased potassium concentration stimulates nephron Na-K-ATPase activity resulting in potassium movement into the tubular lumen and exertion. The renin–angiotensin–aldosterone system is also activated to increase potassium exertion (Fig. 1 gives a brief, simplied, schematic review of the renin–angiotensin–aldosterone system). Finally, increased sodium and water delivery to the distal tubules stimulates the Na-K-ATPase (contributing to potassium excretion) and increased tubular flow (eg, osmotic diuresis) leading to potassium "washout" and elimination [3,4,11–13].

Hypokalemia

Hypokalemia (generally defined as a serum potassium less than 3.6 mEq per liter) is an exceptionally common electrolyte abnormality encountered in clinical practice. Over 20% of hospitalized patients have been reported to

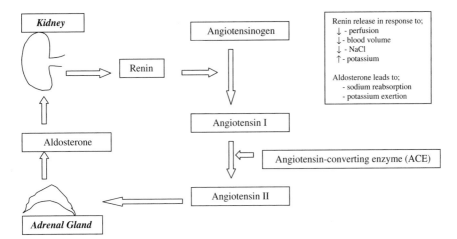

Fig. 1. Renin–angiotensin–aldosterone system (simplified schematic).

have some degree of hypokalemia [14]. A significant fraction of these patients have serum potassiums less than 3 mEq per liter. Patients taking diuretics, particularly thiazides, are at particular risk for hypokalemia. Hypokalemia is also frequently seen in trauma patients, with some centers reporting a 45% to 68% incidence on admission [15,16]. In these patients, hypokalemia is associated with higher injury severity scores and lower glasgow coma scores [16,17].

Hypokalemia has shown to be associated with an increased risk of essential hypertension, ischemic and hemorrhagic stroke, dysrhythmias, and deaths and hospital admissions due to heart failure and cardiovascular events [2,18,19]. Recently, it has been recommended that serum potassium levels be maintained at levels greater than 4.5 mEq per liter for patients with heart failure and patients experiencing an acute myocardial infarction [20].

Clinical manifestations of hypokalemia

The signs and symptoms of hypokalemia are primarily related to changes in the ratio of extracellular to intracellular potassium and its impact on the resting electrical potential across cell membranes. A greater decrease in extracellular potassium concentration compared with intracellular concentration, leads to hyperpolarization of cell membranes and prolongation of action potential and refractory periods. Increased automaticity and excitability also occur in the cardiac system. The organ systems primarily affected by hypokalemia are: cardiac, skeletal muscle, gastrointestinal, and renal [21] (Table 1).

Although very common, rarely is the diagnosis of hypokalemia considered until the results of laboratory tests are known. The majority of hypokalemic patients have serum potassium levels of 3.0 to 3.5 mEq per liter and are asymptomatic. Occasionally, vague symptoms of tiredness and minimal muscle weakness may be reported [2,22]. Moderately hypokalemic patients (serum potassium levels of 3.0 to 2.5 mEq per liter) may demonstrate significant proximal muscle weakness [22]. Cranial muscles are typically spared, and the lower limbs are more affected than the upper

Table 1
Organ system effects of hypokalemia

Cardiac	Dysrhythmias
	Conduction defects
	Increased likelihood of dysrhythmias due to digitalis
Skeletal muscle	Weakness
	Paralysis
	Rhabdomyolysis
	Fasiculations and tetany
Gastrointestinal	Ileus
Renal	Nephrogenic diabetes insipidus
	Metabolic alkalosis

limbs [5,22]. Other vague symptoms including constipation may also be reported. Severely hypokalemic patients (serum potassium levels below 2.5 mEq per liter) may develop rhabdomyolysis, myoglobinuria, an ascending symmetric paralysis with a clear sensorium, and even respiratory arrest [2]. Central nervous system symptoms, although reported, are more likely the result of acid-base changes or other coexisting abnormalities [22]. Symptoms are not only associated with the degree of hypokalemia found, but also the rapidity with which it developed.

Electrocardiograph changes may be present and reflect hypokalemia's effects on myocardial cell membranes (Table 2). The merging of a U-wave with the T-wave may falsely appear to result in the appearance of QT interval prolongation. Giant U-waves may occur, and may be mistaken for peaked T-waves. These large U-waves, however, have a broader base than true for peaked T-waves [23]. Unfortunately, the presence or absence of electrocardiographic changes is not predictive of hypokalemia or of its severity.

Patients without heart disease rarely demonstrate any significant cardiac abnormalities due to hypokalemia. This is not the case for patients with left ventricular hypertrophy, cardiac ischemia, or heart failure [2,20,24]. Numerous studies have demonstrated an increased incidence of ventricular dysrhythmias in patients with underlying heart disease, including acute myocardial infarction, and even mild hypokalemia [2,20,24]. Hulting [25] studied patients with acute myocardial infarction and found the risk of ventricular fibrillation to be nearly five times greater for those with a serum potassium of less than 3.9 mEq per liter. Hypokalemia also increases the potential for digoxin toxicity and associated dysrhythmias.

Hypokalemia has a number of effects on renal function. Patients may present with symptoms of polyuria and polydypsia due to impaired ability to concentrate the urine and a resulting picture of nephrogenic diabetes insipidus [26]. Persistent metabolic alkalosis may occur as the result of the decreased ability of the kidney to excrete bicarbonate and citrate, increased ammoniagenesis, and increased collecting duct proton secretion [26,27]. Hypokalemia may also contribute to persistent metabolic alkalosis by increasing urinary chloride excretion and causing serum hypochloremia [26].

Table 2
Electrocardiographic changes associated with hypokalemia

Increased P-wave amplitude
Prolonged PR interval
Apparent QT interval prolongation
Reduction in T-wave amplitude
T-wave inversion
ST segment depression
U-waves

From Webster A, Brady W, Morris F. Recognising signs of danger: ECG changes resulting from an abnormal serum potassium concentration. Emerg Med J 2002;19:74–7.

Etiologies of hypokalemia

The etiology of hypokalemia, for a given patient, falls into three broad categories: insufficient potassium intake, transcellular shift of potassium from the extracellular to intracellular compartments, or excessive potassium loss. The renal and gastrointestinal systems are the primary sites of excess potassium loss from the body (Fig. 2).

Inadequate potassium intake

Inadequate intake of potassium is an exceedingly rare cause of hypokalemia. The minimum daily dietary requirement for potassium is considered to be 1.6 g to 2 g (40 to 50 mEq) per day with the usual dietary intake being 2.1 g to 3.4 g per day [8,24]. If potassium intake is less than 40 mEq per day for a prolonged period, hypokalemia may develop. The elderly, especially those living alone or with disabilities, are more likely to have a potassium-poor diet and to develop hypokalemia on this basis [24]. Hypokalemia is occasionally seen in those individuals who habitually eat clay. The clay binds potassium, making it unavailable for absorption.

Transcellular potassium shifts

The movement of potassium from the extracellular compartment into cells is a relatively uncommon cause of clinically significant hypokalemia. Importantly, although the serum potassium concentration may be low, the amount of total body potassium may be normal. Aggressive potassium administration may result in severe hyperkalemia once the underlying cause

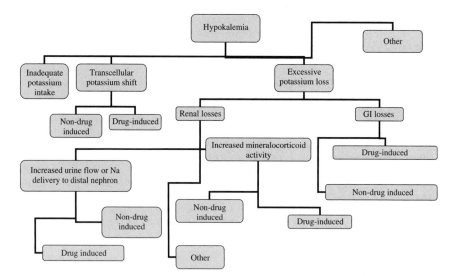

Fig. 2. Etiologies of hypokalemia.

is addressed. Transcellular shifts may be the result of medications or other nondrug causes.

Drug-induced potassium shifts

A large number of medications can cause transcellular potassium shifts [2]. The β_2 sympathomimetic agonists are probably the most studied of these drugs. These drugs increase the movement of sodium into cells in exchange for hydrogen protons and results in an increased intracellular sodium concentration. As a result, the Na-K-ATPase is driven to move sodium out and potassium into cells, resulting in a fall of extracellular potassium concentrations [21]. The degree and duration of hypokalemia varies with the agent used. Interestingly, a study in primates has suggested that the tremor frequently seen with the use of these agents is associated with hypokalemia [28]. Hypokalemia may also occur in patients with a high level of circulating catecholamines, probably via the same mechanism.

Other common medications causing transcellular shifts include phosphodiesterase inhibitors (eg, theophylline and caffeine), insulin, barium poisoning, and verapamil overdose [2,26].

Nondrug-induced potassium shifts

A variety of disorders can cause movement of potassium into cells. Both metabolic and respiratory alkalosis can contribute to hypokalemia due to the exchange of extracellular potassium for intracellular hydrogen ions. The administration of glucose or insulin may cause a decline in serum potassium as insulin stimulates cellular uptake of potassium. Rare causes of severe hypokalemia with paralysis include familial periodic paralysis (typically citizens of Western countries), thyrotoxic periodic paralysis (males of Asian descent), sporadic periodic paralysis (Asian descent), and hypernatremic hypokalemic paralysis. Hypokalemia and paralysis due to transcellular shift should be suspected when no evidence of a total body deficit of potassium is found and there is no acid-base disorder present [29].

Excessive loss of potassium

The most common cause of hypokalemia is the excessive loss of potassium, either in the stool or via urine. Losses from the skin are rare except in the readily identifiable conditions of extensive burns or large volumes of sweat production.

Gastrointestinal losses

Potassium losses via the gastrointestinal tract are likely the second most common cause of hypokalemia in developed countries, and results primarily from losses in the stool [2,4]. Normally, only about 10% of total potassium excretion (~ 10 mEq) each day is via stool. Any cause of increased stool volumes will increase the amount of potassium lost and can result in hypokalemia if the intake of potassium is not increased.

Vomiting and nasogastric suctioning, by themselves, do not cause significant potassium loss as the normal gastric fluid only contains 5 to 10 mEq per liter. However, if aldosterone levels increase because of associated volume loss, an increase in potassium excretion in the urine will occur. In addition, an associated metabolic alkalosis will contribute to increased urinary potassium loss and transcellular shifting of extracellular potassium, again contributing to the development of hypokalemia [4].

Renal losses

Hypokalemia due to increased potassium loss in the urine is probably the most common cause of hypokalemia in developed countries.

Potassium losses due to increased urinary flow or delivery of sodium to distal nephron

Diuretics are the most common drug-related cause of hypokalemia. Thiazide and loop diuretics both increase sodium and chloride delivery to the distal collecting duct, which results in increased potassium secretion and chloride depletion. The incidence of hypokalemia for patients on diuretics may be up to 56%, and the time to development of hypokalemia is quite variable [30].

Osmotic diuresis from poorly controlled diabetes mellitus or the use of mannitol or saline diuresis to treat hypercalcemia may also cause increased renal potassium loss due to increased urine flow and potassium secretion. Administration of high doses of some antibiotics, such as penicillin or its derivatives, also increase the delivery of sodium to the distal nephron and increase potassium secretion [2].

Rare causes of hypokalemia due to increased distal sodium delivery include Type I and Type II renal tubular acidosis (RTA), Gitelman's syndrome, and Bartter's syndrome [5]. In these disorders, although due to different mechanisms, increased delivery of sodium to the distal nephron causes increased potassium secretion. RTA is one of the few disorders in which hypokalemia and metabolic acidosis occur [4].

Increased mineralocorticoid activity

Aldosterone is the primary hormonal regulator of renal potassium secretion. Increased aldosterone levels lead to an increased number of open sodium pores and increased Na-K-ATPase activity in the nephrons and, as a result, increased potassium secretion into the urine.

Primary hyperaldosteronism is the result of a unilateral adrenal adenoma, bilateral adrenal hyperplasia, or rarely an adrenocortical carcinoma [2]. Secondary hyperaldosteronism is the outcome of the normal response to a variety of disease states causing decreased intravascular volume and decreased renal perfusion or to increased renin production. Both result in increased potassium wasting by the kidneys. Other rare causes of aldosteronism include Cushing's syndrome (adrenal, pituitary, or ectopic tumor production of adrenocorticotropic hormone) and congenital adrenal hyperplasia [2].

Several drugs and dietary supplements may cause presentations suggestive of hyperaldosteronism. Life-threatening hypokalemia has been reported in a patient treated with high-dose hydrocortisone [31]. Gluco-corticoids with mineralocorticoid activity and in high doses may saturate 11 β-hydoxysteroid dehydrogenase in the renal cortical collecting ducts. Excess steroid then binds with the mineralocorticoid receptor and produces the same effects as aldosterone [31]. Licorice containing glycyrrhizic acid, although no longer made in the United States, is still found in a variety of herbal teas, chewing tobaccos, sweeteners, and other compounds produced internationally. An active metabolite of licorice, glycyrrhetenic acid, binds to the mineralocorticoid receptor [32]. It also inhibits 11 β-hydoxysteroid dehydrogenase, creating an apparent cortisol excess that also binds to the mineralocorticoid receptor. The findings are similar to that of primary hyperaldosteronism [32].

Other renal etiologies of potassium loss

Hypomagnesemia frequently occurs in many patients who are also at risk for hypokalemia (eg, patients with congestive heart failure and on diuretics, alcoholics). One study of patients with congestive heart failure found 23% of the patients to be hypokalemic and 17% to be hypomagnesemic [33]. Fifty percent of the hypokalemic patients were hypomagnesemic and 67% of the hypomagnesemic patients also were hypokalemic [33]. Renal potassium wasting is common in hypomagnesemic patients and the hypokalemia cannot be reversed until the magnesium deficit is corrected [2]. The mechanism by which a magnesium deficit causes renal potassium wasting is unknown.

Treatment of hypokalemia

Hypokalemia rarely occurs as an isolated condition. In many cases, corrections of other abnormalities (eg, hypovolemia) must take precedence over repletion of serum potassium. Underlying causes of the hypokalemia, such as hypomagnesemia, must also be addressed.

After the initial priorities of airway, breathing, and circulation are addressed a search for the etiology of the hypokalemia should be made. In most cases, a thorough history and physical examination reveal the cause (eg, severe diarrhea, use of diuretics without potassium supplementation). If the etiology is still unclear, additional laboratory tests that will assist in the diagnosis include (1) serum sodium, chloride, bicarbonate, creatinine, and glucose; (2) arterial blood gas; and (3) spot urine measurements of sodium, potassium, chloride, and creatinine. Using the additional laboratory data, the etiology of the hypokalemia may be sorted into one of several categories (Table 3). To be complete, samples should also be sent for determination of plasma renin and aldosterone levels, although they usually will not be available in the ED.

The decision to correct hypokalemia should be based on the clinical state of the patient. Most patients who are asymptomatic and have mild hypokalemia (3.5 to 3.0 mEq per liter) do not require urgent correction, although they should be advised to eat a diet rich in potassium [27]. Potassium supplementation may be required if the hypokalemia persists. However, patients with acute myocardial infarction are an exception, due to the increased risk of ventricular dysrhythmias in the presence of even mild hypokalemia. It is recommended that the serum potassium be maintained above 4.5 mEq per liter in this population [20].

Patients with moderate to severe hypokalemia (<3.0 mEq/L) or those who are symptomatic with significant electrocardiogram changes, dysrhythmias, severe weakness, or paralysis require more urgent potassium replacement. The choice of route and formulation is dependent on the severity of the symptoms and underlying conditions (Table 4).

Table 3
Diagnostic approach to etiology of hypokalemia

Laboratory abnormalities	Etiology
Hypokalemia and normal acid-base state and UK\Ucreat < 2	Transcellular shift (eg, thyrotoxic periodic paralysis, familial periodic paralysis)
Hypokalemia and normal gap metabolic acidosis and (UNa + UK)-UCl ≥ -10	Gastrointestinal losses of potassium (eg, diarrhea or other gut fluid high in bicarbonate
Hypokalemia and normal gap metabolic acidosis and (UNa + UK)-UCl ≤ -10 and UK\Ucreat > 2	Renal-mediated potassium loss due to renal tubular acidosis, drug induced RTA, ureteral diversion
Hypokalemia and metabolic alkalosis and UCl < 20 mEq\L	Gastrointestinal loss of potassium due to vomiting, NG suctioning
	Diuretics (UCl measure after diuretic effect resolved)
Hypokalemia and metabolic alkalosis and UCl > 20 mEq\L	Diuretics (UCl measured during diuretic effect)
	Increased mineralocorticoid effect

Abbreviations: UCl, chloride; UK, potassium; UNa, sodium; Ucreat, creatinine.
Adapted from Ref. [34]. Whittier WL, Rutecki GW. Primer on clinical acid-base problem solving. Dis Mon 2004;50:117–62 and Lin SH, Chiu JS, Hsu CW, et al. A simple and rapid approach to hypokalemic paralysis. Am J Emerg Med 2003;21:487–91.

Table 4
Treatment of hypokalemia

Formulation	Dose and rate	Indication
Oral potassium chloride (multiple formulations)	20–80 mEq/d in divided doses	Nonurgent correction and/or maintenance
Oral potassium liquid	40–60 mEq/dose: serum potassium should be followed to determine dosing interval	Rapid elevation for patients requiring urgent, but not emergent correction.
Intravenous potassium chloride	20–40 mEq/h serum potassium should be reassessed after 60 mEq	Patients with severe symptoms (eg, dysrhythmias, paralysis) or unable to tolerate oral dosing

Adapted from Kim GH, Han JS. Therapeutic Approach to Hypokalemia. Nephron 2002;92(Supp. 1):28–32.

Special care must be taken in the treatment of patients with low serum potassium due to transcellular potassium shifts. These patients may not have significant total body potassium deficits. Rebound hyperkalemia can occur as the cause of the transcellular shift is corrected and if aggressive potassium replacement has been given [29,35].

Hyperkalemia

Although hypokalemia is a more common clinical disorder, hyperkalemia is generally more serious and less well tolerated [2,6]. A total body potassium depletion of 200 to 400 mEq will reduce the serum concentration by about 1 mEq/L, whereas an excess of only 100 to 200 mEq will increase the serum potassium concentration by about 1 mEq/L [6]. With this in mind, it's understandable that increases in the total body potassium content can result in a rapid and potentially life-threatening hyperkalemia.

Case

A 40-year-old male presented to the ED with a chief complaint of profound weakness. He had noticed some mild weakness, generalized malaise, and mild nausea for 2 days but this marked weakness developed suddenly on the morning of admission. He was unable to weight bear, and had to slide himself along the floor to call a neighbor, and was brought in by ambulance.

Until 3 weeks ago, the patient had been healthy with no known medical problems and had not seen a doctor "for years," when he suffered a small acute myocardial infarction. On that admission, hypertension (218/138 on arrival) and hypercholesterolemia were diagnosed and the patient was started on enalapril (Vasotec) 20 mg twice a day, metolprolol (Lopressor) 50 mg twice a day, pravastatin (Pravachol) 20 mg daily, aspirin 81 mg daily, and clopidogrel (Plavix) 75 mg daily.

On arrival in the ED for the current visit, the patient complained of severe, bilateral weakness in the lower extremities greater than the upper extremities, lower extremity numbness and "tingling," and nausea. He denied any chest pain or shortness of breath. His vital signs were; pulse 67, respirations 20, blood pressure 154/83, temperature 97.4°F (36.3°C). On physical examination, his head/neck, lung, and cardiac exam was unremarkable. His abdominal exam revealed mild diffuse tenderness and the neurologic exam was remarkable for nonfocal generalized weakness greater in the lower extremities, with normal sensation. When compared with a prior electrocardiogram, changes included "peaked" T-waves, PR interval increase from 126 millisecond to 172 millisecond and QRS duration increase from 92 millisecond to 120 millisecond (Fig. 3). Laboratory results included serum potassium = 9.1 mmol/L, sodium = 127 mmol/L, CO_2 venous = 15 mmol/L, glucose = 95 mg/dL, blood urea nitrogen (BUN) = 31 mg/dL, and creatinine = 1.5 mg/dL. (BUN and creatinine on the prior admission were 11 mg/dL and 1.0 mg/dL, respectively).

The patient was treated with calcium gluconate 10 mL of a 10% solution (1 g) intravenously (IV), regular insulin 10 units IV, glucose 50 mL of 50% dextrose (25 g) IV, and sodium polystyrene sulfonate (Kayexalate) 30 g orally. After approximately 1 hour, the patient was feeling improved and repeat labs included potassium = 7.8 mmol/L and glucose = 64 mg/dL. An additional 25 mL of 50% dextrose (12.5 g) IV was given.

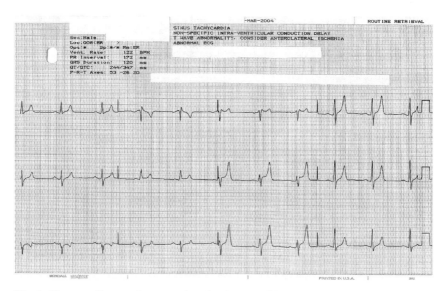

Fig. 3. Electrocardiogram demonstrating the changes of hyperkalemia. ECG from Case #2 demonstrating peaked T-wave, QRS duration prolongation, and PR interval lengthening when compared with an earlier ECG.

In this case, the patient's impaired cardiac conduction and weakness are typical symptoms of both hypo- and hyperkalemia; however, the ECG suggests hyperkalemia.

Hyperkalemia is defined as a level > 5.5 mmol/L [5,7]. Some further divide hyperkalemia into: minimal, 5.5 to 6.5 mmol/L with only minor electrocardiographic changes; moderate, 6.6 to 8.0 mmol/L with ECG changes limited to peaking of T-waves; and severe, >8.0 mmol/L or any level with a widened QRS complex, atrioventricular (AV) block, or ventricular dysrhythmia [36]. Readers are reminded that serious complications do not strictly correlate with a given level, and are related more to the rate of rise in the potassium level, the affect on cardiac conduction, and the underlying cause than on the exact serum potassium concentration [5,7].

Clinical manifestations of hyperkalemia

As with hypokalemia, the organ systems affected are cardiac, neuromuscular, and gastrointestinal. Patients often complain of only vague feelings of not feeling well, gastrointestinal symptoms, or generalized weakness [10]. The most serious concern is impaired cardiac conduction with risk of sudden death from asystole or ventricular fibrillation [4,6,7]. Neuromuscular signs and symptoms include muscle cramps, weakness, paralysis, paresthesias, and decreased deep tendon reflexes [4,37].

Usually, severe symptoms do not occur until potassium levels reach 7.0 mmol/L or above, but there are many individual patient variables, and a rapid rate of rise is more dangerous than a slowly rising level [8,36,38]. In the ED it may be impossible to know if the hyperkalemia is acute or more stable and chronic.

Physicians are unable to use the ECG alone to predict which patients might have hyperkalemia or how high the level might be [1,5,7,39,40]. However, typical ECG changes in a patient with hyperkalemia, increases the urgency for treatment. The "classic" ECG changes associated with hyperkalemia are well described [3–7,40–42]. The earliest changes, often beginning with levels above 6.5 mEq/L, are "peaked," or "tented" T-waves, which are most prominent in the precordial leads. With further rise in serum levels, there is diminished cardiac excitability manifested by flattening of the P-wave, PR interval lengthening, and the eventual disappearance of the P-wave. The QRS duration becomes prolonged, progressing to a "sine wave" appearance, and finally ending in ventricular asystole or fibrillation with levels 8 to 10 mmol/L [3–7,40–42].

Etiologies of hyperkalemia

As with hypokalemia, hyperkalemia results from an imbalance of normal potassium handling. This imbalance can develop from increased potassium load, transcellular shifting of potassium, or decreased potassium elimination

(Table 4). In addition to "real" disease, one other fairly common cause for elevated potassium readings is "pseudohyperkalemia," which is discussed below.

Pseudohyperkalemia

This may be more common than true hyperkalemia, and occurs when potassium is unexpectedly released from cells either at the time of phlebotomy or after collection [4,5]. Traumatic hemolysis during venipuncture or in vitro hemolysis is the most common cause of psyedohyperkalemia being reported in 20% of all blood samples with an elevated potassium level [6]. The laboratory will generally report a "slightly hemolyzed" specimen as a clue to explain the hyperkalemia [4]. Another cause is potassium released from muscle cells distal to a tourniquet with fist clenching during phlebotomy. [3,6,12,43]. This can be avoided by not having the patient clench their fist, limiting tourniquet time, or releasing the tourniquet after the needle enters the vein. Finally, potassium can be released from white blood cells or platelets, after blood is drawn, in patients with severe leukocytosis (white blood cell count $> 50,000-100,000/mm^3$ or thrombocytosis (platelet counts $> 500,000-1$ million/mm^3). If this is suspected, recheck the potassium from a tube of unclotted blood [5,12]. The possibility of pseudohyperkalemia should always be considered if unexpected hyperkalemia is found in an asymptomatic patient with otherwise normal electrolytes and acid-base balance [5,6,12].

Decreased potassium excretion

The large majority of cases of hyperkalemia (over 80%) occur when potassium excretion is impaired by a medical condition or medications in a patient with some degree of underlying renal dysfunction [3,5,12,11]. Most patients with decreased ability to excrete potassium compensate and reach a steady state of normal serum potassium concentration until some second event tips the balance [5]. This second event could be decreased perfusion, infection, obstruction, or a new medication [3,11].

On a physiologic level, there are two possible problems. First is diminished sodium and water delivery to the distal collecting system. This might occur with advanced renal failure or if there is real or effective circulating volume depletion as seen with hypovolemia, dehydration, or severe heart failure. The second possibility is reduced effectiveness or concentration of aldosterone [5,11,44]. We will discuss each of these two possibilities.

Acute or chronic renal failure

Although all the possible causes of renal failure are beyond the scope of this article, any condition that leads to worsening renal insufficiency or renal failure can result in hyperkalemia. There must be adequate blood flow for glomerular filtration and some amount of urinary tubular flow, to the distal collecting tubule, for potassium secretion to occur. When the glomerular filtration rate falls below about 10 mL/min or about 1 L/d, this can lead to hyperkalemia [6]. Patients with *acute* renal failure are at greater risk for life-threatening complications from hyperkalemia as the potassium level is rising more rapidly, before the body has a chance to develop compensatory mechanisms.

Hypoaldosteronism

A more common renal cause for hyperkalemia than *complete* renal failure is renal insufficiency with development of hypoaldosteronism [4,7,10]. This is a condition of relatively well-preserved glomerular filtration rate but decreased aldosterone levels. There are multiple medical causes and hypoaldosterone-inducing medications that play a role in the susceptible patient (see Box 1) [1–3,11]. Hypoaldosteronism can be subdivided by the accompanying renin levels as low, normal, or high [10].

Hyporeninemic hypoaldosteronism results from impaired renin levels ultimately resulting in hypoaldosteronism. Several conditions are associated with defective renin production, including damage to the juxtaglomerular apparatus, dysfunction of sympathetic innervation, and inhibition of prostaglandin synthesis [11]. The classic patient is an elderly diabetic patient with mild to moderate renal insufficiency; however, any condition that damages or limits normal renal production of renin can result in hyporeninemia (see Box 1) [4,7]. The best examples of medications implicated in causing hyporeninemic hypoaldosteronism associated hyper-kalemia are nonsteriodal anti-inflammatory drugs (NSAIDs). NSAIDs can cause hyperkalemia by decreasing glomerular filtration rate, increasing sodium retention, but primarily by suppressing renin output via inhibition of prostaglandins [7,11]. Patients at increased risk for developing hyper-kalemia with NSAID use include the elderly, those with serum creatinine concentration greater than 1.2 mg/dL, patients with congestive heart failure, or those using diuretics [11]. The selective cyclooxygenase-2 inhibitors have been reported to cause severe hyperkalemia by the same mechanism as the traditional NSAIDs [45,46].

Hypereninemic hypoaldosteronism occurs when there is lack of aldoste-rone production. In adrenal insufficiency (Addison's Disease), the adrenal glands do not produce enough aldosterone. Medications disrupting the renin–angiotensin–aldosterone system include angiotensin converting en-zyme inhibitors (eg, captopril, enalapril, lisinopril), angiotensin receptor blockers (eg, irbesartan, losartan, valsartan) and heparin. Identifying patients at risk for developing hyperkalemia before starting these medications is difficult. Hyperkalemia can occur in patients with only modest renal insufficiency, and may not be predicted by the pretreatment

Box 1. Causes of hyperkalemia

Pseudohyperkalemia
- Hemolysis
- Distal to tourniquet or with fist clenching
- Marked leukocystosis (white blood cell count >50,000 mm^3)
- Marked thrombocystosis (platelets >1 million mm^3)

Decreased potassium elimination
Acute or chronic decreased glomerular filtration rate (5–10 mL/min)
   1. Acute or chronic renal failure
Hyopaldosteronism
   1. With low renin levels (hyporeninemic hypoaldosteronism)
- Elderly
- Diabetic
- Interstitial nephritis
- Obstructive uropathy
- Systemic lupus erythematosus (SLE)
- Amyloidosis
- AIDS
- Nonsteroidal anti-inflammatory drugs
   2. With high renin levels (hyperreninemic hypoaldosteronism)
- Addison's Disease
- Angiotensin converting enzyme inhibitors
- Angiotension receptor blockers
- Heparin
End-organ resistance to aldosterone (normal or elevated aldosterone)
- SLE
- Sickle cell anemia
- Obstructive uropathy
- Transplantation
- Potassium-sparing diuretic—spironolactone
Sodium channel blockade
- Potassium-sparing diuretics—amiloride, triamterene
- Trimethoprim (blocks sodium reabsorption)
- Pentamidine (blocks sodium reabsorption)

Increased potassium load
- Potassium supplements
- Dietary salt substitutes
- Potassium penicillin
- Massive blood transfusion
- Poisoning e.g. potassium chloride water softener pellet ingestion

Transcellular shifting
- Insulin deficiency
- Rhabdomyolysis/increased tissue catabolism
- Acidosis
- Hypertonicity
- Exercise
- Hyperkalemic periodic paralysis
- Drugs
   1. Non-selective beta-blockers (inhibits Na-P-ATPase pump)
   2. Digitalis toxicity (inhibits Na-P-ATPase pump)
   3. Succinylcholine (membrane leak)

Modified from Zull DN. Disorders of potassium metabolism. Emerg Med Clin North Am 1989;7(4):771–94; with permission and data from Gennari FJ. Disorders of potassium homeostasis: hypokalemia and hyperkalemia. Crit Care Clin 2002;18(2):273–88 and Linas SL. The patient with hypokalemia or hyperkalemia. In: Schrier RW, editor. Manual of Nephrology, 5th ed. Philadelphia: Lippincott Williams & Wilkins; 2000.

serum creatinine level [11,47,48]. Heparin reduces aldosterone synthesis, and can lead to hyperkalemia in about 7% of patients treated for 3 or more days [4,7,11,49].

End-organ resistance to aldosterone

In addition to hypoaldosterone states, *normal or elevated aldosterone* may be seen when the kidneys develop end-organ resistance to aldosterone [5,10]. Conditions such as obstructive uropathy, sickle cell anemia, systemic lupus erythematous, and renal transplantation predispose to hyperkalemia by this mechanism [10]. The classic medication example is the potassium-sparing diuretic spironolactone (Aldactone), which competitively binds to the aldosterone receptor [11].

Sodium channel blockade

Finally, several medications cause hyperkalemia by inhibiting the sodium channels in the kidney, which leads to sodium excretion and potassium retention. The potassium-sparing diuretics amiloride (Midamor) and triamterene (Dyrenium) work by this mechanism [4,7,11]. An often overlooked possible cause of hyperkalemia by this mechanism are the antibiotics trimethoprim-sulfamethoxazole (Bactrim, Septra) (trimethoprim component) and pentamidine (Pentam), which also block sodium channels [7,11,50].

Use of potassium-sparing diuretics has increased since the results of the 1999 randomized aldactone evaluation study (RALES), which demonstrated a 30% mortality reduction when low dose spironolactone (average dose was 26 mg every day) was added to standard treatment for severe congestive heart failure [51]. The incidence of serious hyperkalemia ($K^+ > 6.0$ mmol/L) in this study occurred in only 2% [51]. However, several reports of life-threatening and fatal hyperkalemia have subsequently been reported [48,52–54].

Increased potassium load

In patients with normal renal function, hyperkalemia from excess potassium load is very uncommon. Possible causes include potassium supplement overdose, massive blood transfusions with hypoperfusion, or accidental overdose ingestion of potassium chloride crystals used in water softeners [6,55]. A more common scenario is gradual total body potassium accumulation in a patient with impaired kidney function. Dietary salt substitutes, potassium supplements, penicillin potassium therapy, and drinking "potassium softened" water may cause hyperkalemia in the predisposed patient [6,55,56].

Transcellular shifting

Redistribution of potassium from the intracellular to the extracellular space is another etiology of hyperkalemia. Insulin is a key hormone for promoting potassium uptake into cells by stimulating the Na-K-ATPase as described earlier. Insulin deficiency, in diabetes mellitus, can lead to hyperkalemia because of lack of transcellular uptake [3,12]. Cell breakdown and increased tissue catabolism can release large amounts of potassium into the circulation. Examples include rhabdomyolysis, massive hemolysis (eg, transfusion reaction), resolving hematoma, catabolic states, or tumor lysis syndrome after chemotherapy initiation [4,6,10].

Although acidosis is frequently described as contributing to hyperkalemia, clinically, there is an inconsistent response in respiratory acidosis and there is a limited response in organic acidosis (ie, lactic acidosis and ketoacidosis) as these organic acids tend to move across membranes with the hydrogen ion [3,4,6,10,12]. Hypertonicity may lead to hyperkalemia by two mechanisms: loss of intracellular water, resulting in an increased intracellular potassium concentration, favoring a gradient for potassium to move out of cells; and as water exits the cell, potassium is swept along with, "solvent drag" [12]. The most common cause of hyperosmolarity is hyperglycemia in uncontrolled diabetes mellitus [3]. Other conditions with hypertonicity are hypernatremia and hypertonic mannitol. Hyperkalemic Periodic Paralysis [3,12] is a rare autosomal dominant disorder in which a sudden rise in serum potassium levels results in transient weakness or paralysis. This often occurs during rest after strenuous exercise or after a large potassium-containing meal. Treatment with insulin, glucose, and a beta-adrenergic agonist may be clinically indicated if the patient has severe weakness with respiratory compromise.

Finally, medications can disrupt the normal intracellular/extracellular potassium ratio. Nonselective beta-blockers (eg, propranolol) can interfere with the Na-K-ATPase, inhibiting potassium uptake into cells [3,7,11]. Generally, this effect is minimal and seems less likely to occur with selective beta-1 blockers such as atenolol or metoprolol [12]. Digoxin inhibits the Na-K-ATPase in a dose-dependent fashion and at toxic levels, potassium transport into cells is impaired, and can cause hyperkalemia [3,7,11]. Succinylcholine may cause a rapid, transient hyperkalemia from intracellular leak. This occurs most commonly in patients with specific underlying conditions, such as major burns, neuromuscular injury, or prolonged immobilization [7].

Emergency department management of hyperkalemia

The risk of severe complications and the urgency for treatment of hyperkalemia is determined by individual patient conditions including presenting symptoms, overall hemodynamic status, kidney function, underlying medical conditions, patient medications, rapidity of potassium rise, serum potassium level, acid-base status, ECG findings, and so on [7,11,36]. Because of the wide variety of factors to consider, treatment cannot be based on serum potassium levels alone, and there are no clear guidelines for admission versus ED treatment versus outpatient treatment [7]. Some suggest that if patients have stable or slowly rising serum potassium levels of 6.5 mmol/L or less and minimal or no ECG changes, then they could be treated as outpatients [36]. Another suggestion is that patients with moderate hyperkalmia (6.5–8.0 mmol/L), ECGs that are normal or have changes limited to peaked T-waves only, and have an identified and manageable cause of hyperkalemia, can be treated in the ED, observed for a short period of time, and sent home [36]. Finally, others suggest that because life-threatening arrhythmias are more likely with rapidly rising levels and the time course of the hyperkalemia is often not known, then all patients with serum potassiums >6.0 mEq/L should be considered at risk for life-threatening arrhythmias and treated [3,11].

The following management suggestions are offered. Patients require immediate treatment and continuous cardiac monitoring with extended observation if levels are rising rapidly, if levels are 7.0 mmol/L or above, if they have severe muscle weakness, if they have marked electrocardiographic changes (more that just peaked-T waves), if they have acute deterioration of renal function, or if they have significant coexisting medical problems [7,11,36]. Asymptomatic patients with stable or slowly rising levels between 6.0 to 6.5 mmol/L, no ECG changes of hyperkalemia, and an identifiable and manageable etiology, can be treated in the ED with exchange resin alone, observed for a short time, and sent home. Last, asymptomatic patients with stable levels below 6.0 mmol/L and an identifiable/manageable etiology can be treated with diet or medication changes as an outpatient [2,4,7,38].

There is a four-pronged approached to the acute management of severe hyperkalemia; cardiac membrane stabilization, reducing plasma potassium concentrations by moving potassium from the extracellular to the intracellular space, removing potassium from the body, and determining cause and preventing recurrence [7,11,57] (Table 5).

Membrane stabilization

Calcium is used to *temporarily* antagonize and stabilize the cardiac membrane from the effects of hyperkalemia. It is indicated in patients with significant ECG abnormalities (ie, loss of P-waves and prolonged QRS duration) and when it is potentially dangerous to wait 30 to 60 minutes for other therapies to take affect [6,38]. Calcium gluconate is generally used, and Table 5 gives dosing. The calcium dose can be repeated in 10 minutes [4,5,7]. Calcium *chloride* can also be used with 10 mL of a 10% solution providing three times the elemental calcium than that of 10 mL of 10% calcium *gluconate*. This higher dose of calcium, theoretically, may be beneficial in patients with marked cardiovascular compromise and instability [6].

There are several cautions with calcium use. First, *calcium can potentiate digitalis toxicity* [4,5,7,40]. If it is necessary to give calcium to a patient

Table 5
Treatment of hyperkalemia

Medication	Dose and route	Onset	Duration
Membrane stabilizing			
Calcium Gluconate (caution: digoxin toxic pt.)	10 mL of 10% solution, may repeat once in 5–10 min (children, 0.5 mL/kg IV)	1–3 min	20–60 min
Transcellular potassium shifting			
Insulin, regular AND Glucose (if serum glucose <250 mg/dL) (caution: monitor glucose)	10 units IV with 50 mL of 50% solution (consider following with $D_{10}W$ infusion at 50 mL/h) OR 10 units in 500 mL of $D_{10}W$ over 1 h (children, insulin 0.1 units/kg with $D_{25}W$ infusion 2 mL/kg (0.5 g/kg over 30 min)	10–20 min	2–4 h
Albuterol (nebulized) (caution: pts with severe coronary artery disease)	10–20 mg in 4 mL saline nebulized over 20 min (children, 2.5 mg if <25 kg or 5 mg if >25 kg)	20–30 min	2–4 h
$NaHCO_3$ (Only in metabolic acidosis)	50–100 mEq IV over 5 min (children, 1–2 mEq/kg IV)	<30 min	1–2 h
Elimination of potassium			
Sodium polystyrene sulfonate (caution: give with laxative)	30 g PO, 50 g PR (children, 1–2 g/kg PO or PR)	~2 h (PO) ~1 h (PR)	—
Furosemide	20–40 mg IV (children, 1–2 mg/kg IV)	30–60 min	—
Hemodialysis		minutes	—

Created from data from Refs. [58,59,60].

taking digitalis, it is recommended that the calcium be added to 100 mL of D_5W and infused over 20 to 30 minutes [7,9,11]. Second, it cannot be given through the same IV line as sodium bicarbonate, as it can precipitate out as a calcium salt. Third, calcium is irritating to tissue, and can cause phlebitis and tissue necrosis if it extravagates. Fourth, repeated doses can lead to hypercalcemia. Finally, calcium is a temporary measure that does not decrease serum potassium levels and must be used with other therapies.

Intracellular shifting

Insulin

The next step in acute management is to shift potassium from the extracellular to the intracellular space. Insulin is the most consistent and reliable treatment (even in patients with end-stage renal disease), and is indicated in all cases of hyperkalemia requiring emergency treatment [7,40] (see Table 5 for different dosing options). Treatment should lower the potassium level by about 0.5 to 1.2 mmol/L in 1 hour [6,7,40]. If glucose levels are below about 250 to 300, then glucose should also be administerd with the insulin to prevent hypoglycemia (typical 50 mL of 50% glucose; 1 ampule or 25 g). Hypoglycemia occurs in 11% to 75% of normoglycemic patients, in 30 to 60 minutes, if they are given less than 25 g of glucose [7,40]. In all patients treated with insulin, close glucose monitoring and if necessary, infusion of 10% dextrose at 50 mL/h or repeat dextrose boluses should be given as needed [7,40].

Beta-2 agonist

Another possible treatment to shift potassium intracellularly is IV or nebulized beta-2 agonists. The nebulized dose is 10 to 20 mg in 4 mL of saline, which is higher that the typical 2.5 to 10 mg every 1 to 4 hours recommended for acute bronchospasm (see Table 5). Side effects may include tachycardia or possible development of angina in susceptible patients [7,38].

Bicarbonate

Another historically suggested treatment is sodium bicarbonate. However, the routine use of sodium bicarbonate is controversial, and has fallen out of favor for several reasons [3,6,7,11,40,61]. First, bicarbonate is most effective in the clinically uncommon condition of *nonanion gap metabolic acidosis* [6]. Bicarbonate is less effective in organic metabolic acidosis (ie, lactic and ketoacidosis) and in patients with renal failure (which is one of the most common causes of hyperkalemia) [6]. Second, bicarbonate will precipitate with calcium if given in the same line. Finally, patients could receive a large amount of sodium, a concern in heart failure and renal failure patients [7]. In Ahee and Crowe's [42] review of the efficacy of various treatments for hyperkalemia, they cited four studies showing no reduction in serum potassium within 60 minutes after sodium bicarbonate treatment. So it seems, in the most "clinically common" cases of hyperkalemia, there appears to be little or no value in routinely adding sodium bicarbonate, and this treatment should be reserved for selective cases of nonanion gap metabolic acidosis [2,7,11,40,61].

It must be remembered that these steps to shift potassium to the intracellular space are also only *temporary* measures. Most cases of hyperkalemia are caused by a total body potassium excess and this excess potassium must be removed.

Enhancing clearance

Sodium polystyrene sulfonate (Kayexalate)

Sodium polystyrene sulfonate (Kayexalate) is an exchange resin that works across the gastrointestinal mucosa [7,38]. Each gram of resin will remove about 1 mEq of potassium by exchanging it with about 2 mEq of sodium [3,4,7,38,62]. This can be give orally or as a retention enema (see Table 5 for dosing). The oral dose can be repeated every 2 to 4 hours and the rectal dose every 1 to 2 hours [4,7,38,62]. This treatment may cause sodium retention, edema, and exacerbation of congestive heart failure in patients with severe cardiac dysfunction.

Diuretics

Loop (eg, furosemide [Lasix] and bumetanide [Bumex]) and thiazide diuretics can be used to increase renal tubular flow and potassium elimination. However, the patient must have an adequately functioning kidney, and this is obviously a limiting factor for patients with chronic renal failure. In other patients (particularly those with hyporeninemic hypo-aldosteronism) this is an effective additional treatment [7].

Hemodialysis

Finally, the most definitive and effective method of rapidly lowering the serum potassium is hemodialysis, which can lower levels by as much as 1.2 to 1.5 mEq/h [5,7,38,40]. This is indicated in patients when the above treatments are ineffective or in cases of severe rapidly rising serum potassium levels. Because hemodialysis only affects the extracellular component, small amounts of the total body potassium content may be removed and rebound hyperkalemia may occur in 1 to 2 hours [4,7].

Addressing underlying cause

Finally, treating the underlying conditions, changing medications or altering diets may be indicated. If the cause is not apparent, further evaluation for worsening renal function, determining renin and aldosterone levels, checking cortisol levels, calculating the transtubular potassium gradient, and so on, are indicated [57].

Summary

Regarding hyperkalemia, several closing comments are offered. First, in the area of causation, the majority of patients that develop hyperkalemia have some underlying renal dysfunction. Medications are frequently associated with the development of acute hyperkalemia, especially in patients predisposed by age, medical condition, other medication use, or kidney disorders.

Next in the area of diagnosis, the "classic" ECG changes in a patient with hyperkalemia indicate need for emergent treatment but the ECG by itself is not a consistent predictor of the presence or severity of hyperkalemia.

Finally, in the area of treatment, rapidly rising levels are more serious than slowing rising levels, and the most consistent response to treatment, in all types of patients, is with insulin and glucose. Remember to monitor for hypoglycemia. Routine bicarbonate therapy is not indicated, and should be reserved for patients with nonanion metabolic acidosis. Finally, inhaled albuterol is perhaps an underused treatment.

Hypokalemia and hyperkalemia are frequently encountered in the ED and are the result of disturbances in potassium intake, potassium secretion, and transcellular shifts. An understanding of these disturbances is helpful, and guides appropriate management and prevention of significant morbidity and even death. Presenting symptoms tend to be vague, and generally affect the cardiac, neuromuscular, and gastrointestinal systems.

References

[1] Acker CG, Johnson JP, Palevsky PM, et al. Hyperkalemia in hospitalized patients: cause, adequacy of treatment, and results of an attempt to improve physician compliance with published therapy guidelines. Arch Intern Med 1998;158:917–24.

[2] Gennari FJ. Current concepts: hypokalemia. N Engl J Med 1998;339(7):451–8.

[3] Gennari FJ. Disorders of potassium homeostasis: hypokalemia and hyperkalemia. Crit Care Clin 2002;18(2):273–88.

[4] Zull DN. Disorders of potassium metabolism. Emerg Med Clin North Am 1989;7(4):771–94.

[5] Mandal AK. Hypokalemia and hyperkalemia. Med Clin North Am 1997;81(3):611–39.

[6] Marino PL. Potassium. In: The ICU book. 2nd edition. Baltimore: Williams & Wilkins; 1998.

[7] Mount DB, Zandi-Nejad K. Disorders of potassium balance. In: Brenner BM, editor. Brenner & Rector's the kidney. 7th edition. Philadelphia: Elsevier; 2004. p. 997–1040.

[8] Dietary Reference Intakes for Water. Potassium, sodium, chloride, and sulfate. Washington (DC): National Academy of Sciences. Available at: http://www.nap.edu/openbook/0309091691/html. Accessed May 28, 2004.

[9] Potassium Imbalances. In: Metheny NM, editor. Fluid & electrolyte balance: nursing considerations. 4th edition. Philadelphia: Lippincott Williams & Wilkins; 2000.

[10] Linas SL. The patient with hypokalemia or hyperkalemia. In: Schrier RW, editor. Manual of nephrology. 5th edition. Philadelphia: Lippincott Williams & Wilkins; 2000.

[11] Perazella MA, Mahnensmith RL. Hyperkalemia in the elderly: drugs exacerbate impaired potassium homeostasis. J Gen Intern Med 1997;12:646–56.

[12] Rose BD. Causes of hyperkalemia. UpToDate [on-line]. Version 12.1. Wellesley (MA). Available at: www.uptodate.com. Accessed April 20, 2004.

[13] Brewster UC, Perazella MA. The renin–angiotensin–aldosterone system and the kidney: effects on kidney disease. Am J Med 2004;116(4):263–72.

[14] Paice BJ, Paterson KR, Onyanga-Omara F, et al. Record linkage study of hypokalemia in hospitalized patients. Postgrad Med J 1986;62:187–91.

[15] Vanek VW, Seballos RM, Chong D, et al. Serum potassium concentrations in trauma patients. South Med J 1994;87:41–6.

[16] Beal AL, Scheltema KE, Beilman GJ, et al. Hypokalemia following trauma. Shock 2002;18:107–10.

[17] MacDonald JS, Atkinson CC, Mooney DP. Hypokalemia in acutely injured children: a benign laboratory abnormality. J Trauma 2003;54:197–8.

[18] Smith NL, Lemaitre RN, Heckbert SR, et al. Serum potassium and stroke risk among treated hypertensive adults. Am J Hypertens 2003;16:806–13.

[19] Cohen HW, Shantha M, Alderman MH. High and low serum potassium associated with cardiovascular events in diuretic-treated patients. J Hypertens 2001;19:1315–23.

[20] Macdonald JE, Struthers AD. What is the optimal serum potassium level in cardiovascular patients? J Am Coll Cardiol 2004;43:155–61.

[21] Lin SH, Davids MR, Halperin ML. Hypokalaemia and paralysis. Q J Med 2003;96:161–9.
[22] Riggs JE. Neurologic manifestations of electrolyte disturbances. Neurol Clin 2002;20: 227–39.
[23] Webster A, Brady W, Morris F. Recognising signs of danger: ECG changes resulting from an abnormal serum potassium concentration. Emerg Med J 2002;19:74–7.
[24] Cohn JN, Kowey PR, Whelton PK, et al. New guidelines for potassium replacement in clinical practice. Arch Intern Med 2000;160:2429–36.
[25] Hulting J. In-hospital ventricular fibrillation and its relation to serum potassium. Acta Med Scand Suppl 1981;647:109–16.
[26] Rastergar A, Soleimani M. Hypokalaemia and hyperkalaemia. Postgrad Med J 2001;77: 759–64.
[27] Kim GH, Han JS. Therapeutic approach to hypokalemia. Nephron 2002;92(Suppl 1):28–32.
[28] Tesfamariam B, Waldron T, Seymour AA. Quantitation of tremor in response to beta-adrenergic receptor stimulation in primates: relationship with hypokalemia. J Pharmacol Toxicol Methods 1998;40:201–5.
[29] Lin SH, Chiu JS, Hsu CW, et al. A simple and rapid approach to hypokalemic paralysis. Am J Emerg Med 2003;21:487–91.
[30] Blanning A, Westfall JM. How soon should serum potassium levels be monitored for patients started on diuretics? J Fam Pract 2001;50:207–8.
[31] Tsai WS, Wu CP, Hsu YJ, et al. Life-threatening hypokalemia in an asthmatic patient treated with high-dose hydrocortisone. Am J Med Sci 2004;327:152–5.
[32] Satko SG, Burkart JM. Hypokalemia associated with herbal tea ingestion. Nephron 2001; 87:97–8.
[33] Milionis HJ, Alexandrides GE, Liberopoulos EN, et al. Hypomanesemia and concurrent acid-base and electrolyte abnormalities in patients with congestive heart failure. Eur J Heart Fail 2002;4:167–73.
[34] Whittier WL, Rutecki GW. Primer on clinical acid-base problem solving. Dis Mon 2004;50: 117–62.
[35] Tassone H, Moulin A, Henderson SO. The pitfalls of potassium replacement in thyrotoxic periodic paralysis: a case report and review of the literature. J Emerg Med 2004;26:157–61.
[36] Charytan D, Goldfarb DS. Indications for hospitalization of patients with hyperkalemia. Arch Intern Med 2000;160(11):1605–11.
[37] Gibbs MA, Wolfson AB, Tayal VS. Electrolyte disturbances. In: Marx JA, editor. Rosen's emergency medicine: concepts and clinical practice. 5th edition. St. Louis (MO): Mosby, Inc.; 2002. p. 1724–44.
[38] Rose BD. Treatment of hyperkalemia. UpToDate [on-line]. Version 12.1. Wellesley (MA). Available at: www.uptodate.com. Accessed April 20, 2004.
[39] Wrenn KD, Slovis CM, Slovis BS. The ability of physicians to predict hyperkalemia from the ECG. Ann Emerg Med 1991;20:1229.
[40] Mattu A, Brady WJ, Robinson DA. Electrocardiographic manifestations of hyperkalemia. Am J Emerg Med 2000;18:721–9.
[41] Kuvin JT. Electrocardiographic changes of hyperkalemia: images in clinical medicine. N Engl J Med 1998;338(10):662.
[42] Ahee P, Crowe AV. The management of hyperkalemia in the emergency department. J Accid Emerg Med 2000;17:188–91.
[43] Wiederkehr MR, Moe OW. Factitious hyperkalemia. Am J Kidney Dis 2000;36:1049–53.
[44] Rose BD, Nieman LK, Orth DN. Diagnosis of hyperkalemia and hypoaldosteronism (type 4 RTA). UpToDate [on-line]. Version 12.1. Wellesley (MA). Available at: www.uptodate. com. Accessed April 20, 2004.
[45] Perazella MA, Tray K. Selective cyclooxygenase-2 inhibitors: a pattern of nephrotoxicity similar to traditional nonsteroidal anti-inflammatory drugs. Am J Med 2001;111:64–7.
[46] Hay E, Derazon H, Bukish N, et al. Fatal hyperkalemia related to combined therapy with a COX-2 inhibitor, ACE-inhibitor and potassium rich diet. J Emerg Med 2002;22(4):349–52.

[47] Reardon LC, Macpherson DS. Hyperkelemia in outpatients using angiotensin-converting enzyme inhibitors. How much should we worry? Arch Intern Med 1998;158(1):26–32.

[48] Wrenger E, Müller R, Moesenthin M, et al. Interaction of spironolactone with ACE inhibitors or angiotensin receptor blockers: analysis of 44 cases. BMJ 2003;327:147–9.

[49] Oster JR, Singer I, Fishman LM. Heparin-induced aldosterone suppression and hyperkalemia. Am J Med 1995;98:575–86.

[50] Alappan R, Perazella MA, Buller GK. Hyperkalemia in hospitalized patients treated with trimethoprim-sulfamethoxazole. Ann Intern Med 1996;124:316–20.

[51] Pitt B, Zannad F, Remme WJ, et al. The effect of spironolactone on morbidity and mortality in patients with severe heart failure. N Engl J Med 1999;341(10):709–17.

[52] Berry C, McMurray JJV. Serious adverse events experienced by patients with chronic heart failure taking spironolactone. Heart 2001;85:e8–9.

[53] Schepkens H, Vanholder R, Billiouw JM, et al. Life-theatening hyperkalemia during combined therapy with angiotensin-converting enzyme inhibitors and spironolactone: an analysis of 25 cases. Am J Med 2001;110(6):438–41.

[54] Blaustein DA, Babu K, Reddy A, et al. Estimation of glomerular filtration rate to prevent life-threatening hyperkalemia due to combined therapy with spironolactone and angiotensin-converting enzyme inhibition or angiotensin receptor blockade. Am J Cardiol 2002; 90(6):662–3.

[55] Mosely DS, Osborne B. Ingestion of potassium chloride crystals causes hyperkalemia and hemorrhagic gastritis. Emerg Med New 2003;18–20.

[56] Graves JW. Hyperkalemia due to a potassium-based water softener. N Engl J Med 1998; 339(24):1790.

[57] Gauthier PM, Szerlip HM. Common electrolyte disorders. In: Wachter RM, Goldman L, Hollander H, editors. Hosptial medicine. Philadelphia: Lippincott Williams & Wilkins; 2000.

[58] Foulkes D. Fluids and electrolytes. In: Gunn VL, Nechyba C, editors. The Harriet Lane handbook: a manual for pediatric house offices. 16th edition. Philadelphia: Mosby, Inc.; 2002. p. 242–3.

[59] Schulman SL. Renal failure—acute. In: Schwartz MW, editor. The 5-minute pediatric consult. 3rd edition. Philadelphia: Lippincott Williams & Wilkins; 2003.

[60] Siegel NJ. Fluids, electrolytes, and acid-base. In: Rudolph CD, Rudolph AM, editors. Rudolph's pediatrics. 21st edition. New York: McGraw-Hill; 2003. p. 1653–5.

[61] Ahmed J, Weisberg LS. Hyperkalemia in dialysis patients. Semin Dial 2001;14(5):348–56.

[62] Chmielewski CM. Hyperkalemic emergencies. mechanisms, manifestations, and management. Crit Care Nurs Clin North Am 1998;10(4):449–58.

EMERGENCY
MEDICINE
CLINICS OF
NORTH AMERICA

Emerg Med Clin N Am 23 (2005) 749–770

ELSEVIER
SAUNDERS

Disorders of Water Imbalance

Michelle Lin, MD[a],*, Stephen J. Liu, MD[b],
Ingrid T. Lim, MD[b]

[a]San Francisco General Hospital Emergency Services,
University of California San Francisco, 1001 Potrero Avenue, Suite 1E21,
San Francisco, CA 94110, USA
[b]Stanford-Kaiser Emergency Medicine Residency Program,
701 Welch Road, Building C, Palo Alto, CA 94304-5777, USA

Lightheadedness, nausea, headache, fatigue, and confusion are non-specific symptoms that may be consistent with either hyponatremia or hypernatremia. Such subtle presentations of water imbalance contrast their potentially devastating neurologic sequelae, which may be caused by the disorders themselves or iatrogenically by overly aggressive fluid resuscitation. In the emergency department (ED), two questions frequently arise regarding these conditions. First, when should such a disorder be suspected in a patient? Second, what type of intravenous fluids, if any, should be given and at what rate to correct the water imbalance? To address these issues, a basic understanding of water and sodium cellular physiology is crucial. There are three fundamental principles that will be highlighted.

1. Water freely shifts between the intracellular and extracellular space to maintain osmotic equilibrium. Body fluid can be divided into intracellular and extracellular compartments, separated by a solute-impermeable, but water-permeable, membrane barrier. Water diffuses freely across this membrane barrier, allowing osmolality, defined as the ratio of solute to free water, to remain constant between these two spaces. The predominant effective solute in the extracellular space is sodium, and its serum concentration closely reflects plasma osmolality.
2. A normal kidney will attempt to reabsorb or excrete solute-free water to preserve a normal plasma osmolality of 275 to 290 mOsm/kg. The primary hormone regulating plasma osmolality is arginine vasopressin,

* Corresponding author.
  E-mail address: milin@itsa.ucsf.edu (M. Lin).

0733-8627/05/$ - see front matter © 2005 Elsevier Inc. All rights reserved.
doi:10.1016/j.emc.2005.03.001
emed.theclinics.com

also known as antidiuretic hormone (ADH). It is synthesized in the hypothalamus and released into the systemic circulation by means of the posterior pituitary gland [1]. Despite wide fluctuations in water and sodium intake, the body normally can maintain serum osmolality in a narrow range (275 to 290 mOsm/kg) [2]. Osmoreceptors near the hypothalamus sense plasma osmolality and modulate vasopressin release [3,4]. Vasopressin functions at the distal collecting duct of the kidney to increase water reabsorption in this otherwise relatively water-impermeable section of the nephron [5]. In hypo-osmolar conditions for instance, vasopressin levels fall to a low basal rate to reabsorb less free water, resulting in more dilute urine. In addition to changes in plasma osmolality, hypotension and hypovolemia also may trigger vasopressin release, which potentially may worsen a hypo-osmolar state. Other nonosmotic triggers for vasopressin release include pain, nausea, and acidosis [6,7].

The thirst stimulus provides another crucial, but less sensitive, means for the body to maintain water homeostasis by promoting oral intake of free water. Similar to vasopressin release, thirst also can be triggered by hypotension and hypovolemia [8].

3. Rapid transcellular shift of water can lead to cellular damage, particularly in the central nervous system (CNS). In a normal steady-state environment, free water diffuses in and out of the intracellular space to maintain osmotic equilibrium. With the significant fluid shifts associated with hyponatremia and hypernatremia, however, major cellular volume changes can lead to cell damage and cell death, particularly in the CNS, resulting in irreversible neurologic injury. As an initial compensatory mechanism to preserve cellular volume, there is a rapid shift of sodium, potassium, chloride, and water either out of brain cells in hyponatremia or into brain cells in hypernatremia. After 48 to 72 hours, a slower adaptive phase takes effect. Cells mobilize organic osmolytes, comprised mostly of amino acids, to continue efforts to maintain normal cellular volume. As depicted in Fig. 1, the initial and gradual flux of electrolytes and osmolytes, respectively, along with free water, helps preserve cell volume and thus cellular viability.

Knowledge of the acute and delayed compensatory mechanisms for hyponatremia and hypernatremia dictates the conservative practice guide-lines on therapeutic management. Irreversible CNS damage can result not only from the initial water imbalance, but also iatrogenically from overly aggressive fluid resuscitation. Excessively rapid correction of hyponatremia or hypernatremia can lead to extreme cellular volume changes and cellular damage (see Fig. 1). Only in patients with severe neurologic symptoms should more rapid fluid resuscitation be instituted, because the risk of primary neurologic injury outweighs the risk of potential iatrogenic

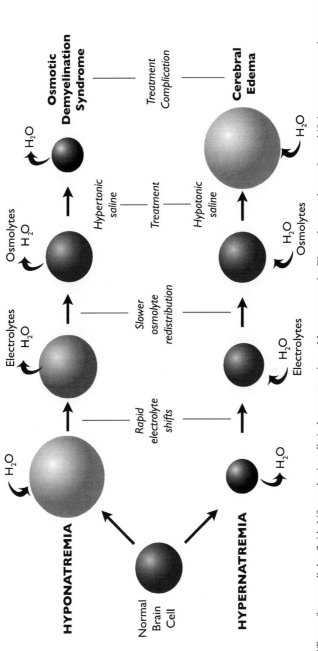

Fig. 1. Effects of transcellular fluid shifts on brain cells in hyponatremia and hypernatremia. Electrolytes and osmolytes shift in response to a hypo-osmolar and hyperosmolar extracellular environment, respectively, to preserve normal cellular volume. Overly aggressive fluid resuscitation can result in complications, such as osmotic demyelination syndrome and cerebral edema.

complications. In patients without severe symptoms, however, more cautious and slower correction of the water imbalance allows osmolytes to return to their normal physiologic state [9,10].

Hyponatremia

Hyponatremia is defined as a serum sodium concentration less than 135 mEq/L. The most common electrolyte abnormality found in hospitalized patients, it is associated with several diseases and surgical and medical treatments. Depending on the criteria used for the definition of hyponatremia, it has an incidence of about 1% in the US population [11] and becomes more prevalent with increasing age. In community-residing patients over 65 years old without an acute illness, 7% were found to have a serum sodium concentration of 137 mEq/L or less [12]. The oldest and frailest of patients are especially prone to acute and chronic hyponatremia [13–15]. Particularly in acute and symptomatic cases, hyponatremia can result in significant mortality, with death rates as high as 17.9% [16–18]. It is unclear whether the high mortality is caused by the hyponatremia itself, the underlying disease process, or the sequelae of overly aggressive hyponatremia management.

Emergency department presentation

The signs and symptoms of hyponatremia depend not only on the absolute serum sodium level, but also on the rate of serum sodium decline. Chronically hyponatremic individuals may be asymptomatic while, in contrast, acutely hyponatremic patients may be quite symptomatic with only mild hyponatremia. Those at the extremes of age are less tolerant of hyponatremia.

The symptoms of hyponatremia are nonspecific and are related primarily to its effects on the CNS. Most patients with a serum sodium concentration greater than 125 mEq/L are relatively asymptomatic [19]. Initial findings include nausea, headache, myalgia, generalized malaise, and depressed deep tendon reflexes as the sodium concentration falls below 125 to 130 mEq/L. This is followed by mental status changes, such as lethargy, confusion, disorientation, agitation, depression, psychosis, and eventually seizures, coma, and death as the sodium concentration falls below 115 to 120 mEq/L [15,20–22] Cerebral edema may occur, especially with rapid reductions in serum sodium concentrations. Individuals at higher risk for developing significant cerebral edema include postoperative patients, premenopausal women [21], and older patients taking a thiazide diuretic [23].

Classification

Hyponatremic patients should be categorized first into hyperosmolar, iso-osmolar, and hypo-osmolar states as summarized in Fig. 2.

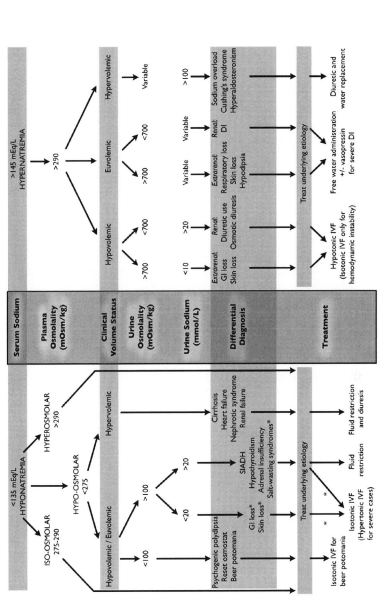
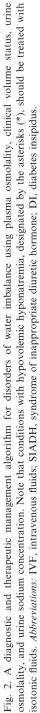

Fig. 2. A diagnostic and therapeutic management algorithm for disorders of water imbalance using plasma osmolality, clinical volume status, urine osmolality, and urine sodium concentration. Note that conditions with hypovolemic hyponatremia, designated by the asterisks (*), should be treated with isotonic fluids. *Abbreviations:* IVF, intravenous fluids; SIADH, syndrome of inappropriate diuretic hormone; DI, diabetes insipidus.

Osmolality can be measured by osmometry or calculated by the following formula:

$$\text{Plasma osmolality} = [2 \times \text{Na (mEq/L)}] + \frac{\text{Glucose (mg/dL)}}{18} + \frac{\text{BUN (mg/dL)}}{2.8}$$

Hyperosmolar hyponatremia

Hyponatremic patients can have a high plasma osmolality (greater than 290 mOsm/kg) from the increased concentration of an effective solute in the extracellular fluid compartment. This creates an osmotic gradient, which drives water from the intracellular to the extracellular space, leading to a lower, diluted serum sodium concentration. Classically, severe hyperglycemia produces such a dilutional hyponatremic state. The effective serum sodium content can be determined by a calculation correction factor. Quantitatively, the measured sodium concentration decreases approximately 1.6 mEq/L for every 100 mg/dL rise in serum glucose concentration. Because this relationship follows a nonlinear pattern, the correction factor has been quoted to range between 1.4 and 2.4 mEq/L, with the higher-end correction factor more applicable for serum glucose levels greater than 400 mg/dL [24,25]. Less common causes of hyperosmolar hyponatremia include mannitol, sorbitol, maltose, and radiocontrast administration [26,27].

Iso-osmolar hyponatremia

Hyponatremia with a normal plasma osmolality (275 to 290 mOsm/kg) occurs as a result of either pseudohyponatremia or transurethral prostatic resection syndrome. Pseudohyponatremia, a laboratory artifact, occurs with severe hypertriglyceridemia and paraproteinemia. Because an excess of large nonaqueous molecules, such as lipids or proteins, occupy a greater portion of the serum, there is a corresponding decrease in total sodium content per unit volume of serum. This laboratory artifact is now fairly obsolete with the replacement of flame emission spectrophotometry instruments with more modern direct potentiometry instruments that use sodium ion-specific electrodes [28].

Transurethral prostatic resection syndrome causes dilutional hyponatremia when massive volumes of sodium-free irrigant, such as glycine or sorbitol, are systemically absorbed intraoperatively. These patients can have a normal or low plasma osmolality. The exact mechanism remains unclear [29].

Hypo-osmolar hyponatremia

Most instances of hyponatremia are associated with a low osmolality (less than 275 mOsm/kg), reflecting a net gain of free water. Patients can be classified according to their total-body volume state (hypovolemia, euvolemia, hypervolemia).

Hypovolemic hyponatremia (sodium loss exceeds free water loss). In hypovolemic patients, sodium depletion exceeds total body water (TBW) volume depletion. Thirst and vasopressin release are triggered by the decrease in effective arterial volume. This leads to water gain and retention, further contributing to the hypo-osmolar state. Checking the urinary sodium concentration may assist in diagnostic and therapeutic management decisions.

A low urinary sodium concentration (less than 20 mEq/L) suggests extrarenal sodium and water losses, because the kidneys are reabsorbing sodium appropriately. Causes include gastrointestinal (GI) disorders, such as vomiting or diarrhea, or severe burns. These patients represent the most common cause for hyponatremia found in ED patients [18]. In contrast, a high urinary sodium concentration (greater than 20 mEq/L) reflects renal sodium and water losses. This generally is caused by a sodium-wasting nephropathy (polycystic kidney disease, chronic pyelonephritis), hypoaldosteronism, or diuretic use. Thiazide diuretics are among the most common causes for symptomatic hyponatremia, especially in elderly women [20].

Euvolemic hyponatremia (free water gain and negligible sodium loss). Adrenal insufficiency and hypothyroidism can cause euvolemic hyponatremia occasionally. The most common cause, however, is the syndrome of inappropriate antidiuretic hormone secretion (SIADH). It is, in fact, the most common case for hyponatremia in hospitalized patients [16]. Vasopressin is released from the posterior pituitary or an ectopic site inappropriately, resulting in decreased free water excretion. The diagnostic criteria for SIADH include: hypo-osmolar hyponatremia, inappropriately concentrated urine (greater than 100 mOsm/kg), clinical euvolemia, and normal adrenal, thyroid, cardiac, hepatic, and renal function.

Causes of SIADH can be categorized into four major groups: malignancy, pulmonary disease, CNS disease, and pharmacologic use (Table 1). Among malignancies, small-cell lung cancer is the most common cause of SIADH. Approximately 15% to 32% of small-cell lung cancer patients experience hyponatremia caused by ectopic production of vasopressin by tumor cells [30–32]. Also in the category of pulmonary disease, the most common cause of severe hyponatremia in patients with pneumonia is *Legionella pneumophila* [42].

In contrast to SIADH patients who excrete concentrated urine, euvolemic patients also may present with maximally dilute urine (less than 100 mOsm/kg), as in the case of psychogenic polydipsia, reset osmostat, and beer potomania. Psychogenic polydipsia, or compulsive water drinking, is found predominantly in the psychiatric population, particularly in individuals with schizophrenia. These patients often drink over 15 L of water a day, overwhelming their kidneys' maximum capability to excrete free water. This leads to dilutional hyponatremia [51]. Reset osmostat is a chronic condition where vasopressin osmoreceptors have a lower threshold to trigger vasopressin release. This has been associated with quadriplegia (effective

Table 1
Causes of syndrome of inappropriate antidiuretic hormone secretion [30–50]

Category	Cause of SIADH
Malignancy	Bronchogenic (especially small-cell lung cancer)
	Head and neck
	CNS
	Pancreas
	Hematopoietic system
Pulmonary disease	Pneumonia (especially if caused by *Legionella pneumophila*)
	Empyema
	Tuberculosis
	Aspergillosis
	Advanced chronic obstructive pulmonary disease
	Bronchiolitis in infants
CNS disease	Meningitis
	Encephalitis
	Brain abscess
	Cerebrovascular accident
	Trauma
	Recent trans-sphenoidal surgery
Pharmacologic	Selective serotonin uptake inhibitors (SSRIs)
	Tricyclic antidepressants
	Phenothiazines
	Antineoplastic agents
	Antiepileptics (carbemazepine, valproate acid)
	Oral hypoglycemic drugs (chlorpropamide, metformin)
	Nonsteroidal anti-inflammatory drugs
	3,4-methylenedioxymethamphetamine (MDMA, ecstasy)

volume depletion from blood pooling in the lower extremities), psychosis, tuberculosis, and chronic malnutrition [52]. Beer potomania is a unique complication of chronic alcoholism. When alcoholics, who already have low dietary sodium and nutritional stores, ingest large quantities of low-sodium beer with minimal food intake, the kidneys produce maximally dilute urine in the effort to retain sodium. Drinking beer in excess of 4 L per day surpasses the kidneys' ability to maintain iso-osmolarity, leading to water retention and hyponatremia [53].

Hypervolemic hyponatremia (free water gain exceeds sodium gain). Hyponatremia in the setting of an increased TBW volume occurs in edematous states including congestive heart failure, hepatic cirrhosis, nephrotic syndrome, and renal failure. These diseases represent total-body fluid overload but, in actuality, low effective arterial volume. Intravascular depletion triggers vasopressin release and thirst. The intake and retention of water exceeds the intake of sodium, leading to dilutional hyponatremia. The degree of hyponatremia is usually proportional to the severity of the underlying illness.

Emergency department evaluation

Patients, especially high-risk patients, should be evaluated for hyponatremia in the ED if they exhibit nonspecific or neurological symptoms. Risk factors include (1) extremes of age; (2) recent initiation of a diuretic, especially a thiazide; (3) a history of malignancy; (4) pulmonary or CNS disease; (5) recent surgical procedure, especially gynecologic or prostatic surgery; and (6) psychiatric disease.

The physical exam should focus not only on the neurological exam but also the determination of the patient's clinical volume status. Tachycardia, orthostatic hypotension, dry mucous membranes, decreased skin turgor, and sunken eyes are all signs of hypovolemia. A meta-analysis study, however, found that in patients with vomiting, diarrhea, or decreased oral intake, few physical findings were useful in distinguishing hypovolemia from euvolemia [54]. Signs of hypervolemia include edema, ascites, pulmonary rales, and increased jugular venous distention.

The initial laboratory workup of a hyponatremic patient includes the determination of other serum electrolytes, renal function, plasma and urine osmolality, and urine sodium concentration. Obtaining initial, pretreatment urine tests may be helpful, because ED therapy may alter subsequent test results.

Emergency department management

The two primary goals of ED therapy are to initiate the treatment of the underlying condition and to restore normal serum osmolality without causing an iatrogenic complication. Based on the patient's plasma osmolality and clinical volume status, the patient can be classified into one of the subgroups shown in Fig. 2. For hyperosmolar and iso-osmolar patients, immediate correction of the hyponatremia is unnecessary. Instead, reversal of the underlying disorder, such as hyperglycemia or hyperlipidemia, is sufficient.

Because hypovolemic patients often appear euvolemic [54], the algorithm in Fig. 2 initially groups the two classes together when evaluating hypoosmolar hyponatremia. Urine osmolality and urine sodium concentration further narrow the differential diagnosis. Specifically, if the urine osmolality is less than 100 mOsm/kg, these patients are euvolemic, because they demonstrate maximally dilute urine. Causes include psychogenic polydipsia, reset osmostat, and beer potomania. Alternatively, if the urine osmolality is greater than 100 mOsm/kg, and the urine sodium is less than 20 mEq/L, these patients are hypovolemic from extra-renal sodium and water losses, such as from the GI tract or skin. If the urine osmolality is greater than 100 mOsm/kg, and urine sodium is greater than 20 mEq/L, these patients may be hypovolemic (from renal water loss) or euvolemic (from SIADH, hypothyroidism, or adrenal insufficiency).

Treatment is based on the patient's volume status. Hypovolemic patients have decreased whole-body sodium stores in addition to free water loss.

Regardless of whether free water loss occurred renally or extrarenally, these patients require either oral or intravenous sodium administration. Isotonic saline is the ideal intravenous fluid for concurrent salt and water repletion. Once the patient has reached a clinically euvolemic state, there no longer is a physiologic stimulus for vasopressin release, allowing excess free water to be excreted and further self-correction of hyponatremia. Thus, once hypovolemia is corrected, isotonic intravenous fluids should be changed to a hypotonic fluid, such as 0.45% saline, to avoid correcting the serum sodium concentration too quickly.

In contrast, euvolemic and hypervolemic patients should be treated by water restriction. Total daily free water intake initially should be limited to 800 to 1000 mL. Concurrent administration of a loop diuretic to promote free water excretion may be necessary with significant fluid overload or when the urine is extremely concentrated (greater than 500 mOsm/kg) [55,56]. Uniquely, patients with beer potomania, despite being euvolemic, should be treated with isotonic fluid resuscitation to replenish low sodium stores.

Treatment complication: osmotic demyelination syndrome

The rate of fluid resuscitation for hyponatremia is based on the patient's symptomatology. The risks of hyponatremia-induced cerebral edema must be weighed against the therapeutic risk of developing osmotic demyelination syndrome (ODS).

Physiologically, cerebral edema results from the osmotic movement of water into brain cells in the setting of hypo-osmolarity. ODS, previously termed central pontine myelinolysis, occurs when water moves too rapidly out of brain cells during administration of relatively hypertonic saline solutions. This rapid cellular dehydration originally was identified in the pons, but now has been observed in other areas of the brain [57,58]. Classically, these patients present with a deteriorating mental status and progressive neurological deficits, such as pseudobulbar palsies and spastic quadriparesis, after a transient period of improvement with fluid administration. ODS typically occurs after 1 to 6 days of treatment. It is associated with a dismal prognosis and has no effective treatment [59]. For unclear pathophysiologic reasons, chronic alcoholism and malnutrition have been associated with the development of ODS [60]. From a practical perspective, acutely intoxicated patients with a history of chronic alcoholism who may be "sleeping it off" in the ED, should have their intravenous fluids closely monitored while awaiting sobriety. Because these patients may have chronic hyponatremia from cirrhosis, a rapid rise in serum sodium concentration caused by large-volume fluid administration (4 to 5 L) should be avoided.

Fluid resuscitation rate

Many ED patients initially receive an empiric 500 mL bolus of 0.9% normal saline (154 mEq/L sodium) before their laboratory results reveal a hyponatremic state. Because the clinical presentation of hyponatremia and hypernatremia is similar, hypertonic saline should not be administered empirically before laboratory confirmation. Doing so would worsen a potential hypernatremic state significantly.

For documented hyponatremic patients with significant neurological symptoms, such as seizures, severe altered mental status, or coma, aggressive therapy is necessary to avoid permanent neurological deficits and even death from cerebral edema. The high likelihood of cerebral edema outweighs the risk of possible ODS. In these patients, the target rate of correction is 1.5 to 2 mEq/L per hour with 3% hypertonic saline for the first 3 to 4 hours, or more briefly, if symptoms improve. The maximum rise of serum sodium concentration should not exceed 10 mEq/L in the first 24 hours. Patients with acute (less than 48 hours duration) hyponatremia tolerate a faster increase in sodium concentration, because the brain tissue has not yet fully recruited osmolytes. These patients are usually extremely symptomatic and should have their serum sodium concentration increased by 1.5 to 2 mEq/L per hour to reach a goal sodium concentration of 120 mEq/L. Other concomitant electrolyte imbalances such as hypokalemia also should be corrected.

Fig. 3 provides a practical formula to calculate the volume of hypertonic fluid resuscitation needed. This equation estimates the effect of 1 L of an intravenous fluid on serum sodium concentration. For example, in a 60 kg elderly woman who presents with significant altered mental status and a sodium concentration of 110 mEq/L, hypertonic saline should be instituted immediately in the ED. One liter of 3% saline (513 mEq/L sodium) will increase the serum sodium concentration by approximately 14 mEq/L, as calculated by $(513-110)/[(0.45 * 60) + 1]$. Thus, to increase the serum sodium concentration by 2 mEq/L in the first hour, one-seventh of the liter (143 mL) should be given.

For hyponatremic patients with mild symptoms, the risk of ODS outweighs the risk of cerebral edema. These patients tend to have chronic (greater than 48 hours duration) hyponatremia. ODS very rarely develops if sodium correction is limited to 0.5 mEq/L per hour (approximately 500 mL per hour of 0.9% saline in a 70 kg elderly male) with a maximum sodium increase of 10 to 12 mEq/L over 24 hours [59–64]. Regardless of symptom severity, performing frequent neurological exams is essential to assess for the early iatrogenic development of ODS.

Hypernatremia

Hypernatremia is defined as a serum sodium concentration greater than 145 mEq/L. It is characterized by a deficit of TBW relative to total-body sodium and can result from either net water loss, or, less commonly, from hypertonic sodium gain. Regardless of the cause, the primary problem is inadequate water intake, which can be secondary to a defective thirst

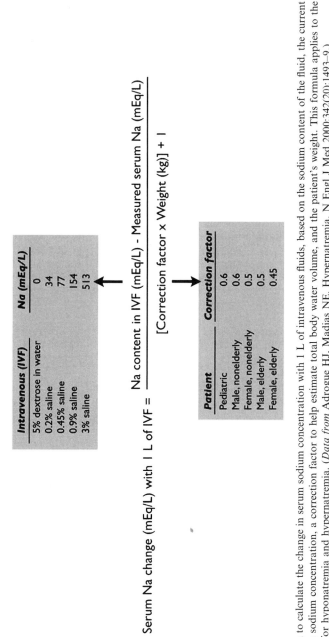

Fig. 3. Formula to calculate the change in serum sodium concentration with 1 L of intravenous fluids, based on the sodium content of the fluid, the current measured serum sodium concentration, a correction factor to help estimate total body water volume, and the patient's weight. This formula applies to the treatment plan for hyponatremia and hypernatremia. (*Data from* Adrogue HJ, Madias NE. Hypernatremia. N Engl J Med 2000;342(20):1493–9.)

mechanism or a lack of access to fluid. This can be accompanied by a low, normal, or high total-body sodium content.

The incidence of hypernatremia ranges from 0.3% to 1% [65]. It is almost never found in an alert patient with a normal thirst mechanism and access to water. Hence, hypernatremia occurs in very young, elderly, debilitated, or altered patients. The body's two main defense mechanisms against hypernatremia, thirst and stimulation of vasopressin release, are diminished after age 60 [66,67]. Unlike hypernatremia in outpatients, hypernatremia that develops in the hospital is usually iatrogenic, resulting from inadequate or inappropriate fluid prescription in the setting of increased water losses [68].

In adults, acute hypernatremia and chronic hypernatremia have been associated with significant mortality as high as 75% and 60%, respectively [69]. In acutely hypernatremic children, mortality rates as high as 20% have been published, with two-thirds of survivors suffering neurologic sequelae. In contrast, chronic hypernatremia in children only results in 10% mortality [70,71]. Similar to hyponatremia, it is difficult to distinguish whether these high mortality rates are caused by the hypernatremia itself, the underlying disease process, or the sequelae of hypernatremia treatment [72].

Emergency department presentation

Most patients with hypernatremia are either very young or very old. Infants can present with tachypnea, muscle weakness, restlessness, a characteristic high-pitched cry, insomnia, or lethargy interspersed with irritability [73]. Hypernatremia in infants rarely results in shock, because extracellular fluid and plasma volume are preserved until dehydration is severe (greater than 10% loss of body weight). At that time, skin turgor becomes reduced, and the abdominal skin may feel doughy [74].

In adults, early symptoms of hypernatremia may be nonspecific and overshadowed by concomitant illness. They might be especially subtle in the elderly patient. Patients with mild hypernatremia may be asymptomatic or exhibit anorexia, nausea, or vomiting. Similar to hyponatremia, the principal clinical manifestations of hypernatremia arise in the CNS. In hypernatremia, intracellular water shifts into the hypertonic extracellular compartment, resulting in cellular dehydration and neurologic symptoms including weakness, altered mental status, agitation, irritability, lethargy, seizures, stupor, and coma. CNS symptomatology correlates with the degree of elevation of the serum sodium concentration [74].

In chronic hypernatremia, neurologic symptoms are much less pronounced, because the brain adapts over time, initially with electrolyte shifts [75] and later with the intracellular influx of osmolytes [9,76]. With long-standing hypernatremia, neurologic deficits, especially in the pediatric population, may be irreversible [71]. Muscle twitching, hyper-reflexia, spasticity, tremor, asterixis, chorea, and ataxia are common [70].

Classification

Hypernatremia can be classified according to the clinical volume status (hypovolemia, euvolemia, hypervolemia) of the patient.

Hypovolemic hypernatremia (free water loss exceeds sodium loss)

The causes for hypotonic fluid loss can be classified into either extrarenal or renal loss. Extrarenal loss can occur through the skin as with profuse sweating, burns, or skin diseases such as pemphigus vulgaris. Alternatively, loss can occur through the GI tract as with diarrhea (especially in the pediatric population), nasogastric suctioning, vomiting, and third-spacing (eg, ileus, pancreatitis or bowel obstruction). Interestingly, multiple-dose activated charcoal administration is associated with a 6% incidence of hypernatremia and 0.6% incidence of severe hypernatremia (serum sodium concentration greater than 155 mEq/L) [77]. In all cases of extrarenal fluid loss, the urinary sodium concentration is low (less than 10 mEq/L), and the urine osmolality is concentrated appropriately (greater than 700 mOsm/kg).

Renal loss of fluid can occur with diuretic use or severe osmotic diuresis from mannitol administration, severe glucosuria in diabetics, or elevated urea in the setting of postobstructive diuresis [78–80]. The urinary sodium concentration usually is elevated (greater than 20 mEq/L), and the urine is isotonic or hypotonic (less than 700 mOsm/kg). Regardless of renal or extrarenal causes, hypovolemic hypernatremia develops in the setting of severe volume loss, and patients usually display signs of hypovolemia such as flat neck veins, orthostatic hypotension, tachycardia, poor skin turgor, and dry mucous membranes.

Euvolemic hypernatremia (free water loss)

These patients have pure water loss without signs of hypovolemia. Patients appear euvolemic despite water loss, because most of the water is lost from the intracellular space. Free water loss can result from extrarenal or renal causes.

Extrarenal loss of free water can occur from insensible losses through the skin or respiratory system. Although water loss can reach several liters per day, most people will not become hypernatremic unless they have impaired thirst or restricted access to water. The urine will be concentrated (greater than 700 mOsm/kg), because the resultant hyperosmolarity stimulates vasopressin release. Another cause of extrarenal loss of free water is primary hypodipsia, which results from the destruction of thirst centers in the hypothalamus, caused by multiple disorders, including hypothalamic tumors, granulomatous diseases, vascular abnormalities, and trauma [6]. These patients will be oliguric, and their urine osmolality will be elevated. Essential hypernatremia is a variant of primary hypodipsia. It is a condition characterized by an upward resetting of the osmotic thresholds for thirst and vasopressin release, while the response to hemodynamic stimuli remains normal [81].

In contrast, renal loss of free water yields hypotonic urine (less than 700 mOsm/kg and often less than 200 mOsm/kg) because of central or nephrogenic diabetes insipidus (DI). Pure water loss in DI results from decreased vasopressin secretion caused by diseases of the hypothalamic-pituitary axis (central DI) or decreased renal tubular responsiveness to vasopressin (nephrogenic DI). Consequently, patients with DI will present with a urine osmolality lower than the plasma osmolality. Even in the most severe forms of DI, however, hypernatremia does not develop unless there is a concomitant defect in thirst or restricted access to water.

Central DI can occur from cerebral trauma, granulomatous disease, hypophysectomy, infection, stroke, or tumors, but approximately 50% of cases are idiopathic. Patients present with polyuria (3 to 15 L per day), secondary polydipsia, and dilute urine. With exogenous vasopressin treatment, these patients will regain the ability to concentrate their urine.

In nephrogenic DI, the collecting ducts are resistant to vasopressin, and thus exogenous vasopressin administration has little effect. In the ED, prescription drugs, such as lithium, foscarnet, clozapine, loop diuretics, demeclocycline, and amphotericin B should be considered as potential culprits [82]. The World Health Organization's database of adverse drug effects lists lithium as the most common cause of drug-induced nephrogenic DI, followed by foscarnet and clozapine [83]. Other causes include acute and chronic renal failure, obstructive uropathy, hypercalcemia, hypokalemia, and sickle cell disease [84].

Hypervolemic hypernatremia (sodium gain)

Hypernatremia from pure sodium overload is rare and frequently iatrogenic. This can be seen in excessive sodium bicarbonate administration during cardiopulmonary resuscitation [85], overcorrection of hyponatremia with hypertonic saline, hypertonic dialysate in peritoneal and hemodialysis, and hypertonic enteral or parenteral hyperalimentation [68]. Noniatrogenic etiologies include various mineralocorticoid deficiencies, salt water near-drownings [86], ingestion of improperly prepared infant formula [87], and ingestion of salt tablets [88]. All of these patients will have significant naturesis with a urine sodium concentration greater than 100 mEq/L. Such rapid and massive increases in sodium load may result in pulmonary edema.

Emergency department evaluation

Patients should be evaluated for hypernatremia in the ED if they exhibit nonspecific or neurological symptoms and any of the following high-risk characteristics: (1) restricted access to water or impaired thirst mechanism, such as for those in extremes of age, chronic debilitated, or altered; (2) CNS disease, including malignancy, trauma, and infection that may cause central DI; and (3) use of medications that may cause nephrogenic DI, such as lithium, foscarnet, clozapine, loop diuretics, demeclocycline, and amphotericin B.

Evaluation of the hypernatremic patient closely resembles that of the hyponatremic patient. The physical exam should focus on the patient's clinical volume status to help determine the underlying cause for hypernatremia and the neurological exam to guide therapy. Laboratory evaluation should include assessment of other serum electrolytes, renal function, urine osmolality, and urine sodium concentration. Additionally, checking creatine kinase levels should be considered, because acute cellular dehydration and cell death outside the CNS system may cause rhabdomyolysis [89].

There should be a low threshold to obtain head CT imaging in severely hypernatremic patients. Rapid brain parenchymal dehydration from hypernatremia may cause a mechanical traction on dural veins and venous sinuses. This traction can cause tears and result in subcortical and subarachnoid hemorrhages, subdural hematomas, and venous sinus thromboses [87].

Emergency department management

The two primary goals of ED therapy are to initiate treatment of the underlying condition and restore normal serum osmolality without causing an iatrogenic complication. Upon determining that a patient is hypernatremic, clinical volume status should be assessed. Determination of the urine sodium concentration and urine osmolality narrows the differential diagnosis. Treatment is based on the patient's volume status, as summarized in Fig. 2.

In a hypovolemic patient, volume resuscitation for a hemodynamically unstable patient should be accomplished with isotonic 0.9% saline. Once the patient is hemodynamically stable, intravenous fluids should be changed to a hypotonic 0.45% saline solution, because isotonic saline resuscitation in the absence of hemodynamic compromise may cause fluid overload while only minimally decreasing the serum sodium concentration.

The euvolemic patient requires pure water replacement with intravenous hypotonic saline or free water. When using dextrose-containing solutions, the glucose should be monitored closely, because hyperglycemia worsens hyperosmolarity and can lead to osmotic diuresis. For significantly hypernatremic patients in whom central DI is considered, 5 to 10 units of aqueous vasopressin should be given subcutaneously every 3 to 4 hours. The administration of vasopressin is preferable to desmopressin, a long-acting vasopressin analog. Monitoring serum sodium and urine-specific gravity initially every 2 to 4 hours minimizes the risk of overcorrection and consequent potential water intoxication. An increasing urine-specific gravity indicates a response to vasopressin.

The hypervolemic patient has excess sodium, which requires naturesis with loop diuretics and free water replacement. For patients with severe renal failure, naturesis is achieved by dialysis.

Treatment complication: cerebral edema. The challenge in the management of hypernatremia, similar to hyponatremia, is determining the rate of sodium and water correction. Acute hypernatremia that has developed over a few hours (eg, iatrogenic sodium loading) can be corrected rapidly, because the compensatory intracellular influx of osmolytes has not occurred yet.

Most cases of hypernatremia in the ED, however, occur over a chronic (greater than 48-hour duration) time span. Lowering the plasma osmolality with hypotonic fluids too rapidly will cause the osmotic shift of water into brain cells, leading to iatrogenic cerebral edema and the potential sequelae of seizures, permanent brain injury, and death [90].

Fluid resuscitation rate. Because of the risk of cerebral edema, current practice guidelines recommend lowering the serum sodium concentration by 0.5 to 1 mEq/L per hour, with a maximum decrease of 10 mEq/L per 24-hour period [91]. No more than half of the water deficit should be replaced within the first 24 hours, with the remainder corrected over the next 1 to 2 days [92].

In reality, most ED patients will have received a 500 mL bolus of 0.9% normal saline (154 mEq/L sodium) before being diagnosed with hypernatremia. This is an appropriate initial approach to fluid management until after laboratory results return. As with hypertonic saline, given that symptoms of hyponatremia and hypernatremia are similar, empiric administration of hypotonic saline should be avoided, because these undifferentiated patients could have either extreme of water imbalance.

Fig. 3, applicable also for fluid resuscitation calculations in hyponatremic patients, provides an equation to translate hypernatremia treatment recommendations into clinical practice. For instance, in an elderly 80 kg man with a serum sodium concentration of 160 mEq/L, administering 1 L of 0.45% saline (77 mEq/L sodium) will cause a sodium decrease by approximately 2 mEq/L, in the absence of insensible water losses. This was determined by calculating $(77-160)/[(0.5 * 80) + 1]$. Thus, to decrease the patient's serum sodium concentration by 0.5 mEq/L in the first hour, one-quarter of the fluid volume (250 mL) should be administered.

Frequent neurological exams should be performed to assess for clinical deterioration, because transient improvement followed by deterioration in the neurological status suggests the development of iatrogenic cerebral edema and requires temporary cessation of water replacement.

Summary

Because of the nonspecific signs and symptoms associated with disorders of water imbalance, emergency physicians must maintain a high index of suspicion for hyponatremia and hypernatremia, especially in patients at greater risk for these electrolyte disorders. Classifying patients based on their clinical volume status, serum and urine osmolality, and urine sodium concentration helps to identify the cause of the water imbalance and to tailor treatment. Specifically, important laboratory tests to order include a serum and urine sodium concentration, serum and urine osmolality, other electrolyte concentrations, and renal function tests. Choosing the appropriate type of intravenous fluid and calculating the initial fluid resuscitation rate require careful weighing of risks and benefits associated with cellular volume changes in the CNS. Correcting serum sodium concentration too slowly or too rapidly may have devastating consequences. It is essential to monitor serum sodium levels frequently, as often as every 2 to 4 hours initially, during therapy to prevent ODS in hyponatremic patients and cerebral edema in hypernatremic patients. Promising studies involving aquaretics, which are vasopressin receptor antagonists that promote free water excretion, may play a role soon.

Pitfalls

There are several potential pitfalls when treating patients with disorders of water imbalance. These include:

- Not evaluating high-risk patients for disorders of water imbalance (eg, hyponatremia frequently is associated with diuretic use and malignancy, and hypernatremia is associated with lithium use)
- Using inappropriate intravenous fluids for resuscitation (eg, for hyponatremia, isotonic saline should be used, and hypertonic 3% saline should be reserved for only those with severe neurologic symptoms. For hypernatremia, hypotonic fluid should be used, and isotonic saline should be reserved for only those with hemodynamic compromise.)
- Correction of hyponatremia or hypernatremia more rapidly than 0.5 to 1.0 mEq/L/hr can lead to ODS or cerebral edema, respectively. The maximum change in serum sodium concentration should be approximately 10 mEq/L over a 24-hour period. As a rough estimation for patients weighing 70 kg, hyponatremia usually requires 450 to 550 mL per hour of isotonic 0.9% saline, while hypernatremia usually requires 200 to 300 mL per hour of hypotonic 0.45% saline to correct the serum sodium concentration by approximately 0.5 mEq per hour. Further, for hyponatremic patients with significant neurologic symptoms such as seizures, usually 150 to 250 mL of hypertonic 3% saline should be administered in the first hour to increase the serum sodium concentration by 2 mEq.
- Not performing frequent neurological exams during fluid resuscitation can lead to the undetected development of ODS in hyponatremic patients and cerebral edema in hypernatremic patients.

Acknowledgments

The authors wish to thank Dr. Esther L. Langmack for her generous assistance with manuscript preparation.

References

[1] Abramow M, Beauwens R, Cogan E. Cellular events in vasopressin action. Kidney Int Suppl 1987;21:S56–66.

[2] Zerbe RL, Henry DP, Robertson GL. Vasopressin response to orthostatic hypotension. Etiologic and clinical implications. Am J Med 1983;74(2):265–71.

[3] Dunn FL, Brennan TJ, Nelson AE, et al. The role of blood osmolality and volume in regulating vasopressin secretion in the rat. J Clin Invest 1973;52(12):3212–9.

[4] McKinley MJ, Mathai ML, McAllen RM, et al. Vasopressin secretion: osmotic and hormonal regulation by the lamina terminalis. J Neuroendocrinol 2004;16(4):340–7.

[5] Berliner RW, Levinsky NG, Davidson DG, et al. Dilution and concentration of the urine and the action of the antidiuretic hormone. Am J Med 1958;24(5):730–44.

[6] Robertson GL. Antidiuretic hormone. Normal and disordered function. Endocrinol Metab Clin North Am 2001;30(3):671–94.

[7] Wood CE, Chen HG. Acidemia stimulates ACTH, vasopressin, and heart rate responses in fetal sheep. Am J Physiol 1989;257(2 Pt 2):R344–9.

[8] Zerbe RL, Robertson GL. Osmoregulation of thirst and vasopressin secretion in human subjects: effect of various solutes. Am J Physiol 1983;244(6):E607–14.

[9] Lien YH, Shapiro JI, Chan L. Study of brain electrolytes and organic osmolytes during correction of chronic hyponatremia. Implications for the pathogenesis of central pontine myelinolysis. J Clin Invest 1991;88(1):303–9.

[10] Videen JS, Michaelis T, Pinto P, et al. Human cerebral osmolytes during chronic hyponatremia. A proton magnetic resonance spectroscopy study. J Clin Invest 1995;95(2):788–93.

[11] Al-Salman J, Kemp D, Randall D. Hyponatremia. West J Med 2002;176(3):173–6.

[12] Caird FI, Andrews GR, Kennedy RD. Effect of posture on blood pressure in the elderly. Br Heart J 1973;35(3):527–30.

[13] Miller M, Morley JE, Rubenstein LZ. Hyponatremia in a nursing home population. J Am Geriatr Soc 1995;43(12):1410–3.

[14] Kleinfeld M, Casimir M, Borra S. Hyponatremia as observed in a chronic disease facility. J Am Geriatr Soc 1979;27(4):156–61.

[15] Ellis SJ. Severe hyponatraemia: complications and treatment. QJM 1995;88(12):905–9.

[16] Anderson RJ, Chung HM, Kluge R, et al. Hyponatremia: a prospective analysis of its epidemiology and the pathogenetic role of vasopressin. Ann Intern Med 1985;102(2):164–8.

[17] Tierney WM, Martin DK, Greenlee MC, et al. The prognosis of hyponatremia at hospital admission. J Gen Intern Med 1986;1(6):380–5.

[18] Lee CT, Guo HR, Chen JB. Hyponatremia in the emergency department. Am J Emerg Med 2000;18(3):264–8.

[19] Arieff AI, Llach F, Massry SG. Neurological manifestations and morbidity of hyponatremia: correlation with brain water and electrolytes. Medicine (Baltimore) 1976;55(2):121–9.

[20] Ashraf N, Locksley R, Arieff AI. Thiazide-induced hyponatremia associated with death or neurologic damage in outpatients. Am J Med 1981;70(6):1163–8.

[21] Ayus JC, Wheeler JM, Arieff AI. Postoperative hyponatremic encephalopathy in menstruant women. Ann Intern Med 1992;117(11):891–7.

[22] Moritz ML, Ayus JC. The pathophysiology and treatment of hyponatraemic encephalopathy: an update. Nephrol Dial Transplant 2003;18:2486.

[23] Sonnenblick M, Friedlander Y, Rosin AJ. Diuretic-induced severe hyponatremia: Review and analysis of 129 reported patients. Chest 1993;103(2):601–6.

[24] Katz MA. Hyperglycemia-induced hyponatremia—calculation of expected serum sodium depression. N Engl J Med 1973;289(16):843–4.

[25] Hillier TA, Abbott RD, Barrett EJ. Hyponatremia: evaluating the correction factor for hyperglycemia. Am J Med 1999;106(4):399–403.

[26] Aviram A, Pfau A, Czaczkes JW, et al. Hyperosmolarity with hyponatremia, caused by inappropriate administration of mannitol. Am J Med 1967;42(4):648–50.
[27] Palevsky PM, Rendulic D, Diven WF. Maltose-induced hyponatremia. Ann Intern Med 1993;118(7):526–8.
[28] Maas AHJ, Siggaard-Anderson O, Weisberg HF, et al. Ion-selective electrodes for sodium and potassium: a new problem of what is measured and what should be reported. Clin Chem 1985;31:482–5.
[29] Agarwal R, Emmett M. The post-transurethral resection of prostate syndrome: therapeutic proposals. Am J Kidney Dis 1994;24(1):108–11.
[30] Johnson BE, Chute JP, Rushin J, et al. A prospective study of patients with lung cancer and hyponatremia of malignancy. Am J Respir Crit Care Med 1997;156(5):1669–78.
[31] Sorensen JB, Andersen MK, Hansen HH. Syndrome of inappropriate secretion of anti-diuretic hormone (SIADH) in malignant disease. J Intern Med 1995;238(2):97–110.
[32] Klein LA, Rabson AS, Worksman J. In vitro synthesis of vasopressin by lung tumor cells. Surg Forum 1969;20:231–3.
[33] Talmi YP, Hoffman HT, McCabe BF. Syndrome of inappropriate secretion of arginine vasopressin in patients with cancer of the head and neck. Ann Otol Rhinol Laryngol 1992;101(11):946–9.
[34] Cullen MJ, Cusack DA, O'Briain DS, et al. Neurosecretion of arginine vasopressin by an olfactory neuroblastoma causing reversible syndrome of antidiuresis. Am J Med 1986;81(5):911–6.
[35] Marks LJ, Berde B, Klein LA, et al. Inappropriate vasopressin secretion and carcinoma of the pancreas. Am J Med 1968;45(6):967–74.
[36] Eliakim R, Vertman E, Shinhar E. Syndrome of inappropriate secretion of antidiuretic hormone in Hodgkin's disease. Am J Med Sci 1986;291(2):126–7.
[37] Belton K, Thomas SH. Drug-induced syndrome of inappropriate antidiuretic hormone secretion. Postgrad Med J 1999;75(886):509–10.
[38] Cusick JF, Hagen TC, Findling JW. Inappropriate secretion of antidiuretic hormone after transsphenoidal surgery for pituitary tumors. N Engl J Med 1984;311(1):36–8.
[39] Anderson RJ, Pluss RG, Berns AS, et al. Mechanism of effect of hypoxia on renal water excretion. J Clin Invest 1978;62(4):769–77.
[40] Chabot F, Mertes PM, Delorme N, et al. Effect of acute hypercapnia on alpha atrial natriuretic peptide, renin, angiotensin II, aldosterone, and vasopressin plasma levels in patients with COPD. Chest 1995;107(3):780–6.
[41] Rose CE Jr, Anderson RJ, Carey RM. Antidiuresis and vasopressin release with hypoxemia and hypercapnia in conscious dogs. Am J Physiol 1984;247:127–34.
[42] Stout JE, Yu VL. Legionellosis. N Engl J Med 1997;337(10):682–7.
[43] Liu BA, Mittmann N, Knowles SR, et al. Hyponatremia and the syndrome of inappropriate secretion of antidiuretic hormone associated with the use of selective serotonin reuptake inhibitors: a review of spontaneous reports. CMAJ 1996;155(5):519–27.
[44] Fabian TJ, Amico JA, Kroboth PD, et al. Paroxetine-induced hyponatremia in the elderly due to the syndrome of inappropriate secretion of antidiuretic hormone (SIADH). J Geriatr Psychiatry Neurol 2003;16(3):160–4.
[45] Kimelman N, Albert SG. Phenothiazine-induced hyponatremia in the elderly. Gerontology 1984;30(2):132–6.
[46] Wagner AM, Brunet S, Puig J, et al. Chlorambucil-induced inappropriate antidiuresis in a man with chronic lymphocytic leukemia. Ann Hematol 1999;78(1):37–8.
[47] Ishii K, Aoki Y, Sasaki M, et al. Syndrome of inappropriate secretion of antidiuretic hormone induced by intra-arterial cisplatin chemotherapy. Gynecol Oncol 2002;87(1):150–1.
[48] Garrett CA, Simpson TA Jr. Syndrome of inappropriate antidiuretic hormone associated with vinorelbine therapy. Ann Pharmacother 1998;32(12):1306–9.

[49] Kadowaki T, Hagura R, Kajinuma H, et al. Chlorpropamide-induced hyponatremia: incidence and risk factors. Diabetes Care 1983;6(5):468–71.

[50] Hartung TK, Schofield E, Short AI, et al. Hyponatraemic states following 3,4-methylenedioxymethamphetamine (MDMA, ecstasy) ingestion. QJM 2002;95(7):431–7.

[51] Riggs AT, Dysken MW, Kim SW, et al. A review of disorders of water homeostasis in psychiatric patients. Psychosomatics 1991;32(2):133–48.

[52] Robertson GL, Aycinena P, Zerbe RL. Neurogenic disorders of osmoregulation. Am J Med 1982;72(2):339–53.

[53] Fenves AZ, Thomas S, Knochel JP. Beer potomania: two cases and review of the literature. Clin Nephrol 1996;45(1):61–4.

[54] McGee S, Abernethy WB III, Simel DL. The rational clinical examination. Is this patient hypovolemic? JAMA 1999;281(11):1022–9.

[55] Decaux G, Waterlot Y, Genette F, et al. Treatment of the syndrome of inappropriate secretion of antidiuretic hormone with furosemide. N Engl J Med 1981;304(6):329–30.

[56] Hantman D, Rossier B, Zohlman R, et al. Rapid correction of hyponatremia in the syndrome of inappropriate secretion of antidiuretic hormone: An alternative treatment to hypertonic saline. Ann Intern Med 1973;78(6):870–5.

[57] Adams RD, Victor M, Mancall EL. Central pontine myelinolysis: a hitherto undescribed disease occurring in alcoholics and malnourished patients. AMA Arch Neurol Psychiatry 1959;81(2):154–72.

[58] Gocht A, Colmant HJ. Central pontine and extrapontine myelinolysis: a report of 58 cases. Clin Neuropathol 1987;6(6):262–70.

[59] Sterns RH, Riggs JE, Schochet SS Jr. Osmotic demyelination syndrome following correction of hyponatremia. N Engl J Med 1986;314(24):1535–42.

[60] Sterns RH, Cappuccio JD, Silver SM, et al. Neurologic sequelae after treatment of severe hyponatremia: a multicenter perspective. J Am Soc Nephrol 1994;4(8):1522–30.

[61] Cluitmans FH, Meinders A. Management of severe hyponatremia: rapid or slow correction? Am J Med 1990;88(2):161–6.

[62] Sterns RH. Severe symptomatic hyponatremia: treatment and outcome. A study of 64 patients. Ann Intern Med 1987;107(5):656–64.

[63] Norenberg MD, Leslie KO, Robertson AS. Association between rise in serum sodium and central pontine myelinolysis. Ann Neurol 1982;11(2):128–35.

[64] Brunner JE, Redmond JM, Haggar AM, et al. Central pontine myelinolysis and pontine lesions after rapid correction of hyponatremia: a prospective magnetic resonance imaging study. Ann Neurol 1990;27(1):61–6.

[65] Long CA, Marin P, Bayer AJ, et al. Hypernatremia in an adult in-patient population. Postgrad Med J 1991;67(789):643–5.

[66] Phillips PA, Rolls BJ, Ledingham JG, et al. Reduced thirst after water deprivation in healthy elderly men. N Engl J Med 1984;311(12):753–9.

[67] Rowe JW, Shock NW, DeFronzo RA. The influence of age on the renal response to water deprivation in man. Nephron 1976;17(4):270–8.

[68] Snyder NA, Feigal DW, Arieff AI. Hypernatremia in elderly patients: a heterogeneous, morbid, and iatrogenic entity. Ann Intern Med 1987;107(3):309–19.

[69] Janz T. Sodium. Emerg Med Clin North Am 1986;4(1):115–30.

[70] Riggs JE. Neurologic manifestations of electrolyte disturbances. Neurol Clin 2002;20(1):227–39.

[71] Macaulay R, Watson M. Hypernatremia in rats as a cause of brain damage. Arch Dis Child 1967;42(225):485–91.

[72] Palevsky PM. Hypernatremia. Semin Nephrol 1998;18(1):20–30.

[73] Adrogue HJ, Madias NE. Hypernatremia. N Engl J Med 2000;342(20):1493–9.

[74] Conley SB. Hypernatremia. Pediatr Clin North Am 1990;37(2):365–72.

[75] Ayus JC, Krothapalli RK, Arieff AI. Treatment of symptomatic hyponatremia and its relation to brain damage. A prospective study. N Engl J Med 1987;317(19):1190–5.

[76] Trachtman H, Barbour R, Sturman JA, et al. Taurine and osmoregulation: taurine is a cerebral osmoprotective molecule in chronic hypernatremic dehydration. Pediatr Res 1998; 23(1):35–9.

[77] Dorrington CL, Johnson DW, Brant R. Multiple Dose-Activated Charcoal Complication Study Group. The frequency of complications associated with the use of multiple-dose activated charcoal. Ann Emerg Med 2003;41(3):370–7.

[78] Gennari FJ, Kassirer JP. Osmotic diuresis. N Engl J Med 1977;291(14):714–20.

[79] Gipstein RM, Boyle JD. Hypernatremia complicating prolonged mannitol diuresis. N Engl J Med 1965;272:1116–7.

[80] Craig JC, Grigor WG, Knight JF. Acute obstructive uropathy—a rare complication of circumcision. Eur J Pediatr 1994;153(5):369–71.

[81] DeRubertis FR, Michelis MF, Davis BB. Essential hypernatremia. Report of three cases and review of the literature. Arch Intern Med 1974;134(5):889–95.

[82] Kumar S, Berl T. Sodium. Lancet 1998;352(9123):220–8.

[83] Bendz H, Aurell M. Drug-induced diabetes insipidus: incidence, prevention and management. Drug Saf 1999;21(6):449–56.

[84] Holtzman EJ, Ausiello DA. Nephrogenic diabetes insipidus: causes revealed. Hosp Pract 1994;29(3):89–93.

[85] Mattar JA, Weil MH, Shubin H, et al. Cardiac arrest in the critically ill. II. Hyperosmolar states following cardiac arrest. Am J Med 1974;56(2):162–8.

[86] Modell JH. Serum electrolyte changes in near-drowning victims. JAMA 1985;253(4):557.

[87] Finberg L, Luttrell C, Redd H. Pathogenesis of lesions in the nervous system in hypernatremic states. II. Experimental studies of gross anatomic changes and alterations of chemical composition of the tissues. Pediatrics 1959;23:46–53.

[88] Addleman M, Pollard A, Grossman RF. Survival after severe hypernatremia due to salt ingestion by an adult. Am J Med 1985;78(1):176–8.

[89] Abramovici MI, Singhal PC, Trachtman H. Hypernatremia and rhabdomyolysis. J Med 1992;23(1):17–28.

[90] Arieff AI, Guisado R. Effects on the central nervous system of hypernatremic and hyponatremic states. Kidney Int 1976;10(1):104–16.

[91] Kahn A, Brachet E, Blum D. Controlled fall in natremia and risk of seizures in hypertonic dehydration. Intensive Care Med 1979;5(1):27–31.

[92] Ayus JC, Armstrong DL, Arieff AI. Effects of hypernatraemia in the central nervous system and its therapy in rats and rabbits. J Physiol 1996;492:243–55.

ELSEVIER
SAUNDERS

Emerg Med Clin N Am 23 (2005) 771–787

EMERGENCY
MEDICINE
CLINICS OF
NORTH AMERICA

Differential Diagnosis of Metabolic Acidosis

Jennifer J. Casaletto, MD

Department of Emergency Medicine, Maricopa Medical Center,
2601 East Roosevelt Avenue, Phoenix, AZ 85007, USA

Without enough time to take that first sip of morning coffee, the paramedics roll in with an ill-appearing young adult female who has been vomiting for the last several hours. She is febrile and tachypneic. Her parents state that she has been depressed lately and even contemplated suicide, but seemed to be well at dinner the previous evening. Her initial lab results reveal an anion gap acidosis with a respiratory alkalosis, confirming your diagnostic suspicions. As you turn to discuss the findings with her family, the intern is tugging at your opposite sleeve worriedly reporting, "The patient we thought was suffering from alcoholic ketoacidosis doesn't have any ketones in his urine." As you take a breath to begin your explanation regarding the lack of ketones, a colleague at the clinic calls hoping to transfer a hypertensive, diabetic patient whom he believes has become severely hyponatremic and hyperkalemic secondary to renal tubular acidosis (RTA) synrdome. Desperately trying to recall the differences between RTAs, you find yourself wading through the MUDPILES of metabolic acidosis and HARDUP for answers from your inquisitive intern. Relax, go back to that full coffee, and read on....

Metabolic acidosis is defined as an acidemia created by primary increase in H^+ concentration or reduction in HCO_3^- concentration. Acutely, medullary chemoreceptors compensate for a metabolic acidosis by means of a hyperventilatory response, resulting in a reduction of $PaCO_2$, in attempt to increase the pH to normal. In an isolated metabolic acidosis, the degree of acute respiratory compensation can be predicted based on the following relationship: $PaCO_2 = (1.5 \times [HCO_3^-]) + 8$ (ie, the $PaCO_2$ is expected to decrease 1.5 mmHg for each mmol/L decrease in $[HCO_3^-]$). Chronically, the pH imbalance of a metabolic acidosis is opposed by increased renal reabsorption of HCO_3^-.

E-mail address: jennifercasaletto@hotmail.com

0733-8627/05/$ - see front matter © 2005 Elsevier Inc. All rights reserved.
doi:10.1016/j.emc.2005.03.007   *emed.theclinics.com*

Metabolic acidosis is created by one of three mechanisms: increased production of acids, decreased excretion of acids, or loss of alkali. Clinically, metabolic acidoses are divided into processes resulting in an elevated anion gap and a normal anion gap. The diagnosis and classification of metabolic disturbances are based on nearly simultaneous arterial blood gas and electrolyte panel measurements. Confirm internal consistency of the results by comparing the measured $[HCO_3^-]$ (reported with the electrolyte panel) and the arterial blood gas $[HCO_3^-]$ calculated by the Henderson-Hasselbach equation. These values should agree within 2 mmol/L. A pH of less than 7.35 without an increase in the patient's baseline $PaCO_2$ indicates the presence of a metabolic acidosis. Using the electrolyte panel, calculate the anion gap: $([Na] - [Cl] - [HCO_3])$. A normal anion gap is considered to be 8 plus or minus 4 mmol/L, making the hallmark of an elevated anion gap acidosis an anion gap of greater than 12. The anion gap represents unmeasured plasma anions. Elevation of the anion gap may be caused by a decrease in unmeasured cations (eg, calcium, magnesium, or potassium) or an increase in unmeasured anions.

The two most commonly recognized metabolic acidoses in adult patients are an elevated anion gap acidosis secondary to lactate and a normal anion gap acidosis secondary to prolonged diarrhea. The latter marks the most commonly diagnosed cause of acidosis in pediatric patients.

Elevated anion gap acidoses

The elevation of the anion gap is created by inorganic (eg, phosphate, or sulfate), organic (eg, ketoacids or lactate), or exogenous (eg, salicylates) acids incompletely neutralized by bicarbonate. The most common etiologies of elevated anion gap acidoses can be remembered using the mnemonic MUDPILES: methanol, uremia, diabetic and alcoholic ketoacidosis, paraldehyde, isoniazid or iron, lactate, ethylene glycol, and salicylates (Box 1). A subsegment of these elevated anion gap acidoses are referred to as high-anion gap acidoses, which are defined by the coexistence of an

---

Box 1. Etiologies of elevated anion gap acidosis

Methanol
Uremia
Diabetic, alcoholic, and starvation ketoacidosis
Paraldehyde
Isoniazid and iron
Lactic acidosis
Ethylene glycol
Salicylates

elevated anion gap and a decreased $[HCO_3^-]$. There are four principle etiologies of high-anion-gap acidosis: lactic acidosis, ketoacidosis, ingested toxins, and renal failure.

Methanol

Methanol is widely available in paints, solvents, antifreeze, and fuel for outdoor stoves and torches; therefore an index of suspicion for exposure plays a large part in diagnosing methanol-induced acidosis. Absorption takes place by means of gastrointestinal (GI), dermal, and respiratory routes [1–3]. Methanol is converted to formaldehyde by alcohol dehydrogenase, then to formic acid (formate). The formic acid accumulates, leading to physiologic effects and anion gap acidosis. Signs and symptoms may be delayed for 30 hours or more following exposure [4]. Methanol's toxicity predominantly affects the neurologic, ophthalmologic, and GI systems. The state of inebriation caused by methanol often has elapsed before presentation with neurologic symptoms (such as headache and dizziness) caused by the formate [4]. Agitation, acute mania, amnesia, decreased level of consciousness, and seizures, however, can complicate the initial presentation [1,5–9]. Ophthalmologic complaints may develop as early as 6 hours postexposure or be delayed greater than 24 hours. In two large case series, all patients with acidemia had ophthalmologic complaints [1,10]. Symptoms include blurred vision, photophobia, visual hallucinations, and varying degrees of visual impairment [1,9,11–13]. Examination findings range from normal to retinal edema associated with unreactive pupils and absent vision [1,9,11–13]. GI effects frequently are limited to nausea and vomiting, but may include severe abdominal pain, GI hemorrhage, diarrhea, liver function abnormalities, and pancreatitis [1,7–9,13].

In addition to an anion gap acidosis, methanol toxicity also results in a difference between the measured serum and calculated serum osmolalities, referred to as an osmolal gap. A normal osmolal gap has been defined as less than 10 mOsm/kg. As baseline osmolal gaps vary among patients, however, methanol toxicity cannot be ruled out by the presence of a normal gap [4]. Methanol levels can be measured to further confirm diagnostic suspicion of methanol toxicity; however, such levels are rarely available in real time and only measure methanol that has not been metabolized. Methanol levels greater than 20 mg/dL or less than 20 mg/dL with an accompanying acidosis are considered toxic [4]. Finally, imaging may reveal cerebral edema or basal ganglia hemorrhages or infarcts in severely ill patients with methanol toxicity [14–18].

Uremia

A history of progressive renal disease and elevated serum urea nitrogen (BUN) and creatinine levels are keys to diagnosing elevated gap acidosis as a result of chronic renal failure. Normal anion gap metabolic acidosis accompanies renal insufficiency, and progresses to elevated gap acidosis as the glomerular filtration rate (GFR) decreases and renal failure ensues. With a decrease in GFR comes decreasing filtration and increasing reabsorption of inorganic and organic acids, leading to an increased anion gap [19]. Furthermore, a decreasing number of functioning nephrons results in reduced NH_4 production, resulting in an insufficient amount of NH_4 to buffer the net increase in acids [19,20]. Bicarbonate concentration rarely falls below 15 mmol/L, and the anion gap rarely exceeds 20 mmol/L [19].

Physical manifestations of the uremic syndrome involve multiple systems. Neurologically, daytime drowsiness progresses to obtundation, while distal dysesthesias result from uremia's effects on the peripheral neurologic system. Atherosclerosis and noncardiogenic pulmonary edema predominate among cardiovascular effects. GI manifestations include anorexia with subsequent nausea and vomiting, often progressing to gastritis and peptic ulcer disease. Uremic patients commonly complain of diffuse pruritus; both dystrophic calcifications and changes in skin pigmentation may be present also. Anemia and platelet dysfunction result from uremia. Finally, the endocrinologic effects of uremia encompass insulin resistance, hyper-lipidemia, hyperparathyroidism, and gonadal atrophy with associated dysfunction [20].

Ketoacidoses: diabetic, alcoholic, and starvation

Diabetic ketoacidosis (DKA) encompasses a triad of clinical findings: hyperglycemia, ketonemia, and acidemia. It occurs most often in people with type I diabetes; however, there are occurrences in people with type II diabetes. The latter occurs predominantly in obese, African-American type II diabetics [21,22]. Onset of DKA requires the shortage or absence of insulin coupled with increased levels of glucagon. Most often this state is caused by noncompliance with an insulin regimen or to a period of increased physical stress (eg, infection or surgery). In the face of insulin non-compliance, glucagon levels increase in response to insulin withdrawal. In the face of physical stress, rising levels of epinephrine are thought to stimulate glucagon release. In both scenarios, glucagon leads to the ketoacidotic state by means of two pathways. By means of the first pathway, glucagon initiates gluconeogenesis and impairs peripheral glucose use, resulting in hyperglycemia followed by an osmotic diuresis. By means of the second pathway, glucagon stimulates hepatic oxidation of free fatty acids released from adipose tissue as a result of insulin deficiency. Oxidation of free fatty acids produces ketoacids, β-hydroxybutyrate, and acetoacetate, leading to metabolic acidosis.

Patients suffering from DKA often present with nausea, vomiting, and polyuria that may be associated with abdominal pain. Exam reveals Kussmaul respirations and signs of dehydration. Without treatment, DKA may progress, leading to a decreasing level of consciousness and rarely, circulatory collapse. A case series of 308 patients with nonfatal DKA demonstrated the following common laboratory abnormalities:

- A mean serum glucose of 675 mg/dL, a mean serum sodium of 131 mmol/L (caused by increased intracellular water in the plasma space in response to the hyperglycemia-induced osmolality rise)
- A mean serum potassium of 5.3 mmol/L (secondary to the insulin shortage, which traps potassium in the plasma space)
- A mean serum bicarbonate of 6 mmol/L [23,24]

In addition to the hyperglycemic state, the presence of ketonuria, assessed by the nitroprusside reaction with acetoacetate, helps set the diagnosis of DKA apart from most remaining sources of elevated anion gap acidosis. In the presence of mild hyperglycemia, ketonuria, and an insufficient history of present illness, however, serum dilution followed by ketone testing may be required to differentiate DKA from other ketoacidoses. Patients with DKA have a lower β-hydroxybutyrate to acetoacetate ratio, resulting in positive serum ketone testing at dilutions greater than 2:1, setting them apart from patients with alcoholic or starvation ketoacidosis [25].

The diagnosis of alcoholic ketoacidosis (AKA) is accelerated by the frequently difficult to elicit history of chronic alcoholism, most often including a recent binge followed by an abrupt cessation of alcohol use. As in DKA, glucagon levels are elevated because of insufficient intracellular glucose, leading to ketoacid formation. Clinical presentation is remarkable for vomiting, abdominal pain, and dehydration. In contrast to DKA, serum glucose levels are most often low to normal. Furthermore, the rise in the β-hydroxybutyrate to acetoacetate ratio from 3:1 in DKA to 7:1 in (AKA) results in a nitroprusside test that is more often negative because of the relative lack of acetoacetate [19,25].

Starvation ketoacidosis occurs during fasting in the face of physiologic stress, such as illness, exercise, or pregnancy [26–30]. During this time, starvation-induced absence of insulin stimulates the previously discussed ketogenic pathway, accounting for the pathogenesis of acute starvation ketoacidosis [26]. As in AKA, the serum glucose level is low to normal, and serum ketones may not be found if the nitroprusside test is used, because of a predominance of β-hydroxybutyrate.

Paraldehyde

Several decades ago, paraldehyde was used as a pharmacologic treatment for alcohol withdrawal. In overdose, paraldehyde's clinical picture matches that of a sedative–hypnotic overdose: hypotension, bradypnea, hypothermia, and altered mental status [31]. Ingestion leads to formation of acetic and chloracetic acids, which create the elevated anion gap in the resultant metabolic acidosis [32].

Isoniazid and iron

After being on a steady decline for more than 20 years, the incidence of tuberculosis in the United States rose each year after 1985, until peaking in 1992 [33]. As the primary antituberculin agent for prophylaxis and initial single- and multi-drug therapy of tuberculosis, it seems only logical that isoniazid (INH) usage also rose. Isoniazid toxicity may be acute, indirectly-mediated depletion of pyridoxine or a chronic, directly-mediated, hypersensitivity reaction. It is the former that leads to a relative γ-aminobutyric acid (GABA) deficiency, resulting in refractory generalized, tonic–clonic seizures [34]. Anion gap metabolic acidosis is the product of a rapid, excessive accumulation of lactate during these seizures. The lactate cannot be cleared secondary to INH's inhibition of the formation of nicotinamide adenine dinucleotide (NAD), an essential cofactor in the conversion of lactate to pyruvate [34]. In addition, INH decreases the metabolism of β-hydroxybutyrate, further contributing to the elevated anion gap acidosis [35].

Before the onset of seizures and metabolic acidosis, acute INH overdoses may present with vomiting, diaphoresis, tachycardia, and hypertension occurring within 30 minutes of ingestion [36]. Agitation, altered mental status, and hallucinations have been reported, likely secondary to the decrease in GABA [34]. Associated seizures are generalized, classically prolonged, and refractory to standard antiepileptic therapy [34]. Hemodynamic instability may occur in the patient with seizures and acidosis [36,37].

Similar to INH, iron exhibits a direct and indirect toxicity; however, unlike INH, both types occur with acute overdose in a dose-dependent fashion. Iron mediates direct GI toxicity after its absorption into the vascular walls, resulting in GI cell necrosis and hemorrhage [38]. There is also evidence that iron may act as a direct myocardial toxin [39]. Unbound iron, which remains after transferrin is saturated, creates indirect cellular toxicity. It uncouples mitochondrial oxidative phosphorylation, thereby devastating ATP synthesis. It also forms free radicals, which damage cell membranes by means of lipid peroxidation [40,41]. Impaired ATP synthesis has its most damaging effects on GI, cardiovascular, hepatic, and central nervous system (CNS) cells because of their high metabolic activity. This damage furthers the aforementioned GI hemorrhage and myocardial dysfunction and adds hepatic failure and CNS dysfunction to the realm of iron toxicity [42]. The elevated anion gap consists of lactate produced as a result of hypovolemia, cardiogenic shock, and anaerobic metabolism, and of unbuffered protons produced as a result of free ferric iron hydration.

When considering iron overdose as part of a differential diagnosis, it is hoped that history consistent with iron ingestion or an abdominal radiograph revealing radiopaque tablets can be obtained. Without these hints, diagnosis relies on recognition of the clinical stages of iron poisoning and an elevated iron level drawn 3 to 5 hours postingestion in the presence of an elevated anion gap acidosis. Clinically, iron poisoning takes place in five stages [43]. The elevated anion gap metabolic acidosis is most prominent in stages two through four, corresponding to several hours up to 5 days postingestion. Stage 1 consists of GI symptoms ranging from abdominal pain and vomiting to life-threatening GI hemorrhage. Symptoms begin 1 to 6 hours after an ingestion of greater than 10 to 20 mg/kg of elemental iron and may be delayed with enteric-coated preparations. Stage 2 represents a period of relative stability in which GI symptoms abate; however, subclinical hypoperfusion and metabolic acidosis persist. This stage may last up to 24 hours. Although some patients may recover from stage 2, many who have ingested more than 40 mg/kg progress to the systemic toxicity. The onset of stage 3 occurs 24 to 48 hours postingestion and is characterized by reoccurrence of GI symptoms, hypoperfusion, severe metabolic acidosis, altered mental status, and coagulopathy. Although stage 3 accounts for the highest number of iron poisoning deaths, iron levels are often normal by this stage. Progression to stage 4 is rare; it is marked by acute hepatic failure and encephalopathy. Those who recover from an acute iron overdose, may present subacutely, 2 to 4 weeks postoverdose, in stage 4 with a bowel obstruction caused by GI scarring [42,44].

Lactic acidosis

There are three general categories of lactic acidosis. The L isomer of lactate is most common and what usually is measured when obtaining serum lactate levels. It is also responsible for the first two categories of lactic acidosis referred to as types A and B. These two distinctions refer to those etiologies that produce lactic acidosis by means of tissue hypoxia (type A) and those that are accompanied by normal oxygen delivery (type B). The D isomer is responsible for the third type of lactic acidosis, which occurs in patients with small bowel resection or jejunoileal bypass. The D lactate is formed by colonic bacteria after ingestion of a large carbohydrate load in the face of carbohydrate malabsorption [45]. It cannot be metabolized by lactate dehydrogenase, leading to accumulation that presents clinically with an encephalopathy and elevated anion gap acidosis [46].

Type A lactic acidosis can be the result of hemodynamic shock, severe hypoxemia or anemia, vigorous exercise, mesenteric ischemia, or mitochondrial dysfunction. All types of hemodynamic shock; hypovolemic, septic, cardiogenic, anaphylactic, and spinal shock limit the delivery of oxygen secondary to diminished blood flow to the tissue. It is beyond the scope of this article to discuss the differential diagnosis of shock. Severe hypoxemia caused by such entities as pulmonary disease processes or pulmonary embolism can be identified easily with pulse oximetry or arterial blood gas measurement. Anemia is readily identifiable with the measurement of a hemoglobin or hematocrit. Exercise above the anaerobic threshold, including seizures and hypothermic shivering, results in a relative tissue hypoxia secondary to an unmet increased oxygen demand. Some texts classify seizures as type B acidoses, presumably because of the increased lactate production [19]. Lactic acidosis may be attributed to anaerobic exercise in patients with the appropriate history or with myoglobinuria and elevated creatinine phosphokinase (CPK). Mesenteric ischemia-induced lactic acidosis most often presents in conjunction with abdominal pain out of proportion to exam in a patient population with risk factors for either a low-flow state or an embolic event. Despite the presence of risk factors, abdominal pain, and elevated gap acidosis, imaging or surgery often is required to confirm the diagnosis. Finally, mitochondrial dysfunction can be the consequence of a congenital enzyme defect or, more commonly, mediated by toxins. Examples of the former include mitochondrial encephalopathy with acidosis and stroke (MELAS) and Pearson syndrome, often diagnosed in childhood after extensive genetic evaluation. Examples of the latter include carbon monoxide, which inhibits delivery of oxygen to the mitochondria by means of the binding of hemoglobin, and cyanide, which directly binds and inactivates complex IV of the mitochondrion's electron transport chain. In both scenarios, mitochondrial dysfunction results in lactic acid production caused by the anaerobic metabolism of pyruvate.

Type B lactic acidoses result from an overproduction or decreased hepatic removal of lactate in the face of maintained oxygen delivery to the tissues. The etiologies of type B acidoses are as follows: hypoglycemia/glycogen storage disease, diabetes mellitus, ethanol, hepatic failure, malignancy, and drugs. In the face of hypoglycemia, epinephrine and glucagon are secreted to stimulate the breakdown of glycogen to glucose. In patients with limited or abnormal glycogen stores, however, the amount of glucose generated is not sufficient, and glycolysis ensues, leading to increased pyruvate and lactate. In diabetic patients, low insulin levels reduce the activity of pyruvate dehydrogenase, resulting in increased lactate levels. In addition, there is evidence that the existence of plasma ketones inhibit hepatic uptake of lactate [47]. In the intoxicated patient, ethanol increases the NADH/NAD ratio, favoring the conversion of pyruvate to lactate, instead of glucose. Hepatic failure results in lactic acidosis caused by the liver's failure to remove lactate, either by converting it to carbon dioxide and water or to glucose. Lactic acidosis has been described in cancer patients in the absence of tissue hypoperfusion and other known causes of increased lactate production. Known as lactic acidosis of malignancy, it has been reported in patients with Hodgkin's disease, acute leukemia, and sarcoma [48–50]. Although many common medications are known to cause hyperlactatemia, some of the most pronounced elevated lactate levels are seen in those patients taking biguanides and nucleoside analog reverse transcriptase inhibitors (NRTIs) or those on propofol infusions. Severe, life-threatening lactic acidosis has been associated with biguanides, such as metformin, in two clinical settings: renal insufficiency and overdose [51]. It appears as though prescribed use in uncomplicated noninsulin-dependent diabetes mellitus patients does not pose a risk for severe acidosis. The occurrence of mildly symptomatic to severe lactic acidosis in HIV patients under treatment with NRTI therapy is thought to caused by mitochondrial disruption; however, it thus far has not been be associated with specific clinical scenarios. A recent case review reported female sex to be an independent risk factor for development of lactic acidosis and suggested that duration of NRTI therapy, specific drug use, and genetic predisposition also may be risk factors [52]. Finally, deaths have been reported in children and adults undergoing propofol infusions of greater than 48 hours. Propofol infusion syndrome includes cardiac failure, rhabdomyolysis, severe metabolic acidosis, and renal failure. The metabolic acidosis is thought to be the result of impaired free fatty acid use and mitochondrial activity [53].

Ethylene glycol

Ethylene glycol lowers the freezing point of water, and is therefore most often found in antifreeze, deicing solutions, and brake fluid. As with methanol, a high index of suspicion for exposure plays a large part in the diagnosis of poisoning. Absorption takes place in the GI tract; skin and inhalational exposures are negligible [4]. Ethylene glycol is converted to glycoaldehyde by alcohol dehydrogenase, then to glycolic acid, glyoxylic acid, and oxalic acid [54]. The elevated anion gap acidosis primarily is caused by the accumulation of glycolic acid with minimal assistance from lactic acid [55–57]. Until recently, however, ethylene glycol's toxic effects have been attributed solely to calcium oxalate crystal deposition. Although suggested in the 1970s, the direct toxic effect of ethylene glycol's organic acid metabolites was not demonstrated until recently [58,59]. Signs and symptoms typically occur within 4 to 8 hours of ingestion, but may be prolonged for 12 or more hours if ingested with ethanol [4]. Ethylene glycol's toxicity reveals itself clinically in four stages, with predominant effects on the neurologic, cardiopulmonary, and renal systems. Stage 1 is referred to as the acute neurologic stage in which ethylene glycol results in an inebriated state similar to that of ethanol. Larger ingestions may result in hallucinations, seizures, or coma. Stage 2, the cardiopulmonary stage, begins 12 to 24 hours postingestion and is characterized by hypertension, tachycardia, and tachypnea. Although the tachypnea may occur solely in response to metabolic acidosis, it also may be the harbinger of ensuing pulmonary edema secondary to myocardial depression or direct pulmonary toxicity. In addition, hypocalcemia, secondary to the chelation of calcium by oxalic acid, and myositis, heralded by CPK elevations, may be present. Stage 3, the renal stage, occurs 24 to 72 hours postingestion and is distinguished by flank pain and acute tubular necrosis (ATN) with or without oliguria. Increased degree of acidosis, delay in presentation, and glycolic acid levels predict progression to renal failure more reliably than ethylene glycol levels [59–61]. Stage 4, the delayed neurologic sequelae stage, presents with cranial nerve palsies approximately 1 week after ingestion.

Similar to methanol toxicity, ethylene glycol toxicity classically results in elevated anion and osmolal gaps but cannot be ruled out by the presence of a normal osmolal gap [54]. Additionally, levels greater than 20 mg/dL or less than 20 mg/dL with an accompanying acidosis are considered toxic. Unlike methanol, there are many laboratory-based clues that can further the clinician's diagnostic suspicion of ethylene glycol ingestion [4]. Approximately half of ethylene glycol intoxicated patients exhibit envelope-shaped calcium oxalate dihydrate or needle-shaped calcium oxalate monohydrate crystalluria [55,62]. Both freshly voided urine and fresh emesis with pH greater than 4.5 will fluoresce under a Wood's lamp if fluorescein-containing antifreeze has been ingested [4]. An EKG may demonstrate a prolonged QT interval, providing a clue to ethylene glycol-induced hypocalcemia. Finally, cerebral imaging studies show cerebral edema with decreased attenuation in the basal ganglia, thalami, midbrain, and upper pons [63,64].

Salicylates

Acute and chronic toxicity can result from ingestion of salicylates found in oral medications, either alone or in combination with decongestants, antihistamines, or opioids, and from some skin and teething ointments, sunscreens, and antidiarrheals that contain salicylate compounds. Salicylates create a mixed acid–base disturbance by means of direct stimulation of the medullary respiratory center, leading to respiratory alkalosis, and uncoupling of oxidative phosphorylation, leading to metabolic acidosis. The metabolic acidosis then is amplified by renal bicarbonate excretion in response to increased ventilation, lactic acid accumulation resulting from mitochondrial impairment, ketoacid production caused by salicylate-induced inhibition of Krebs cycle dehydrogenases, and free salicylic acid [65]. Serum salicylate levels peak 2 to 4 hours after an acute ingestion. A level of 30 mg/dL following an acute ingestion is potentially toxic, whereas chronic toxicity may occur even at a therapeutic level of 4 to 6 gm/dL. Clinically, an elevated salicylic acid concentration appears as tachypnea or hyperpnea, caused by direct medullary stimulation, and hyperthermia, caused by the uncoupling of oxidative phosphorylation. Vasoconstriction of the auditory microvasculature generates tinnitus during the initial presentation of toxicity. Vomiting begins 3 to 8 hours postingestion as a result of direct stimulation of the medullary chemoreceptors. Severe dehydration may ensue as a consequence of increased ventilation, vomiting, and hyperthermia. CNS manifestations parallel increasing acidemia, as an increased amount of nonionized salicylic acid results in increased intracellular levels. Increased capillary permeability in the pulmonary and cerebral tissue may result in edema; the mechanism is thought to relate to salicylate's blockade of the cyclooxygenase pathway leading to production of proinflammatory leukotrienes. Rarely, mucosal bleeding results from salicylate's platelet inhibition and depression of hepatic synthesis of factor VII.

The presentation of salicylism, characterized by hyperthermia, altered level of consciousness, pulmonary edema, and shock in the face of a mixed acid–base disorder may present a diagnostic dilemma or even point directly toward a septic etiology without the available history implicating an acute or chronic salicylate overdose. Although tinnitus may point the clinician in the correct direction early in the course of toxicity, this history is often unavailable. Thus a high index of suspicion must be maintained in the face of an anion gap acidosis. The urine ferric chloride test provides a timely and simple way to check for the presence of salicylates at the bedside. It is performed by placing a few drops of 10% ferric chloride solution in a patient's urine, which will indicate the presence of salicylates by turning purple immediately [66]. Although it does not give a quantitative result and cannot confirm toxicity, a negative result indicates that the metabolic disturbances are unlikely the result of salicylates. An elevated serum salicylate level is required to confirm toxicity in the case of an acute overdose, while persistent symptoms and associated laboratory abnormalities may indicate the presence of chronic overdose in the face of mildly elevated serum salicylate levels.

Hyperchloremic or normal anion gap acidoses

The presence of a hyperchloremic or normal anion gap acidosis occurs by means of an excessive loss of HCO_3^- or an inability to excrete H^+. HCO_3^- can be lost from the GI tract or from the kidneys, whereas, the inability to excrete H^+ is a result of renal failure. More recent literature advocates calculation of a urinary anion gap (UAG) to aid in differentiating etiologies of an existing hyperchloremic acidosis. Although a negative UAG suggests GI HCO_3^- loss, a positive UAG indicates inability to excrete H^+ [67]. In hyperchloremic acidosis, the increase in $[Cl^-]$ equals the decrease in $[HCO_3^-]$. Conditions in which this relationship does not exist must be classified as mixed acid–base disorders. The etiologies of a hyperchloremic or normal anion gap acidosis can be remembered by the mnemonic HARD UP: hyperalimentation, acetazolamide, renal tubular acidoses and renal insufficiency, diarrhea and diuretics, ureterostomy, and pancreatic fistula (Box 2). Diarrheal and renal etiologies are by far the most common.

Hyperalimentation

Hyperchloremic acidosis results from parenteral hyperalimentation administered without a sufficient amount of bicarbonate or bicarbonate-yielding solutes, such as lactate or acetate [68]. Protons are released from synthetic, positively charged amino acids (eg, arginine, lysine, or histidine)

Box 2. Etiologies of normal anion gap acidosis

Hyperalimentation
Acetazolamide (carbonic anhydrase inhibitors)
Renal tubular acidosis and renal insufficiency
Diarrhea and diuretics
Ureteroenterostomy
Pancreatic fistula

---

in hyperalimentation mixtures as they are metabolized. In the face of a relative bicarbonate deficiency, these protons cannot be buffered, leading to a normal anion gap acidosis.

Acetazolamide (and carbonic anhydrase inhibitors)

Acetazolamide may be used in the treatment of high altitude sickness, glaucoma, hyperuricemia, and hypokalemic periodic paralysis. It therefore should be suspected as an etiology of normal gap metabolic acidosis in patients with history of such illnesses and laboratory findings remarkable for an increased $[Cl^-]$ and decreased $[HCO_3^-]$. Acetazolamide and other carbonic anhydrase inhibitors work as proximal tubule diuretics by blocking the catalytic dehydration of luminal carbonic acid. This blockade prevents the proximal reabsorption of sodium bicarbonate. Acetazolamide's blockade of HCO_3^- reabsorption does not cause a severe metabolic acidosis because of HCO_3^- reabsorption at more distal nephron sites and decreased filtration of HCO_3^- in the presence of metabolic acidosis [69].

Renal tubular acidoses and renal insufficiency

Type 1 renal tubular acidosis (RTA), or distal RTA, most often occurs as a secondary distal RTA in association with a systemic inflammatory illness such as Sjögren's syndrome or multiple myeloma. Rarely, it can be an inherited disorder, a result of chronic renal transplant rejection, or drug-induced [19]. Type 1 RTA is a consequence of the failure of one or both of the collecting duct proton pumps (H^+-ATPase and H^+ K-ATPase) to excrete H^+. The failure of these pumps results in the inability to acidify the urine below a pH of 5.5. The elevated urinary pH does not allow adequate trapping of NH_4 in the collecting duct. Hence, the clinical findings of a type 1 or distal RTA include: hypokalemia, hyperchloremic acidosis, low urinary NH_4, and urine pH greater than 5.5. Chronic toluene abuse and lithium, pentamidine, and rifampin use produce a type 1 RTA with similar findings [19,69,70]. Amphotericin B use produces a picture clinically consistent with type 1 RTA by means of an alteration in distal nephron permeability that allows leakage of H^+ from lumen to blood, thereby destroying the pH gradient and reducing net H^+ secretion [71].

Type 2 RTA, or proximal RTA, also is referred to as Fanconi syndrome. Proximal RTA is found most commonly in children. In adults, it usually is associated with multiple myelomas, in which increased excretion of immunoglobulin light chains injures the proximal tubule epithelium, or use of carbonic anhydrase inhibitors. Physiologically, generalized proximal tubular dysfunction leads to bicarbonaturia until steady state is reached, and persistent proteinuria, glycosuria, aminoaciduria, and phosphaturia. Unlike type 1 RTA, urinary pH is appropriately acidic because of a steady state in which the amount of $[HCO_3^-]$ filtered does not exceed that which can be reabsorbed distally. Enhanced Cl^- reabsorption, stimulated by volume contraction, results in hyperchloremia. In untreated patients, serum $[HCO_3^-]$ is low, reaching a nadir of 15 to 18 mEq/L. The rate of K excretion is proportional to the HCO_3^- delivery to the distal nephron, leading to an associated hypokalemia.

The diagnosis of type 2 RTA relies on the recognition of a chronic hyperchloremic metabolic acidosis accompanied by acidic urine, hypokalemia, and a low fractional excretion of HCO_3^-. With infusion of sodium bicarbonate, bicarbonaturia ensues, and the urine becomes alkaline. A further diagnostic clue is the large amounts of exogenous HCO_3^- required to correct plasma $[HCO_3^-]$.

Hyperchloremic metabolic acidosis occurs in 50% of patients with hyporeninemic hypoaldosteronism, also known as type 4 RTA [69]. This syndrome occurs in older patients with interstitial renal disease, hypertension, diabetes mellitus, and concurrent congestive heart failure [68,69]. Distal tubular damage produces diminished rates of Na absorption, H^+ secretion, and K secretion. A clinical triad of hyponatremia, hyperkalemia, and hyperchloremic acidosis is the hallmark of this disorder. Diuretics such as triamterene, spironolactone, and amiloride create a similar syndrome [68].

As discussed previously, renal failure results in an elevated anion gap uremic acidosis, secondary to decreased filtration of acids and decreased ammoniagenesis. Early in renal disease, however, when the GFR is between 20 and 50 mL per minute, a hyperchloremic acidosis is present because of the decreased ability of the kidneys to compensate with adequate HCO_3^- reabsoprtion.

Diarrhea and diuretics

The most common normal anion gap acidosis results from the GI HCO_3^- loss that accompanies diarrhea. Stool contains large amounts of HCO_3^- in addition to the organic ions that are absorbed and converted to HCO_3^-; both are lost with diarrhea. Stool contains a greater amount of sodium relative to chloride, resulting in a diarrhea-induced relative hyperchloremia.

Hypokalemia exists in large part because of the large quantities of K lost from stool, but also from a hypovolemia-induced hyper-renin–hyper-aldosterone state that enhances renal K secretion. Although acidic urine production would be anticipated in the face of such a metabolic acidosis, urine produced in conjunction with diarrheal illness more often has a pH of 6.0 or higher [72]. Increased urine pH occurs in the face of metabolic acidosis and hypokalemia because of increased renal NH_4 synthesis and excretion. With a concurrent history of diarrhea, it is this fact that allows hyperchloremic metabolic acidosis of GI origin to be differentiated from that of RTA.

As mentioned previously, diuretics such as triamterene, spironolactone, and amiloride interfere with distal tubular Na absorption, H^+ secretion, and K secretion, resulting in a hyperkalemic, hyperchloremic metabolic acidosis resembling that of type 4 RTA [68].

Ureteroenterostomy and enterostomy

Although now rare, ureteroenterostomy (surgical insertion of the ureters into the bowel) was the first form of diversion to be popularized for patients with exstrophy. This style of diversion results in hyperchloremic metabolic acidosis, because the urine reaching the colon is alkalinized by colonic bicarbonate secretion in exchange for chloride [68]. Other types of enterostomies, tube drainage, and fistulae that result in loss of HCO_3^- rich intestinal and biliary fluid also result in normal gap metabolic acidosis.

Pancreatic fistula

External pancreatic fistulas occur as a consequence of surgical therapy for chronic pancreatitis or pseudocyst, whereas internal fistulas occur mainly in the setting of chronic pancreatitis after rupture of a pseudocyst [73]. The fluid from an internal fistula may track to the peritoneal cavity or pleural space, a diagnosis that can be established by documenting high levels of amylase within the respective fluid. In either scenario, HCO_3^- rich pancreatic fluid is diverted from the bowel where normal HCO_3^- reabsorption occurs. This loss of HCO_3^- results in a normal gap metabolic acidosis.

Summary

Although the presence and etiology of a metabolic acidosis in a tachypnic, dehydrated patient with a sweet odor on his or her breath and complaints of vomiting and polyuria is obvious, the physician is rarely so fortunate. More often, a metabolic acidosis must be confirmed by means of a simultaneous arterial blood gas and an electrolyte panel. Serum anion gap must be calculated to differentiate between an elevated gap and normal gap acidosis.

The applicable mnemonic must be recalled, and each etiology examined and considered or rejected as a possibility in the given clinical scenario. As in nearly every etiology discussed in this article, the key to diagnosis can be found with a careful history and a high index of suspicion for toxic exposure.

References

[1] Bennet IL, Cary FH, Mitchell GL, et al. Acute methyl alcohol poisoning: a review based on experiences in an outbreak of 323 cases. Medicine 1953;32(4):431–63.

[2] Frenia ML, Schauben JL. Methanol inhalation toxicity. Ann Emerg Med 1993;22(12): 1919–23.

[3] Kahn A, Blum D. Methyl alcohol poisoning in an 8-month-old boy: an unusual route of intoxication. J Pediatr 1979;94(5):841–3.

[4] Ford MD, McMartin K. Ethylene glycol and methanol. In: Ford MD, Delaney KA, Ling LJ, et al, editors. Clinical toxicology. Philadelphia: WB Saunders; 2001. p. 757–67.

[5] Gonda A, Gault H, Churchill D, Hollomby D. Hemodialysis for methanol intoxication. Am J Med 1978;64(5):749–58.

[6] Keyvan-Larijarni H, Tannenberg AM. Methanol intoxication: comparison of peritoneal dialysis and hemodialysis treatment. Arch Intern Med 1974;134(2):293–6.

[7] Naraqi S, Dethlefs RF, Slobodniuk RA, et al. An outbreak of acute methyl alcohol intoxication. Aust N Z J Med 1979;9(1):65–8.

[8] Shahangian S, Ash KO. Formic and lactic acidosis in a fatal case of methanol intoxication. Clin Chem 1986;32(2):395–7.

[9] Swartz RD, Millman RP, Billi JE, et al. Epidemic methanol poisoning: clinical and biochemical analysis of a recent episode. Medicine 1981;60(5):373–82.

[10] Dethlefs R, Naraqi S. Ocular manifestations and complications of acute methyl alcohol intoxication. Med J Aust 1978;2(10):483–5.

[11] Greiner JV, Pillai S, Limaye SR, et al. Sterno-induced methanol toxicity and visual recovery after prompt hemodialysis. Arch Ophthalmol 1989;107(5):643.

[12] Ingemansson SO. Clinical observations on ten cases of methanol poisoning with particular reference to ocular manifestations. Acta Opthalmol 1984;62(1):15–24.

[13] Jacobsen D, Webb R, Collins TD, et al. Methanol and formate kinetics in late diagnosed methanol intoxication. Med Toxicol 1988;3(5):418–23.

[14] Aquilonius SM, Askmark H, Enoksson P, et al. Computerized tomography in severe methanol intoxication. BMJ 1978;2(6142):929–30.

[15] Chen JC, Schneiderman JF, Wortzman G. Methanol poisoning: bilateral putaminal and cerebellar cortical lesions on CT and MR. J Comput Assist Tomogr 1993;15(3):522–4.

[16] Hantson P, Duprez T, Mahieu P. Neurotoxicity to the basal ganglia shown by MRI following poisoning by methanol and other substances. J Toxicol Clin Toxicol 1997;35(2):151–61.

[17] Mittal BV, Desai AP, Kahde KR. Methyl alcohol poisoning: an autopsy study of 28 cases. J Postgrad Med 1991;37(1):9–13.

[18] Phang PT, Passerini L, Mielke B, et al. Brain hemorrhage associated with methanol poisoning. Crit Care Med 1988;16(2):137–40.

[19] DuBose TB Jr. Acidosis and alkalosis. In: Fauci AS, Braunwald E, Isselbacher KJ, et al, editors. Harrison's principles of internal medicine. 14th edition. New York: McGraw-Hill; 1998. p. 277–83.

[20] Bailey JL, Mitch WE. Pathophysiology of uremia. In: Brenner BM, editor. The kidney. 7th edition. Philadelphia: Elsevier; 2004. p. 2139–43.

[21] Kitabchi A, Wall BM. Management of diabetic ketoacidosis. Am Fam Physician 1999;60(2): 455–64.

[22] Umpierrez GE, Kelly JP, Navarette JE, et al. Hyperglycemic crises in urban blacks. Arch Intern Med 1997;157:669–75.

[23] Beigelman PM. Severe diabetic ketoacidosis. 482 episodes in 257 patients; experience of three years. Diabetes 1971;20(7):490–500.

[24] Foster DW. Diabetes mellitus. In: Fauci AS, Braunwald E, Isselbacher KJ, et al, editors. Harrison's principles of internal medicine. 14th edition. New York: McGraw-Hill; 1998. p. 2071–2.

[25] Umpierrez GE, DiGirolamo M, Tuvlin JA, et al. Differences in metabolic and hormonal milieu in diabetic- and alcohol-induced ketoacidosis. J Crit Care 2000;15(2):52–9.

[26] Owen OE, Capiro S, Reichard GA Jr, et al. Ketosis of starvation: a revisit and new perspectives. Clin Endocrinol Metab 1983;12(2):359–79.

[27] Toth HL, Greenbaum LA. Severe acidosis caused by starvation and stress. Am J Kidney Dis 2003;42(5):E16–9.

[28] Koeslag JH, Noakes TD, Sloan AW. Post-exercise ketosis. J Physiol 1980;301:79–90.

[29] Rudolf MC, Sherwin RS. Maternal ketosis and its effects on the fetus. Clin Endocrinol Metab 1983;12(2):413–28.

[30] Mahoney CA. Extreme gestational starvation ketoacidosis: case report and review of pathophysiology. Am J Kidney Dis 1992;20(3):276–80.

[31] Ford MD, Delaney KA, Ling LJ, et al, editors. Clinical toxicology. Philadelphia: WB Saunders; 2001.

[32] Disney JD. Acid–base disorders. In: Marx JA, Hockberger RS, Walls RM, editors. Rosen's emergency medicine concepts and clinical practice. 5th edition. St. Louis (MO): Mosby; 2002. p. 1718–9.

[33] Centers for Disease Control and Prevention. Trends in tuberculosis—United States, 1998–2003. MMWR Morbid Mortal Wkly Rep 2004;53(10):209–14.

[34] Henry GC, Haynes S. Isoniazid and other antituberculosis drugs. In: Ford MD, Delaney KA, Ling LJ, et al, editors. Clinical toxicology. Philadelphia: WB Saunders; 2001. p. 439–41.

[35] Pahl MV, Jaziri NG, Ness R, et al. Association of beta hydroxybutyric acidosis with isoniazid intoxication. J Toxicol Clin Toxicol 1984;22(2):167–76.

[36] Brown A, Mallet M, Fiser D, et al. Acute isoniazid intoxication: reversal of CNS symptoms with large doses of pyridoxime. Pediatr Pharmacol 1984;4(3):199–202.

[37] Hankins DG, Saxena K, Faville RJ Jr, et al. Profound acidosis caused by isoniazid ingestion. Am J Emerg Med 1987;5(2):165–6.

[38] Roberts RJ, Nayfield S, Soper R, et al. Acute iron intoxication with intestinal infarction managed in part by small bowel resection. Clin Toxicol 1975;8(1):3–12.

[39] Tenenbein M, Kopelow ML, deSa DJ. Myocardial failure and shock in iron poisoning. Hum Toxicol 1988;7(3):281–4.

[40] Mills KC, Curry SC. Acute iron poisoning. Emerg Med Clin North Am 1994;12(2):397–413.

[41] Robotham JL, Lietman PS. Acute iron poisoning. A review. Am J Dis Child 1980;134(9):875–9.

[42] Tenenbein M. Iron. In: Ford MD, Delaney KA, Ling LJ, et al, editors. Clinical toxicology. Philadelphia: WB Saunders; 2001. p. 305–9.

[43] Banner W Jr, Tong TG. Iron poisoning. Pediatr Clin North Am 1986;33(2):393–409.

[44] Velez LI, Delaney KA. Heavy metals. In: Marx JA, Hockberger RS, Walls RM, editors. Rosen's emergency medicine concepts and clinical practice. 5th edition. St. Louis (MO): Mosby; 2002. p. 2151.

[45] Uribiarri J, Oh MS, Carroll HJ. D-lactic acidosis: a review of clinical presentation, biochemical features, and pathophysiologic mechanisms. Medicine 1998;77(2):73–82.

[46] Gauthier PM, Szerlip HM. Metabolic acidosis in the intensive care unit. Crit Care Clin 2002; 18(2):289–308.

[47] Metcalfe HK, Monson JP, Welch SG, et al. Inhibition of lactate removal by ketone bodies in rat liver: evidence for a quantitatively important role of plasma membrane lactate transporter in lactate metabolism. J Clin Invest 1986;78(3):743–7.

[48] Nadiminti Y, Wang JC, Chou SY, et al. Lactic acidosis associated with Hodgkin's disease. N Engl J Med 1980;303(1):15–7.

[49] Roth GJ, Porte D Jr. Chronic lactic acidosis and acute leukemia. Arch Intern Med 1970; 125(2):317–21.

[50] Kachel RG. Metastatic reticulum cell sarcoma and lactic acidosis. Cancer 1975;36(6): 2056–9.

[51] Chang CT, Chen YC, Fang JT, et al. Metformin-associated lactic acidosis: case reports and literature review. J Nephrol 2002;15(4):398–402.

[52] Arenas-Pinto A, Grant AD, Edwards S, et al. Lactic acidosis in HIV-infected patients: a systematic review of published cases. Sex Transm Infect 2003;79(4):340–3.

[53] Vasile B, Rasulo F, Candiani A, et al. The pathophysiology of propofol infusion syndrome: a simple name for a complex syndrome. Intensive Care Med 2003;29(9):1417–25.

[54] White SR, Kosnik J. Toxic alcohols. In: Marx JA, Hockberger RS, Walls RM, editors. Rosen's emergency medicine concepts and clinical practice. 5th edition. St. Louis (MO): Mosby; 2002. p. 2127–33.

[55] Jacobsen D, Ovrebo S, Ostborg J, et al. Glycolate causes the acidosis in ethylene glycol poisoning and is effectively removed by hemodialysis. Acta Med Scand 1984;216(4):409–16.

[56] Blakeley KR, Rinner SE, Knochel JP. Survival of ethylene glycol poisoning with profound acidemia. N Engl J Med 1993;328(7):515–6.

[57] Gabow PA, Clay K, Sullivan JB, et al. Organic acids in ethylene glycol intoxication. Ann Intern Med 1984;105(1):16–20.

[58] Parry MF, Wallach R. Ethylene glycol poisoning. Am J Med 1974;57(1):143–50.

[59] Brent J, McMartin K, Phillips S, et al. Fomepizole for the treatment of ethylene glycol poisoning. Methylpyrazole for Toxic Alcohols Study Group. N Engl J Med 1999;340(11):832–8.

[60] Karlson-Stiber C, Persson H. Ethylene glycol poisoning: experiences from an epidemic in Sweden. J Toxicol Clin Toxicol 1992;30(4):565–74.

[61] Sabeel AI, Kurkaus J, Lindholm T. Intensified dialysis treatment of ethylene glycol intoxication. Scand J Urol Nephrol 1995;29(2):125–9.

[62] Leikin JB, Toerne T, Burda A, et al. Summertime cluster of intentional ethylene glycol ingestions. JAMA 1406;278(17):1406.

[63] Zeiss J, Velasco ME, McCann KM, et al. Cerebral CT of lethal ethylene glycol intoxication with pathologic correlation. AJNR Am J Neuroradiol 1989;10(2):440–2.

[64] Morgan BW, Ford MD, Follmer R. Ethylene glycol ingestion resulting in brainstem and midbrain dysfunction. J Toxicol Clin Toxicol 2000;38(4):445–51.

[65] Seger DL, Murray L. Aspirin and nonsteroidal agents. In: Marx JA, Hockberger RS, Walls RM, editors. Rosen's emergency medicine concepts and clinical practice. 5th edition. St. Louis (MO): Mosby; 2002. p. 2076–8.

[66] Donovan JW, Akhtar J. Salicylates. In: Ford MD, Delaney KA, Ling LJ, et al, editors. Clinical toxicology. Philadelphia: WB Saunders; 2001. p. 275–80.

[67] Batlle DC, Hizon M, Cohen E, et al. The use of urinary anion gap in the diagnosis of hyperchloremic metabolic acidosis. N Engl J Med 1988;318(10):594–9.

[68] Kokko JP. Fluids and electrolytes. In: Goldman L, Bennett JC, editors. Cecil textbook of medicine. 21st edition. St. Louis (MO): Mosby; 2000. p. 562.

[69] Brenner BM, editor. The kidney. 7th edition. Philadelphia: Elsevier; 2004.

[70] Colucciello SA, Tomaszewski C. Substance Abuse. In: Marx JA, Hockberger RS, Walls RM, editors. Rosen's emergency medicine concepts and clinical practice. 5th edition. St. Louis (MO): Mosby; 2002. p. 2537.

[71] DuBose TD Jr, Caflisch CR. Validation of the difference in urine and blood CO_2 tension during bicarbonate loading as an index of distal nephron acidification in experimental models of distal renal tubular acidosis. J Clin Invest 1985;75(4):1116–23.

[72] Halperin ML, Goldstein MB, Richardson RMA, et al. Distal renal tubular acidosis syndromes: a pathophysiological approach. Am J Nephrol 1985;5(1):1–8.

[73] Forsmark CE. Chronic pancreatitis. In: Feldman M, Friedman LS, Sleisenger MH, editors. Sleisenger & Fordtran's gastrointestinal and liver disease. 7th edition. Philadelphia: Elsevier; 2002. p. 965.

ELSEVIER
SAUNDERS

EMERGENCY
MEDICINE
CLINICS OF
NORTH AMERICA

Emerg Med Clin N Am 23 (2005) 789–813

Disorders of Fuel Metabolism: Medical Complications Associated with Starvation, Eating Disorders, Dietary Fads, and Supplements

Bryan S. Judge, MD*, Bernard H. Eisenga, PhD, MD

DeVos Children's Hospital Regional Poison Center, 1300 Michigan NE Suite 203, Grand Rapids, MI 49503, USA

The number of obese people in the United States is of staggering proportions, with millions of Americans affected [1]. Each year in the United States billions and billions of US dollars are spent on weight loss regimens as well as direct health care costs related to obesity [2,3]. Furthermore, weight loss and exercise regimens, and dietary fads and supplements tend to influence those who are not truly obese, for instance, body mass index of 30 or higher [1,2]. On the other hand, there are certain groups of individuals such as prisoners of war, refugees, those afflicted by anorexia or bulimia nervosa, competitive athletes, and neglected children or elderly persons who are subjected to inadequate nutrient intake, which places them at risk for malnutrition. Consequently, many of these individuals may develop physiologic derangements that can adversely impact their health.

Due to the popularity of diet regimens and supplements, an increasing number of individuals undergoing bariatric surgery [4], anorexia and bulimia nervosa affecting approximately 1% and 3% of the US population, respectively [5–7], and with malnutrition as a threat to certain at-risk individuals, it would behoove the emergency physician to be cognizant of complications that can occur in these patients. As clinicians, we often think of disorders of fuel metabolism as inherited defects of metabolism (ie, inborn errors of metabolism); however, these disorders occur in multiple forms and are most often acquired. This article will primarily focus on the medical complications of disorders of fuel metabolism as they relate to

* Corresponding author.
E-mail address: bryan.judge@spectrum-health.org (B.S. Judge).

0733-8627/05/$ - see front matter © 2005 Elsevier Inc. All rights reserved.
doi:10.1016/j.emc.2005.03.011

states of abnormal fuel intake (starvation, eating disorders, fad diets), abnormal fuel expenditure (endurance athletes, hypermetabolic states), and dietary supplementation.

Disorders associated with abnormal intake

Malnutrition states

Malnutrition is a global problem, but not often encountered in the United States. However, through a survey performed by the Community Childhood Hunger Identification Project it was estimated that 5.5 million children under the age of 12 years in the United States fulfilled the definition of "hungry" as used in its surveys [8]. Furthermore, certain groups of the population are considered at-risk for malnutrition such as preschool-aged children, adult women, and the elderly [9]. States of malnutrition may also occur in a variety of individuals such as soldiers who are prisoners of war or undergoing vigorous training, competitive athletes, patients with immuno-compromised states or chronic debilitating diseases, and persons with eating disorders or undergoing strict diets [5,10]. Serious health consequences can arise quickly in these individuals because they tend to have reduced adiposity, and thus increasingly rely on body protein stores as an important alternative source of energy [11,12].

Starvation is a malnutrition state that results due to insufficient caloric intake. The human body's response to starvation is complex, and there are several physiologic adaptations that occur to prevent the breakdown of lean body mass and augment fat metabolism [13]. This includes the production of "stress" hormones (glucagon, epinephrine, and cortisol) that stimulate lipolysis and ketogenesis to maintain adequate plasma glucose concentrations through gluconeogenesis. As a result of these adaptations humans experience a reduction in body weight, body cell mass, body fat, total and resting energy expenditure, protein synthesis and degradation, and insulin release [10]. These changes can subsequently be reversed with appropriate caloric intake.

For simplicity, starvation can be broken down into three separate phases [11]. During Phase I, which encompasses the first few days of inadequate nutrient intake, hepatic glycogen stores are depleted to sustain glucose levels, while amassed lipids are liberated to undergo oxidation and help curb the breakdown of muscle. Subsequently, Phase II commences, whereby fat oxidation is increased, production of ketone bodies occur, and lean tissues are partially spared (cardiac and skeletal muscles are catabolized to provide the substrates (amino acids) necessary for glucose production via gluconeogenesis). Ketone bodies are an essential fuel for the central nervous system because they are able to cross the blood–brain barrier, whereas lipids cannot. However, as a consequence of ketone body production metabolic acidosis (starvation ketoacidosis) may develop. Finally, after prolonged starvation, Phase III (terminal starvation) occurs. By this time, up to 50% of body protein stores have been decimated, metabolism of lipids decline, ketone body levels fall; all of which put the starving individual in jeopardy of death.

History has shown that states of malnutrition can have untoward effects on human health. As an example, malnourished troops during the Civil War were prone to developing night blindness and scurvy secondary to deficiency of vitamins A and C, respectively [14]. However, the impact of malnutrition on an individual's health extends beyond the deleterious effects associated with poor vitamin intake. Individuals who are semistarved or starved can also develop mineral deficiencies, weakened cell-mediated and humoral immunity, altered flora, and diminished gastric acidity and mucosal integrity, all of which impair the ability to fight or prevent infection [15]. Furthermore, a starved person can die suddenly due to cardiac dysrhythmias that occur as a consequence of protein wasting in the myocardium [16]. Malnutrition not only has an impact on short-term health, but also on the long-term consequences of health. A recent prospective cohort study by Sparén et al [17] found an increase in systolic and diastolic blood pressure, and mortality from ischemic heart disease and stroke in men who experienced involuntary starvation between the ages of 6 and 28 years during the siege of Leningrad from 1941 to 1944. A complete treatise on the multitude of effects that starvation can impose on humans is outside the scope of this article; however, if the reader is so compelled, they are encouraged to refer to the authoritative text on human starvation by Keys and colleagues [18].

Starvation should not be confused with cachexia, although prolonged starvation can result in cachexia. Cachexia, which translates in Greek to "poor condition," differs significantly from starvation, and is characterized by loss of muscle mass in the setting of a chronic inflammatory disease [10]. Cachexia can occur in patients with AIDS, malignancy, chronic obstructive pulmonary disease, congestive heart failure, rheumatologic disorders, and tuberculosis [19–22]. In contrast to starvation, the nutritional alterations in cachexia include minimal or no change in body weight, and increases in resting energy expenditure, protein degradation, and peripheral insulin resistance; furthermore, adequate feeding does not reverse the changes associated with cachexia [10]. The adverse behavioral, metabolic, and physiologic effects of cachexia are mediated by myriad proinflammatory cytokines that cause an increase in the synthesis of proteins involved in the reply to cellular damage, that is, the acute-phase response [10,23]. Patients with cachexia lose a large amount of lean muscle mass due to increased protein degradation to supply the amino acids necessary to mount an acute phase response. For a comprehensive review of cachexia, please refer to articles by Kotler and Thomas [10,23].

Eating disorders

Eating disorders are a pervasive problem in our society. These disorders include anorexia nervosa, bulimia nervosa, and eating disorder not otherwise specified, and mainly affect young women across all socioeconomic classes [6,7]. Eating disorder not otherwise specified describes those patients who do not fulfill the diagnostic criteria for anorexia nervosa or bulimia nervosa, but who have manifestations of an eating disorder and will not be discussed further. Due to the significant morbidity and mortality that poses a threat to those affected by anorexia nervosa and bulimia nervosa it is imperative that the emergency physician be able to diagnose and treat the medical complications caused by these eating disorders.

Anorexia nervosa

Anorexia nervosa is an eating disorder that is exemplified by an intense fear of becoming obese, distorted perceptions of body image, extreme weight loss (failure to maintain body weight >85% of that expected) and amenorrhea [24]. Anorexia, like other eating disorders can begin subtly, that is, a person who is overweight or discontent with their body image may initially engage in moderate methods to lose weight that ultimately progresses to an obsession with eating and weight loss. Symptoms may not manifest until a patient has lost a significant amount of weight or their abnormal behavior is decisively ingrained.

Upon presentation, anorectics may complain of generalized muscle weakness, amenorrhea, weight loss, irritability, constipation, or syncopal episodes [5–7]. Physical examination findings in patients with anorexia nervosa are typical of malnourishment. They usually appear emaciated from muscle wasting and loss of subcutaneous fat that accentuates bony prominences. Heart rate, blood pressure, and temperature are typically depressed. Findings involving the extremities and skin include acrocyanosis, dry scaly skin, edema, lanugo-like hair, brittle hair and nails, and a yellow discoloration of the palms of the hands and soles of the feet [5].

Complications from anorexia nervosa arise as a consequence of starvation, and can be devastating. Sudden death as a result of cardiac dysrhythmias is a common cause of death [25], and several studies have demonstrated a prolonged QTc interval in malnourished and anorectic individuals [26–29]. An electrocardiogram may also show bradycardia, rightward axis deviation of the QRS, diminished amplitudes of the QRS complex and T wave, ST segment depression, and T-wave flattening; most of these findings having no significant clinical impact [29,30]. Other cardiovascular effects associated with anorexia nervosa include diminished cardiac mass due to protein wasting that can result in systolic and diastolic dysfunction, mitral valve prolapse, and congestive heart failure during refeeding [31–33]. Mortality rates may be as high as 20% [34]; however, a meta-analytic study by Sullivan [35] found a crude mortality rate of 5.9% from all causes of death in subjects with anorexia nervosa.

Amenorrhea is a prominent characteristic of anorexia nervosa, and occurs secondary to a disruption in the release of gonadotropin-releasing hormone from the hypothalamus [6]. Female athletes, particularly those involved in ballet, gymnastics, figure skating, and running, are at risk for amenorrhea [6,7], and may go on to develop the female athlete triad, that is, abnormal eating behaviors, amenorrhea, and osteoporosis [36]. Amenorrhea typically coincides with weight loss; however, in approximately 20% of anorectics and over 50% of normal-weight bulimics amenorrhea may occur before weight loss [7,37]. With appropriate weight gain normal function of the hypothalamic–pituitary–ovarian axis is usually restored and menses resumes; however, amenorrhea may be prolonged in many individuals despite adequate weight gain [38].

The most profound consequence of amenorrhea in anorectics is osteopenia. Reduced bone mass can occur even with a short duration of illness [39], and in one study over 50% of anorectics had a bone mineral density that was greater than 2 standard deviations below normal for age and gender [40]. Although not completely understood, osteopenia in patients with anorexia nervosa most likely develops due to a combination of inadequate nutritional factors, an imbalance of hormonal mediators (cortisol, growth hormone), estrogen deficiency, low body weight, and excessive exercise [6,41]. Furthermore, the degree of osteopenia is dependent upon the duration of amenorrhea and the severity of weight loss [42,43]. In a longitudinal study of anorectic patients, Rigotti and colleagues found a relative risk of 7.1 for nonspine fractures when compared with healthy age-matched females [44]. The most effective approach to combating osteopenia includes a treatment program to encourage weight gain sufficient to resume menses and proper dietary intake [45]; however, osteopenia frequently persists even after appropriate weight gain [46].

Another organ system adversely affected in anorectics is the gastrointes-tinal system; however, complications are less pronounced than those seen in bulimics. Gastrointestinal motility is diminished, and may result in postprandial fullness and pain that can precipitate vomiting [47]. Decreased food intake results in dysfunction of the colon and chronic constipation [48]. Fecal impaction may occur in anorectic patients with severely limited oral intake [49]. Overall, the adverse effects imposed on the gastrointestinal system by anorexia nervosa will resolve over time with appropriate intake of nutrients, dietary fiber, and fluid [50].

Anemia and leukopenia occur commonly in starving individuals, and the incidence of both may be as high as 35% in anorectic patients [18,51]. Thrombocytopenia is less commonly seen with anorexia nervosa, occurring in approximately 10% of patients [52]. A recent case series by Abella and colleagues [53] found abnormal bone marrow in 89% of patients with anorexia nervosa, and that the extent of damage to the bone marrow correlated with the amount of weight loss. These hematologic abnormalities may result in fatigue, and increase the risk for bleeding or infection; however, a small study by Bowers suggests that anorectic patients with leukopenia do not have a propensity for infections [54]. With appropriate nutrition and therapy, the anemia, leukopenia, thrombocytopenia, and bone marrow changes that can result from starvation states is typically reversed [18,51,55].

Bulimia nervosa

Bulimia nervosa is characterized by the large consumption or binges of food at least two times a week over a period of at least 3 months, in which the individual attempts to balance the excess food intake through a variety of purging (diuretics, laxative abuse, vomiting) and nonpurging (over-exercising, fasting) techniques [24]. Episodes of bingeing and purging may occur covertly, and are often coupled with alcohol and substance abuse [56–58]. Bulimics like those with anorexia nervosa are typically in denial about their condition and usually do not seek medical attention until a concerned parent compels them to visit a physician.

Patients with bulimia nervosa may present with complaints of muscle cramps, heartburn, fatigue, bloody diarrhea, bruising, irregular menstrual periods, syncopal episodes, parotid gland swelling, dizziness, generalized abdominal pain, impaired concentration, sore throat, and mouth sores [5–7,59]. On physical examination they may have low, high, or more typically normal body weight, and vital sign determination may reveal bradycardia, hypotension, and hypothermia [5,6]. Further scrutiny may demonstrate calluses over the dorsum of the dominant hand (Russell's sign) from self-induced emesis [58], enlargement of the parotid glands from frequent bingeing that occurs in up to 30% of patients [60], dental enamel erosions that are most prominent on the lingual surface of the upper teeth, which are caused by gastric acid [61], and petechial hemorrhages involving the face or subconjunctiva from recent forceful emesis [59].

Bulimics are at risk for numerous and sometimes life-threatening medical complications. Up to 50% of patients with bulimia nervosa will have electrolyte or fluid disturbances that are secondary to vomiting, abuse of diuretics or laxatives, or dehydration [59]. Hypokalemia has been reported to occur in approximately 14% of bulimics [62], and may contribute to the development of cardiac dysrhythmias, rhabdomyolysis, and impairment of smooth and skeletal muscle function. When hyponatremia is detected it should raise the treating physician's suspicion for (1) excessive water intake by the bulimic patient to curb hunger pangs or "gain weight" before an appointment with a health care provider, (2) abuse of thiazide diuretics that can produce marked sodium depletion, or (3) prolonged purging that results in depletion of total body sodium [5,6]. Other electrolyte abnormalities such as hypocalcemia, hypomagnesemia, and hypophosphatemia occur less commonly [59].

Excessive purging can lead to intravascular volume depletion and dehydration. The body compensates by increasing production of aldosterone, which acts to retain sodium to preserve intravascular volume. This secondary hyperaldosteronism can mimic Bartter's syndrome (pseudo-

Bartter's syndrome) [63]. In patients with total body sodium depletion this mechanism by which the body maintains intravascular volume may be compromised. Other laboratory findings in bulimics include metabolic alkalosis and metabolic acidosis. One study found that over 25% of patients with bulimia had metabolic alkalosis [62]. The metabolic alkalosis results from the loss of gastric acid and volume contraction. Metabolic acidosis can occur in those who abuse laxatives, and is generated from the loss of alkaline fluid from the gastrointestinal tract. In fact, in patients with bulimia the presence of metabolic acidosis may serve as a marker for laxative abuse; however, the lack of this finding on laboratory testing does not rule it out [64].

Gastrointestinal complications are particularly problematic for patients with bulimia. Repeated episodes of bingeing and purging can result in gastrointestinal bleeding, constipation, duodenal and gastric ulcers, delayed gastric emptying, malabsorption syndromes, gastroesophageal reflux, Mallory-Weiss tears, and esophagitis [48,65]. Unusual but important gastrointestinal sequelae associated with bulimia nervosa include esophageal perforation, pancreatitis, and gastric distention culminating in perforation from excessive bingeing [59].

Medication abuse by individuals with eating disorders

To facilitate the purging process some patients with eating disorders may abuse several types of laxatives, diuretics, or syrup of ipecac. Laxative abuse, which accounted for 7% to 15% of cases of diarrhea of undetermined etiology when patients were screened for laxatives [66,67], most commonly causes diarrhea but may cause abdominal cramping, pain with defecation, bloody stools, and if protracted, may lead to fluid and electrolyte disturbances and impair gastrointestinal motility [68]. Chronic abuse of two groups of stimulant laxatives, diphenolic (bisacodyl and phenolphthalein) and anthraquinones (danthron and senna) has been associated with cathartic colon, a state of abnormal colonic function and structure [69,70]. Prolonged use of anthraquinones may cause melanosis coli, a brown–black discoloration of the rectal and sigmoid mucosa visualized during colonoscopy [68]. This discoloration serves only as a marker of chronic anthraquinone ingestion, and debate exists whether the chronic abuse of anthraquinone laxatives increases the risk for colorectal cancer [71,72]. Other complications associated with anthraquinone abuse include clubbing of the fingers (senna) [73], and cholestatic hepatitis (cascara) [74], whereas phenolphthalein has been associated with fixed drug eruptions [75].

Abuse of syrup of ipecac can be significantly more toxic than laxative abuse. Ipecac contains emetine, an alkaloid that induces vomiting and is toxic to cardiac and skeletal muscle [76]. Chronic use of ipecac can result in myopathy, cardiomyopathy, dysrhythmias, and death; patients may initially present with nausea, vomiting, muscle weakness, and myalgias [76–78]. Furthermore, tolerance to the emetic effects of emetine develop with prolonged use, and enhanced systemic absorption can occur in patients who ingest more and more ipecac to achieve the desired clinical effect [76]. Ipecac-induced myopathy is usually reversible with cessation of the drug unless complicated by cardiovascular toxicity or the primary disease, and recovery may take several months [78].

Anorectic and bulimic individuals may also use diuretics to "lose weight" by decreasing body water. However, the chronic use of diuretics and laxatives does not result in net weight loss, but rather the perception of weight loss through a transient decrease in body water [79]. Prescription diuretics that may be abused include loop, potassium-sparing, and thiazide diuretics. Loop diuretic (furosemide, ethacrynic acid) toxicity can result in hypokalemia, hypomagnesemia, metabolic alkalosis, orthostatic hypotesion, and hearing loss [80–82]; toxic effects from thiazide diuretics (chlorothiazide, hydrochlorothiazide) include hypokalemia, hyponatremia, metabolic alkalosis, paresthesias, and pulmonary edema [83–85]; and toxicity of potassium-sparing diuretics (spironolactone, triamterene) can produce hyperkalemia and hyperchloremic metabolic acidosis [86,87].

Nutritional consequences of bariatric surgery

Over 100,000 gastrointestinal surgeries were performed in the United States for severe obesity in 2003 [4]. Patients who undergo these procedures are at risk for several nutritional deficiencies. Iron deficiency anemia occurs commonly in postbariatric surgery patients, and is secondary to malabsorption and maldigestion of dietary iron [88]. A recent study [89] suggested that addition of vitamin C to iron supplements after bariatric surgery is more effective in restoring hemoglobin and ferritin than iron therapy alone. Whereas a prospective, double-blind, randomized study by Brolin et al [88] found that prophylactic iron therapy prevented iron deficiency but was inconsistent in thwarting anemia in menstruating women who had undergone a Roux-en-Y gastric bypass.

Wernicke-Korsakoff syndrome has also been reported in a number of patients who have undergone bariatric surgery [90–92]. Patients who experience excessive vomiting postsurgery are at risk for developing this complication and usually do not develop signs and symptoms (ataxia, confusion, diplopia, ophthalmoplegia, peripheral neuropathy) until several months after the onset of vomiting [93]. Prompt recognition of Wernicke-Korsakoff syndrome and treatment with thiamine before administration of glucose are paramount in preventing the severe and often permanent sequelae associated with this disease.

An important long-term complication of bariatric surgery is the adverse effect that it can impart on the skeletal system. Abnormalities in calcium and vitamin D metabolism that result from gastrointestinal bypass operations can lead to severe metabolic bone disease that may not be detected until years later [94]. A recent study by Coates and colleagues [95] demonstrated that within 3 to 9 months after a laparoscopic Roux-en-Y gastric bypass patients experienced a significant increase in bone resorption and significant decrease in bone mineral content. Patients who have undergone a bariatric procedure should be treated with calcium and vitamin D supplements to protect against hypocalcemia and vitamin D deficiency.

Fad diets

Over the past few years, many Americans have adopted low-carbohydrate diets as a method in which to lose weight. Generally, these regimens promote the consumption of foods high in fat and protein, while limiting intake of carbohydrates. The lack of carbohydrates induces a ketotic state that facilitates weight loss through diuresis. Ketosis and dehydration can result in constipation, fatigue, nephrolithiasis, and orthostatic hypotension [96]. Weight gain recurs with rehydration and appropriate dietary intake. To date, there have been no controlled clinical trials to evaluate the efficacy of low-carbohydrate diets. However, a recent systematic review of low-carbohydrate diets found that they had no significant adverse effect on systolic blood pressure, fasting blood glucose and insulin levels, or serum lipid levels; however, the authors of the review concluded that they were unable to make a recommendation for or against the use of low-carbohydrate diets due to lack of sufficient evidence [97].

Some fad diets are not without risk. In the 1970s, liquid protein diets were a popular way to lose vast amounts of weight. However, several individuals experienced sudden death while on these regimens. Many of the patients had a prolonged QTc, torsades de pointes, ventricular dysrhythmias, or died during refeeding [16,98]. The cause of death from low calorie diets has been proposed to stem from cardiac protein wasting [16], increased myocardial sensitivity to catecholamines [99], and diet-induced QTc prolongation [98], all of which can give rise to fatal dysrhythmias.

Emergency management of the patient with a disorder associated with abnormal intake

Patients with many of the disorders discussed above can present unique therapeutic challenges for the emergency physician. If a patient appears malnourished upon presentation, pertinent information should be obtained regarding their dietary habits, amount of weight loss, past medical history, social situation, medications, and use of supplements. Intravenous access should be established and the patient placed on a cardiac monitor. A comprehensive metabolic panel (including phosphate level), complete blood count, and EKG are prudent to rule out electrolyte disturbances, hematologic abnormalities, and prolonged QTc interval, respectively. Appropriate imaging studies should be tailored for each individual patient if a gastrointestinal complication or fracture is suspected. Patients should also be assessed for any underlying psychiatric illnesses and substance abuse. Indications for hospital admission include severe malnutrition, dehydration, electrolyte disturbances, cardiac dysrhythmias, autonomic instability, failure of outpatient therapy for an eating disorder, uncontrollable bingeing and purging, hazardous social situation, medical complications associated with malnutrition, suicidal ideations, or severe depression [100].

Although it seems logical to administer intravenous fluids and provide nutrition to a severely malnourished individual, the treating physician must use caution when doing so because these patients are at risk for refeeding syndrome. Refeeding syndrome was first described in Japanese prisoners of war shortly after World War II [101]. During starvation insulin secretion is diminished in response to decreased intake of carbohydrates and the body relies on the catabolism of fat and protein for energy. Stores of intracellular phosphate become depleted even though some patients may have normal serum phosphate levels [102]. When starving patients are administered carbohydrates enterally or parenterally, insulin secretion increases and stimulates the cellular uptake of phosphate, which can produce severe hypophosphatemia [103]. As a consequence of hypophosphatemia and refeeding, cells are unable to produce sufficient adenosine triphosphate (ATP) to meet increased metabolic demands, which results in several physiologic derangements [104].

Usually, hypophosphatemia associated with refeeding syndrome occurs within 3 days of beginning feeding [102]. Significant clinical effects from refeeding syndrome include dysrhythmias, respiratory failure, rhabdomyolysis, seizures, coma, congestive heart failure, weakness, hemolysis, hypotension, ileus, metabolic acidosis, and sudden death [102–104]. Refeeding syndrome is preventable, and the role of the emergency physician is to identify patients at risk and avoid overzealous administration of intravenous fluids and nutrition, unless a medical emergency mandates otherwise, for example, hypoglycemia, or hypotension. To circumvent refeeding syndrome malnourished patients should be admitted with consultation from a dietician, electrolytes monitored, phosphate supplemented, and a gradual, progressive feeding regimen instituted [34].

Disorders associated with abnormal fuel expenditure

Several illnesses can produce high nutritional requirements and include bacteremia and sepsis, drug overdose, adverse and idiosyncratic drug reactions, hormonal dysfunction, and neurologic disease. Specific examples are thyrotoxicosis, pancreatitis, sepsis, AIDS wasting syndrome, advanced cancer, burns, salicylate or monoamine oxidase inhibitor intoxication, neuroleptic malignant syndrome, serotonin syndrome, and spastic neurologic disease. All of these conditions produce a hypermetabolic state characterized by increased energy expenditure or increased metabolic rates that ultimately causes increased cellular carbon dioxide.

Early recognition of malignant hyperthermia may be associated with elevated end-tidal carbon dioxide, and may help in the diagnosis of this condition [105]. Excretion of high amounts of carbon dioxide stresses the respiratory system, producing hyperventilation that can often lead to skeletal muscle fatigue and respiratory failure. Respiratory failure can also be characterized by inadequate access to energy substrates or inadequate cellular production of energy equivalents. Inattention to adequate energy replacement can result in underestimation of the necessary energy equivalents for proper cellular function.

Physiologic responses to disease are often characterized by increased production of oxidation byproducts that results in cellular oxidative stress [106]. Oxidative stress produces free radicals that accumulate intracellularly, damaging mitochondria and subsequently inhibits the cellular production of ATP. Free radicals can also produce lipid peroxidation byproducts that in a cyclic fashion augments the production of additional free radicals and other toxic metabolites, all of which are directly toxic to the lung and appear to be significant factors in the development of acute respiratory distress syndrome. Multiple other organ systems can be damaged by free radicals leading to shock and poor cardiac output [106].

Patients suffering from these conditions require judicious replacement of energy substrates to maintain the functions of life. This includes carbohydrates, short chain fatty acids, protein, vitamins, and other micronutrients [107]. Protein catabolism is markedly increased in these disease states, and to maintain lean body mass adequate protein should be made available. For example, it has been estimated that a severely burned patient may require from 6000 to 9000 kcal per day to maintain energy reserves [108]. Protein requirements may be as high as 4 g/kg of body weight per day [108]. Studies have shown a beneficial effect such as increased lean body mass from a combination of arginine, glutamine, and beta-hydroxy-beta-methylbutyrate (HMB) in burn patients and those suffering from cachexia due to advanced cancer and AIDS [109,110]. Enteral nutrition has not been proven to be superior, but it is believed to improve clinical outcome when compared with parenteral nutrition, and should be instituted as early as possible; however, in patients with impaired gastrointestinal function such as short gut syndrome, bowel obstruction, ileus, or pancreatitis, parenteral nutrition may be required [111,112]. In general, nutritional supplementation should be started within a few days after the onset of illness [113].

Dietary supplements

The thrust to excel and win has consumed the world of athletics. Over the last 10 years there has been an explosive growth in the use of over-the-counter dietary supplements by athletes both professional and amateur that are hyped to enhance energy production and improve recovery (ergogenics), enhance stamina, or prevent fatigue and increase muscle mass [114–118]. These include creatine monohydrate, dehydroepiandrostenedione (DHEA), androstenedione, and the methylxanthines (eg, caffeine). Other commonly used supplements include ephedrine or ephedrine-containing products and HMB. Although word-of-mouth appraisals by athletes have touted the ergogenic benefits of many of these compounds, there is little evidence to support the use of most of these products. Arguably, some of these products have undesirable side effects and may actually cause toxicity.

Creatine Monohydrate

One of the most widely used supplements by athletes including professional, amateur, and adolescents is creatine monohydrate [119]. Although creatine monohydrate is primarily used to enhance athletic performance, it has been used in patients with congestive heart failure with variable success, and has been shown to be neuroprotective in animals when administrated before brain injury [120,121]. Studies have demonstrated that creatine monohydrate possesses significant antioxidant and antiinflammatory activity [119,122]. Furthermore, creatine monohydrate may improve serum cholesterol and certain neuromuscular disorders including congenital myopathies, muscular dystrophy, inflammatory myopathies, and amyotrophic lateral sclerosis [120,123,124].

Creatine monohydrate is a naturally occurring compound and cellular energy intermediate that is used for the production of energy for muscle contraction. It is found in all tissues including the liver, pancreas, kidney, and brain, but the highest concentrations are in muscle, which contains about 0.5% creatine monohydrate per gram muscle weight. Creatine monohydrate is formed endogenously, but can also be obtained from exogenous sources. Individuals with high daily meat ingestion can consume upwards of 3 to 5 g of creatine monohydrate per day as 0.2 kg of meat contains approximately 1 g of creatine monohydrate. Creatine monohydrate can be legally obtained over the counter as an oral dietary supplement and recommended doses for promotion of ergogenic effects vary from 3 to 20 g/d. Regimens for enhancement of muscular performance include a loading and maintenance phase, or daily supplementation to achieve the desired ergogenic effects.

After oral administration, creatine monohydrate is absorbed in the intestine and transported in the blood. Creatine monohydrate is excreted unchanged in the urine or metabolized to creatinine before urinary excretion with a total body loss of about 2 g/d. Upon cellular uptake, creatine monohydrate is readily phosphorylated to form creatine phosphate (CP) that can act as an energy intermediate. During anaerobic muscle activity ATP provides the energy necessary for coupling of actin and myosin molecules that results in muscular contraction. ATP is rapidly degraded during this reaction to form ADP. Therefore, CP is an important immediate source of phosphate for the production of ATP, and can facilitate extended muscular contraction. Stores of both ATP and CP are limited, and are available for brief, intense power during anaerobic muscle contraction. Under normal conditions most muscle cells have enough CP to carry on anaerobic muscular activity for approximately 10 seconds, and it takes upwards of 60 seconds to regenerate CP in conditions of anaerobic muscular activity.

Creatine monohydrate has gained popularity over the last 10 years, but had been used by athletes in Eastern Bloc nations including the former Soviet Union for over 20 years [125]. Anecdotal reports from athletes and trainers in these countries exalting the ergogenic effects of creatine monohydrate supplementation, as well as, performance of these athletes in world wide competitions led to the use of creatine monohydrate supplements by athletes in Western nations. Over the last decade several placebo-controlled research studies using blinded and nonblinded subjects have investigated the effects of oral creatine monohydrate supplementation on athletes [126–131]. Why supplement with creatine monohydrate? It has been theorized that by maximizing the cellular stores of creatine monohydrate an individual could perform a more strenuous workload that would ultimately increase muscular strength. A study assessing the efficacy of creatine monohydrate supplementation by athletes has demonstrated a positive effect on workload and enhanced power and strength in untrained subjects; however, creatine monohydrate supplementation has little effect on aerobic performance [132]. Other studies assessing these effects in trained athletes and physically active men are less convincing [133,134].

Short-term administration of creatine monohydrate is generally considered safe and recent long-term data show no significant effect on clinical markers of health in individuals using creatine monohydrate supplements [135]. Safety of usage over periods longer than 21 months has yet to be reported. Because creatine monohydrate is metabolized to creatinine, debate exists regarding the renal toxicity of creatine monohydrate supplements. There have been some case reports of renal dysfunction in subjects using creatine monohydrate; however, a correlation between creatine monohydrate usage and renal impairment has not been demonstrated [136]. Interestingly, there has been a case report of nephrotic syndrome in a male using an anabolic steroid and creatine monohydrate on a long-term basis [137]. In general, the short-term usage of creatine monohydrate is not associated with impairment of renal function.

Most studies assessing the short-term use of creatine monohydrate demonstrate few toxic sequelae. Creatine monohydrate use can cause gastrointestinal upset with some nausea, vomiting, and diarrhea. These effects usually occur in naive users, and generally will resolve over time. Subjects also demonstrate weight gain either due to water retention or skeletal muscle hypertrophy. From assessment of the literature it appears that creatine monohydrate users at risk for significant toxic manifestations are those who have underlying renal dysfunction, those using diuretics, those who become dehydrated either from voluntary water restriction (wrestlers), or those who do not adequately replace fluid loss during exercise.

Oral creatine monohydrate is made by a number of different suppliers, and due to production techniques may contain potentially toxic or carcinogenic contaminants [138]. There is no control by the United States Food and Drug Administration (FDA) over the processing and distribution of oral creatine monohydrate supplements. Theoretically, risks can be minimized by the consumption of adequate amounts of water, limiting use to periods not longer than one to two consecutive months, using a pure product that is not contaminated with potentially toxic components and not exceeding the recommended doses. However, as with many of these over-the-counter supplements caution should be taken when using creatine monohydrate.

Beta-hydroxy-beta-methylbutyrate

HMB is another over-the-counter product that has been subjected to extensive research. HMB is a naturally occurring metabolite of L-leucine and is structurally related to the other branched-chained amino acids L-isoleucine and L-valine. HMB is considered an ergogenic agent that has additional nitrogen-sparing anticatabolic activity. The mechanism of action for HMB is unknown, although it has been hypothesized to involve cholesterol synthesis and membrane repair after strenuous muscle activity [139].

HMB is often used with amino acids or combinations of amino acids and creatine monohydrate. Combinations of HMB, arginine, and glutamine given to patients with cachexia from advanced AIDS, cancer, and burns have shown increases in lean body mass [109,110]. Research has also demonstrated beneficial effects in body composition and protein metabolism in elderly women using HMB, arginine, and lysine [140]. Evaluation of strength gain and fat free mass in untrained collegiate males after HMB supplementation demonstrated increases in both parameters in a dose response fashion [141]. Concomitant use of HMB and creatine monohydrate has shown no adverse effects on all indices of health studied in trained male athletes, and this combination has been shown to synergistically increase lean body mass and muscle strength when combined with a weight-training program [142,143]. Furthermore, 8 weeks of HMB supplementation to healthy untrained collegiate males did not show any adverse effects on hepatic enzyme function, lipid profile, or renal function [144].

Human studies on the use of HMB to promote strength and lean body mass have shown equivocal results [145–147]. A meta-analysis by Nissen and Sharp suggests that HMB supplementation will augment lean body mass and improve strength parameters and another study led by the same authors demonstrated that HMB supplementation is safe in recommended doses and may actually improve objective measures of health such as reductions in systolic blood pressure and total cholesterol [148,149]. Other data suggest HMB supplementation or a combination of HMB and creatine monohydrate to trained athletes is not effective for increasing aerobic power or anaerobic capacity [150]. HMB has been shown to improve lean body mass and strength for untrained or elderly individuals; however, these benefits are less apparent in highly trained individuals [151,152]. Regardless of the debate over the efficacy of HMB for improving lean body mass and strength, supplementation in recommended doses appears to be safe [144]. Additionally, supplementation with high doses of arginine, glutamine or lysine together with HMB appears to be well tolerated and safe, as is use with creatine monohydrate [109,110,140].

Androstenedione

Androstenedione has been banned by many sports organizations including the National Football League, the National Collegiate Athletics Association, and the International Olympic Committee. Recently, the FDA has issued an edict to discontinue manufacture, marketing, and distribution of androstenedione-containing products to companies producing these dietary supplements. Despite this, androstenedione remains a popular supplement among many athletes [132].

Androstenedione is a naturally occurring steroid produced in the adrenal gland, and the gonad and is synthesized from DHEA. Recommended supplemental doses of androstendione are usually 50 to 100 mg/d, although higher doses have been suggested for achieving the desired anabolic effect. The metabolic fate of androstenedione includes the production of testosterone and also estradiol. Commercially produced androstenedione is obtained from microbiologic oxidation of cholesterol or plant phytosterols. Androstenedione is a precursor in the commercial production of testosterone and other anabolic steroids, oral contraceptives, and other hormones. Androstenedione is also available in many over-the-counter dietary supplements.

Androstenedione is rarely used alone but most often in combination with other androgen precursors in a process known as "stacking." "Stacking" requires the use of different androstendione precursors and other substances touted to prevent androstendione metabolism to estradiol. It is believed stacking will promote the ideal conditions for muscle growth and also minimize the estrogen-like side effects well known to be associated with the use of anabolic steroids, such as gynecomastia. Androstendione is also used in combination with growth hormone (hGH) or growth hormone secretagogues.

Androstenedione supplementation will increase plasma testosterone for short periods, but a positive effect on nitrogen retention and increased muscle mass and strength after use of these dietary supplements has not been demonstrated [153–156]. Interestingly, there appears to be downregulation of endogenous testosterone in men who use androstendione supplementation for at least 4 weeks [157]. Androstenedione produces similar side effects to those caused by anabolic steroids including unfavorable changes in serum lipids, aggressive behavior, and may cause serious liver problems [154–156].

DHEA

DHEA is a naturally occurring hormone produced principally in the adrenal cortex. DHEA and its sulfated metabolite DHEAS have weak androgenic activity. DHEA production decreases with age and levels of DHEAS are typically low in chronic disease states such as cancer and AIDS. DHEA does not have significant ergogenic effects because only minute amounts are metabolized to androstendione; therefore, use by athletes is limited. Oral DHEA administration will cause increases in serum levels of DHEA and DHEAS; however, long-term daily administration to men has shown no changes in serum lutenizing hormone levels, follicle stimulating hormone levels, or prostate specific antigen [158]. Although DHEA production declines with age, many of the studies assessing the efficacy of supplemental DHEA have shown conflicting results [159].

DHEA is believed to have significant anti-inflammatory and anti-aging effects. Because of this, DHEA supplementation is believed to be beneficial for use in the elderly. Although DHEA is banned in Canada and the United Kingdom, it is available in the United States and there has been an increase in the use of DHEA by the elderly and middle-aged adults. The recommended dose for supplemental DHEA is 25 to 50 mg/d but, as with androstendione, higher doses have also been recommended.

DHEA supplementation to perimenopausal women has shown no improvement in severity of symptoms, and no differences in lipid profiles were detected between the study groups [160]. However, short-term and long-term administration of DHEA to postmenopausal women has shown positive effects on menopausal symptoms and appears to modulate growth hormone secretion [161–163]. Elderly males given DHEA have not shown an increase in bone turnover rates, and a study by Kawano et al has demonstrated improvement in endothelial function and insulin sensitivity in men given low-dose DHEA supplementation [164,165]. Further investigation is required to address the relevance of these findings.

Both DHEA and androstendione can produce a number of unwanted and undesirable side effects. Supplementation of DHEA or androstenedione in healthy young males has not shown changes in lean body mass, strength, or testosterone levels [166]. Masculine changes in females including clitoromegaly, hirsutism, hair loss, and deepening of the voice have occurred with the use of DHEA. Acne, transient hepatitis, and deceased levels of high-density lipoprotein (HDL) have also been reported.

Dietary stimulants for weight loss and improvement of athletic performance have been used for decades. These stimulants include amphetamine, cocaine, the methylxanthines, and ephedra-containing products. Historically, both amphetamine and cocaine were used to enhance endurance and improve performance and both have been used to enhance weight loss. Due to prominent side effects, including death, both have been banned. Recently, the FDA banned the manufacture and distribution of ephredra-containing products due to the many reports of significant toxicity and death associated with their use.

Ephedra

Ephedra, commonly known as Ma-Huang, is a naturally occurring alkaloid found in a number of plants, including *Ephedra sinensis*. Herbal preparations containing ephedra have been used for centuries in the Far East, for myriad proposed benefits. Athletes have used these preparations to combat fatigue and enhance athletic performance. However, the purported ergogenic effects of ephedra-containing herbs have not been demonstrated in scientific studies. Ephedrine is the active component of the ephedra-containing plants, and is a sympathomimetic that causes the release of both central and peripheral biogenic amines including norepinephrine, epinephrine, and dopamine. The release of these biogenic amines most likely contributes to the stimulation and "perceived" performance enhancement associated with the use of these herbal products.

Ephedrine is used as the starting material in the illicit production of amphetamine and methamphetamine. Ephedrine-containing products have been used in a number of weight loss products. The toxicity associated with the use of these products includes elevations in blood pressure, myocardial infarction, cerebral vascular accidents, and death [167–171]. Although the risk of death is low with use of these products, the associated adverse effects, the unpredictability of individual response, and the use of ephedrine in the production of methamphetamine led to the ban by the FDA [172].

Methylxanthines

The methylxanthines include caffeine, theobromine, and theophylline. These compounds are naturally occurring, and found in coffee beans, tea leaves, and chocolate. These products have been used for centuries, and are commonly consumed on a daily basis. Caffeine is the prototypical methylxanthine, and has been shown to have a significant ergogenic effect with noted improvement in both aerobic and anaerobic activities [115,173,174]. Although extensive research on caffeine has been done, debate continues regarding its ergogenic effects and overall mechanism of action. Caffeine inhibits membrane adenosine receptors, is involved in the deactivation of cellular cyclic adenosine monophosphate (cAMP), and augments the availabilty of fatty acids [115,173–175]. Caffeine has shown to be ergogenic when combined with creatine monohydrate monohydrate and exercise [176].

Caffeine is well tolerated in most individuals, but adverse effects can occur from significant ingestion including insomnia, irritability, premature ventricular contractions, heartburn, and seizures. Caffeine is recognized as safe and is used by many Olympic athletes, because the cutoff permitted in Olympic competition is high [174].

There are numerous agents advertised to improve athletic performance, enhance endurance, increase strength, and decrease the effects of aging. Most of the agents are readily available over the counter, and studies assessing efficacy are lacking or are poorly designed and controlled. Use of these products particularly by adolescents and young adults should be discouraged. Time and further investigation will support or disprove the claims made by the manufacturers of these products. Caution should be the rule when using these supplements.

Summary

Disorders of fuel metabolism occur in many forms. Life-threatening medical complications can arise in individuals who are suffering from a starvation state, eating disorder, fad diet, hypermetabolic state, or the abuse of dietary supplements. Comprehension of these disorders is beneficial, because an emergency physician can anticipate encountering several patients with these disorders throughout their career. It is imperative when confronted with such a patient in the emergency department that the treating physician is able to identify and institute appropriate therapy for the complications associated with these disorders.

References

[1] Flegal KM, Carroll MD, Ogden CL, et al. Prevalence and trends in obesity among US adults, 1999–2000. JAMA 2002;288:1723–7.
[2] Perrone J. Dieting agents and regimens. In: Goldfrank L, Flomenbaum N, Lewin N, et al, editors. Goldfrank's toxicologic emergencies. 7th edition. New York: McGraw-Hill; 2002. p. 2170.
[3] Wolf AM, Colditz GA. Current estimates of the economic cost of obesity in the United States. Obes Res 1998;6:97–106.
[4] Steinbrook R. Surgery for severe obesity. N Engl J Med 2004;350:1075–9.
[5] Comerci GD. Medical complications of anorexia nervosa and bulimia nervosa. Med Clin North Am 1990;74:1293–310.
[6] Golden NH. Eating disorders in adolescence and their sequelae. Best Practice Res Clin Obstet Gynaecol 2003;17:57–73.

[7] Rome ES. Eating disorders. Obstet Gynecol Clin N Am 2003;30:353–77.
[8] Wehler CA, Scott RI, Anderson JJ, et al. Community Childhood Hunger Identification Project: a survey of childhood hunger in the United States. Washington (DC): Food Research and Action Center; 1995.
[9] Rose D, Oliveira V. Nutrient intakes of individuals from food-insufficient households in the United States. Am J Public Health 1997;87:1956–61.
[10] Kotler DP. Cachexia. Ann Intern Med 2000;133:622–34.
[11] Castellini MA, Rea LD. The biochemistry of natural fasting at its limits. Experientia 1992; 48:575–82.
[12] Goodman MN, Lowell B, Belur E, et al. Sites of protein conservation and loss during starvation: influence of adiposity. Am J Physiol Endocrinol Metab 1984;246:E383–90.
[13] Cahill GF Jr. Starvation in man. N Engl J Med 1970;282:668–75.
[14] Bollet AJ. Malnutrition in Civil War armies. Pharos Alpha Omega Alpha Honor Med Soc 2003;66:18–28.
[15] Tomkins A, Watson F. Malnutrition and infection: a review. Geneva (Switzerland): World Health Organization; 1989.
[16] Sours HE, Frattali VP, Brand CD, et al. Sudden death associated with very low calorie weight reduction regimens. Am J Clin Nutr 1981;34:453–61.
[17] Sparen P, Vagero D, Shestov DB, et al. Long term mortality after severe starvation during the seige of Leningrad: prospective cohort study. BMJ 2004;328:11–4.
[18] Keys A, Brozek J, Henschel A, et al. The biology of human starvation. Vols. 1 and 2. Minneapolis: Univ. of Minnesota Press; 1950.
[19] Kotler DP, Wang J, Pierson RN. Body composition studies in patients with the acquired immunodeficiency syndrome. Am J Clin Nutr 1985;42:1255–65.
[20] Roubenoff R, Roubenoff RA, Cannon JG, et al. Rheumatoid cachexia: cytokine-driven hypermetabolism accompanying reduced body cell mass in chronic inflammation. J Clin Invest 1994;93:2379–86.
[21] Shike M, Russell DM, Detsky AS, et al. Changes in body composition in patients with small-cell cancer. The effect of total parenteral nutrition as an adjunct to chemotherapy. Ann Intern Med 1984;101:303–9.
[22] Toth MJ, Gottlieb SS, Goran MI, et al. Daily energy expenditure in free-living heart failure patients. Am J Physiol Endocrinol Metab 1997;272:E469–75.
[23] Thomas DR. Distinguishing starvation from cachexia. Clin Geriatr Med 2002;18: 883–91.
[24] Association American Psychiatric. Diagnostic and statistical manual of mental disorders. 4th edition. Washington (DC): American Psychiatric Association Press; 1994.
[25] Beaumont PJ, Russell JD, Touyz SW. Treatment of anorexia nervosa. Lancet 1993;341: 1635–40.
[26] Cooke RA, Chambers JB, Singh R, et al. QT interval in anorexia nervosa. Br Heart J 1994; 71:69–73.
[27] Corovic N, Durakovic Z. Misigoj-Durakovic: dispersion of the corrected QT interval in the electrocardiogram of the ex-prisoners of war. Int J Cardiol 2003;88:279–83.
[28] Isner JM, Roberts WC, Heymsfield SB, et al. Anorexia nervosa and sudden death. Ann Intern Med 1985;102:49–52.
[29] Swenne I, Larsson PT. Heart risk associated with weight loss in anorexia nervosa and eating disorders: risk factors for QTc interval prolongation and dispersion. Acta Paediatr 1999;88: 304–9.
[30] Mehler PS, Chri Gray M, Schulte M. Medical complications of anorexia nervosa. J Womens Health 1997;6:533–41.
[31] de Simone G, Scalfi L, Galderisi M, et al. Cardiac abnormalities in young women with anorexia nervosa. Br Heart J 1994;71:287–92.
[32] Galetta F, Franzoni F, Prattichizzo F, et al. Heart rate variability and left ventricular diastolic function in anorexia nervosa. J Adolesc Health 2003;32:416–21.

[33] Schocken DD, Holloway JD, Powers PS. Weight loss and the heart. Effects of anorexia nervosa and starvation. Arch Intern Med 1989;149:877–81.

[34] Melchior JC. From malnutrition to refeeding during anorexia nervosa. Curr Opin Clin Nutr Metab Care 1998;1:481–5.

[35] Sullivan PF. Mortality in anorexia nervosa. Am J Psychiatry 1995;152:1073–4.

[36] Yeager KK, Agostini R, Nattiv A. The female athlete triad: disordered eating, amenorrhea, osteoporosis. Med Sci Sports Exerc 1993;25:775–7.

[37] Golden NH, Jacobson MS, Schebendach J, et al. Resumption of menses in anorexia nervosa. Arch Pediatr Adolesc Med 1997;151:16–21.

[38] Copeland PM, Sacks NR, Herzog DB. Longitudinal follow-up of amenorrhea in eating disorders. Psychosom Med 1995;57:121–6.

[39] Schneider M, Fisher M, Weinerman S, et al. Correlates of low bone density in females with anorexia nervosa. Int J Adolesc Med Health 2002;14:297–306.

[40] Bachrach LK, Guido D, Katzman D, et al. Decreased bone density in adolescent girls with anorexia nervosa. Pediatrics 1990;86:440–7.

[41] Treasure J, Serpell L. Osteoporosis in young people. Psychiatr Clin North Am 2001;24: 359–70.

[42] Brooks E, Ogden B, Cavalier D. Compromised bone density 11.4 years after diagnosis of anorexia nervosa. J Womens Health 1998;7:567–74.

[43] Hotta M, Shibasaki T, Sato K, et al. The importance of body weight history in the occurrence and recovery of osteoporosis in patients with anorexia nervosa: evaluation by dual X-ray absorptiometry and bone metabolic markers. Eur J Endocrinol 1998;139:276–83.

[44] Rigotti N, Neer R, Skates S. The clinical course of osteoporosis in anorexia nervosa. JAMA 1991;265:1133–8.

[45] Mehler PS. Osteoporosis in anorexia nervosa: prevention and treatment. Int J Eat Disord 2003;33:113–26.

[46] Hartman D, Crisp A, Rooney B, et al. Bone density of women who have recovered from anorexia nervosa. Int J Eat Disord 2000;28:107–12.

[47] Stacher G, Bergmann H, Wiensnagrotzki S, et al. Primary anorexia nervosa: gastric emptying and antral motor activity in 53 patients. Int J Eat Disord 1992;11:163–72.

[48] Cuellar RE, VanThiel DH. Gastrointestinal consequences of the eating disorders: anorexia nervosa and bulimia. Am J Gastroenterol 1986;81:1113–24.

[49] McClain CJ, Humphries LL, Hill KK, et al. Gastrointestinal and nutritional aspects of eating disorders. J Am Coll Nutr 1993;12:466–74.

[50] Waldholtz BD, Andersen AE. Gastrointestinal symptoms in anorexia nervosa. Gastroenterology 1990;98:1415–9.

[51] Vande Zande VL, Mazza JJ, Yale SH. Hematologic and metabolic abnormalities in a patient with anorexia nervosa. Wis Med J 2004;103:38–40.

[52] Rieger W, Brady JP, Weisberg E. Hematologic changes in anorexia nervosa. Am J Psychiatry 1978;135:984–5.

[53] Abella A, Feliu E, Granada I, et al. Bone marrow changes in anorexia nervosa are correlated with the amount of weight loss and not with other clinical findings. Am J Clin Pathol 2002;118:582–8.

[54] Bowers TK, Eckert E. Leukopenia in anorexia nervosa. Lack of increased risk of infection. Arch Intern Med 1978;138:1520–3.

[55] Steinberg SE, Nasraway S, Peterson L. Reversal of severe serous atrophy of the bone marrow in anorexia nervosa. JPEN J Parenter Enteral Nutr 1987;11:422–3.

[56] Jonas JM, Gold MS, Sweeney D, et al. Eating disorders and cocaine abuse: a survey of 259 cocaine abusers. J Clin Psychiatry 1987;48:47–50.

[57] Killen J, Taylor C, Telch M, et al. Evidence for an alcohol stress link among normal weight adolescents reporting purging behavior. Int J Eat Disord 1987;6:349–56.

[58] Russell G. Bulimia nervosa: ominous variant of anorexia nervosa. Psychol Med 1979;9: 429–48.

[59] Mitchell JE, Sheila MS, de Zwaan M. Comorbidity and medical complications of bulimia nervosa. J Clin Psychiatry 1991;52:13–20.

[60] Ogren FP, Huerter JV, Pearson PH, et al. Transient salivary gland hypertrophy in bulimics. Laryngoscope 1987;97:951–3.

[61] Altshuler BD, Dechow PC, Waller DA, et al. An investigation of the oral pathologies occurring in bulimia nervosa. Int J Eat Disord 1990;9:191–9.

[62] Mitchell JE, Pyle RL, Eckert ED, et al. Electrolyte and other physiological abnormalities in patients with bulimia. Psychol Med 1983;13:273–8.

[63] Ramos E, Hall-Craggs M, Demers LM. Surreptitious habitual vomiting simulating Bartter's syndrome. JAMA 1980;243:1070–2.

[64] Mitchell JE, Hatsukami D, Pyle RL. Metabolic acidosis as a marker for laxative abuse in patients with bulimia. Int J Eat Disord 1987;6:557–60.

[65] Harris RT. Bulimarexia and related serious eating disorders with medical complications. Ann Intern Med 1983;99:800–7.

[66] Bytzer P, Stokholm M, Andersen I, et al. Prevalence of surreptitious laxative abuse in patients with diarrhoea of uncertain origin: a cost benefit analysis of a screening procedure. Gut 1989;30:1379–84.

[67] Perkins SL, Livesey JF. A rapid high-performance thin-layer chromatographic urine screen for laxative abuse. Clin Biochem 1993;26:179–81.

[68] Baker EH, Sandle GI. Complications of laxative abuse. Annu Rev Med 1996;47:127–34.

[69] Geboes K, Bossaert H. Cathartic colon—two case reports. Am J Proctol Gastroenterol Colon Rectal Surg 1980;31:21–4.

[70] Oster JR, Materson BJ, Rogers AI. Laxative abuse syndrome. Am J Gastroenterol 1980;74: 451–8.

[71] Kune GA. Laxative use not a risk for colorectal cancer: data from the Melbourne colorectal cancer study. Z Gastroenterol 1993;31:140–3.

[72] Siegers CP, von Hertzberg-Lottin E, Otte M, et al. Anthranoid laxative abuse—a risk for colorectal cancer? Gut 1993;34:1099–101.

[73] Levine D, Goode AW, Wingate DL. Purgative abuse associated with reversible cachexia, hypogammaglobulinaemia, and finger clubbing. Lancet 1981;1:919–20.

[74] Nadir A, Reddy D, Van Thiel DH. Cascara sagrada-induced intrahepatic cholestasis causing portal hypertension: case report and review of herbal hepatotoxicity. Am J Gastroenterol 2000;95:3634–7.

[75] Zanolli MD, McAlvany J, Krowchuk DP. Phenolphthalein-induced fixed drug eruption: a cutaneous complication of laxative use in a child. Pediatrics 1993;91:1199–201.

[76] Manno BR, Manno JE. Toxicology of ipecac: a review. Clin Toxicol 1977;10:221–42.

[77] Adler AG, Walinsky P, Krall RA, et al. Death resulting from ipecac poisoning. JAMA 1980;243:1927–8.

[78] Palmer EP, Guary AT. Reversible myopathy secondary to abuse of ipecac in patients with major eating disorders. N Engl J Med 1985;313:1457–9.

[79] Bulik CM. Abuse of drugs associated with eating disorders. J Subst Abuse 1992;4:69–90.

[80] Block WD, Shiner PT, Roman J. Severe electrolyte disturbances associated with metolazine and furosemide. South Med J 1978;71:380–1.

[81] Brucato A, Bonati M, Gaspari F. Tetany and rhabdomyolysis due to surreptitious furosemide—importance of magnesium supplementation. J Toxicol Clin Toxicol 1993;31: 341–4.

[82] Ashraf N, Locksley R, Arieff AI. Thiazide-induced hyponatremia associated with death or neurologic damage in outpatients. Am J Med 1981;70:1163–8.

[83] Greenberg A. Diuretic complications. Am J Med Sci 2000;319:10–24.

[84] Hollifield JW, Slaton PE. Thiazide diuretics, hypokalemia and cardiac arrhythmias. Acta Med Scand 1981;647(Supp):67–73.

[85] Kavaru MS, Ahmad M, Amirthalingam KN. Hydrochlorothiazide-induced acute pulmonary edema. Cleve Clin J Med 1990;57:181–4.

[86] Feinfeld DA, Carvounis CP. Fatal hyperkalemia and hyperchloremic acidosis. Association with spironolactone in the absence of renal impairment. JAMA 1978;240:1516.

[87] Gabow PA, Moore S, Schrier RW. Spironolactone-induced hyperchloremic acidosis in cirrhosis. Ann Intern Med 1979;90:338–40.

[88] Brolin RE, Gorman JH, Gorman RC, et al. Prophylactic iron supplementation after Roux-en-Y gastric bypass: a prospective, double-blind, randomized study. Arch Surg 1998; 133:740–4.

[89] Rhode BM, Shustik C, Christou NV, et al. Iron absorption and therapy after gastric bypass. Obes Surg 1999;9:17–21.

[90] Fawcett S, Young GB, Holliday RL. Wernicke's encephalopathy after gastric partitioning for morbid obesity. Can J Surg 1984;27:169–70.

[91] Salas-Salvado J, Garcia-Lorda P, Cuatrecasas G, et al. Wernicke's syndrome after bariatric surgery. Clin Nutr 2000;19:371–3.

[92] Seehra H, MacDermott N, Lascelles RG, et al. Wernicke's encephalopathy after vertical banded gastroplasty for morbid obesity. BMJ 1996;312:434.

[93] Mason EE. Starvation injury after gastric reduction for obesity. World J Surg 1998;22: 1002–7.

[94] Goldner WS, O'Dorisio TM, Dillon JS, et al. Severe metabolic bone disease as a long-term complication of obesity surgery. Obes Surg 2002;12:685–92.

[95] Coates PS, Fernstrom JD, Fernstrom MH, et al. Gastric bypass surgery for morbid obesity leads to an increase in bone turnover and a decrease in bone mass. J Clin Endocrinol Metab 2004;89:1061–5.

[96] Anonymous. The Atkins Diet. Med Lett Drugs Ther 2000;42:52.

[97] Bravata DM, Sanders L, Huang J, et al. Efficacy and safety of low-carbohydrate diets: a systematic review. JAMA 2003;289:1837–50.

[98] Singh BN, Gaarder TD, Kanegae T, et al. Liquid protein diets and torsades de pointes. JAMA 1978;240:115–9.

[99] Drott C, Lundholm K. Cardiac effects of caloric restriction-mechanisms and potential hazards. Int J Obes 1992;16:481–6.

[100] Fisher M, Golden NH, Katzman D, et al. Eating disorders in adolescents: a background paper. J Adolesc Health 1995;16:420–37.

[101] Schnitker MA, Mattman PE, Bliss TL. A clinical study of malnutrition in Japanese prisoners of war. Ann Intern Med 1951;35:69–96.

[102] Marinella MA. The refeeding syndrome and hypophosphatemia. Nutr Rev 2003;61:320–3.

[103] Soloman SM, Kirby DF. The refeeding syndrome: a review. JPEN J Parenter Enteral Nutr 1990;14:90–7.

[104] Berner YN, Shike M. Consequences of phosphate imbalance. Annu Rev Nutr 1988;8: 121–48.

[105] Baudendistel L, Goudsouzian N, Cote C, et al. End-tidal CO2 monitoring. Its use in the diagnosis and management of malignant hyperthermia. Anaesthesia 1984;39:1000–3.

[106] Cotran R, Kumar V, Robbins S. Robbins pathologic basis of disease. 4th edition. Philadelphia: W.B. Saunders; 1989.

[107] Malone AM. Nutritional management of ventilated patients. RT J Respir Care Pract 2001;1–7.

[108] Wesner E, Young EA. Nutrition and internal medicine. In: Stein JH, editor. Internal medicine. 4th edition. St. Louis (MO): Mosby; 1994. p. 500–25.

[109] Clark RH, Feleke G, Din M, et al. Nutritional treatment for acquired immunodeficiency virus-associated wasting using beta-hydroxy beta-methylbutyrate, glutamine, and arginine: a randomized, double-blind, placebo-controlled study. JPEN J Parenter Enteral Nutr 2000; 24:133–9.

[110] May PE, Barber A, D'Olimpio JT, et al. Reversal of cancer-related wasting using oral supplementation with a combination of beta-hydroxy-beta-methylbutyrate, arginine, and glutamine. Am J Surg 2002;183:471–9.

[111] Lipman TO. Bacterial translocation and enteral nutrition in humans: an outsider looks in. JPEN J Parenter Enteral Nutr 1995;19:156–65.

[112] Moore FA, Moore EE, Jones TN, et al. TEN versus TPN following major abdominal trauma—reduced septic morbidity. J Trauma Injury Infect Crit Care 1989;29:916–22.

[113] Bernard GR, Artigas A, Brigham KL, et al. Report of the American-European consensus conference on ARDS: definitions, mechanisms, relevant outcomes and clinical trial coordination. The Consensus Committee. Intensive Care Med 1994;20:225–32.

[114] Bohn AM, Betts S, Schwenk TL. Creatine and other nonsteroidal strength-enhancing aids. Curr Sports Med Rep 2002;1:239–45.

[115] Juhn M. Popular sports supplements and ergogenic aids. Sports Med 2003;33:921–39.

[116] Mesa JL, Ruiz JR, Gonzalez-Gross MM, et al. Oral creatine supplementation and skeletal muscle metabolism in physical exercise. Sports Med 2002;32:903–44.

[117] Pecci MA, Lombardo JA. Performance-enhancing supplements. Phys Med Rehabil Clin N Am 2000;11:949–60.

[118] Racette SB. Creatine supplementation and athletic performance. J Orthop Sports Phys Ther 2003;33:615–21.

[119] Lawler JM, Barnes WS, Wu G, et al. Direct antioxidant properties of creatine. Biochem Biophys Res Commun 2002;290:47–52.

[120] Baker SK, Tarnopolsky MA. Targeting cellular energy production in neurological disorders. Expert Opin Investig Drugs 2003;12:1655–79.

[121] Witte KK, Clark AL, Cleland JG. Chronic heart failure and micronutrients. J Am Coll Cardiol 2001;37:1765–74.

[122] Nomura A, Zhang M, Sakamoto T, et al. Anti-inflammatory activity of creatine supplementation in endothelial cells in vitro. Br J Pharmacol 2003;139:715–20.

[123] Mazzini L, Balzarini C, Colombo R, et al. Effects of creatine supplementation on exercise performance and muscular strength in amyotrophic lateral sclerosis: preliminary results. J Neurol Sci 2001;191:139–44.

[124] Wyss M, Schulze A. Health implications of creatine: can oral creatine supplementation protect against neurological and atherosclerotic disease? Neuroscience 2002;112: 243–60.

[125] Kalinski MI. State-sponsored research on creatine supplements and blood doping in elite Soviet sport. Perspect Biol Med 2003;46:445–51.

[126] Biwer CJ, Jensen RL, Schmidt WD, et al. The effect of creatine on treadmill running with high-intensity intervals. J Strength Cond Res 2003;17:439–45.

[127] Brilla LR, Giroux MS, Taylor A, et al. Magnesium-creatine supplementation effects on body water. Metabolism 2003;52:1136–40.

[128] Brose A, Parise G, Tarnopolsky MA. Creatine supplementation enhances isometric strength and body composition improvements following strength exercise training in older adults. J Gerontol A Biol Sci Med Sci 2003;58:11–9.

[129] Chrusch MJ, Chilibeck PD, Chad KE, et al. Creatine supplementation combined with resistance training in older men. Med Sci Sports Exerc 2001;33:2111–7.

[130] Chwalbinska-Moneta J. Effect of creatine supplementation on aerobic performance and anaerobic capacity in elite rowers in the course of endurance training. Int J Sport Nutr Exerc Metab 2003;13:173–83.

[131] Volek JS, Rawson ES. Scientific basis and practical aspects of creatine supplementation for athletes. Nutrition 2004;20:609–14.

[132] Kreider RB. Effects of creatine supplementation on performance and training adaptations. Mol Cell Biochem 2003;244:89–94.

[133] Delecluse C, Diels R, Goris M. Effect of creatine supplementation on intermittent sprint running performance in highly trained athletes. J Strength Cond Res 2003;17:446–54.

[134] Green JM, McLester JR, Smith JE, et al. The effects of creatine supplementation on repeated upper- and lower-body Wingate performance. J Strength Cond Res 2001;15: 36–41.

[135] Kreider RB, Melton C, Rasmussen CJ, et al. Long-term creatine supplementation does not significantly affect clinical markers of health in athletes. Mol Cell Biochem 2003;244: 95–104.

[136] Farquhar WB, Zambraski EJ. Effects of creatine use on the athlete's kidney. Curr Sports Med Rep 2002;1:103–6.

[137] Revai T, Sapi Z, Benedek S, et al. Severe nephrotic syndrome in a young man taking anabolic steroid and creatine long term. Orv Hetil 2003;144:2425–7.

[138] Brudnak MA. Creatine: are the benefits worth the risk? Toxicol Lett 2004;150:123–30.

[139] Knitter AE, Panton L, Rathmacher JA, et al. Effects of beta-hydroxy-beta-methylbutyrate on muscle damage after a prolonged run. J Appl Physiol 2000;89:1340–4.

[140] Flakoll P, Sharp R, Baier S, et al. Effect of beta-hydroxy-beta-methylbutyrate, arginine, and lysine supplementation on strength, functionality, body composition, and protein metabolism in elderly women. Nutrition 2004;20:445–51.

[141] Gallagher PM, Carrithers JA, Godard MP, et al. Beta-hydroxy-beta-methylbutyrate ingestion, part I: effects on strength and fat free mass. Med Sci Sports Exerc 2000;32:2109–15.

[142] Crowe MJ, O'Connor DM, Lukins JE. The effects of beta-hydroxy-beta-methylbutyrate (HMB) and HMB/creatine supplementation on indices of health in highly trained athletes. Int J Sport Nutr Exerc Metab 2003;13:184–97.

[143] Jowko E, Ostaszewski P, Jank M, et al. Creatine and beta-hydroxy-beta-methylbutyrate (HMB) additively increase lean body mass and muscle strength during a weight-training program. Nutrition 2001;17:558–66.

[144] Gallagher PM, Carrithers JA, Godard MP, et al. Beta-hydroxy-beta-methylbutyrate ingestion, part II: effects on hematology, hepatic and renal function. Med Sci Sports Exerc 2000;32:2116–9.

[145] Kreider RB, Ferreira M, Wilson M, et al. Effects of calcium beta-hydroxy-beta-methylbutyrate (HMB) supplementation during resistance-training on markers of catabolism, body composition and strength. Int J Sports Med 1999;20:503–9.

[146] Nissen S, Sharp R, Ray M, et al. Effect of leucine metabolite beta-hydroxy-beta-methylbutyrate on muscle metabolism during resistance-exercise training. J Appl Physiol 1996;81:2095–104.

[147] Panton LB, Rathmacher JA, Baier S, et al. Nutritional supplementation of the leucine metabolite beta-hydroxy-beta-methylbutyrate (HMB) during resistance training. Nutrition 2000;16:734–9.

[148] Nissen S, Sharp RL, Panton L, et al. Beta-hydroxy-beta-methylbutyrate (HMB) supplementation in humans is safe and may decrease cardiovascular risk factors. J Nutr 2000;130:1937–45.

[149] Nissen SL, Sharp RL. Effect of dietary supplements on lean mass and strength gains with resistance exercise: a meta-analysis. J Appl Physiol 2003;94:651–9.

[150] O'Connor DM, Crowe MJ. Effects of beta-hydroxy-beta-methylbutyrate and creatine monohydrate supplementation on the aerobic and anaerobic capacity of highly trained athletes. J Sports Med Phys Fitness 2003;43:64–8.

[151] Slater G, Jenkins D, Logan P, et al. Beta-hydroxy-beta-methylbutyrate (HMB) supplementation does not affect changes in strength or body composition during resistance training in trained men. Int J Sport Nutr Exerc Metab 2001;11:384–96.

[152] Vukovich MD, Stubbs NB, Bohlken RM. Body composition in 70-year-old adults responds to dietary beta-hydroxy-beta-methylbutyrate similarly to that of young adults. J Nutr 2001; 131:2049–52.

[153] Ballantyne CS, Phillips SM, MacDonald JR, et al. The acute effects of androstenedione supplementation in healthy young males. Can J Appl Physiol 2000;25:68–78.

[154] Broeder CE, Quindry J, Brittingham K, et al. The Andro Project: physiological and hormonal influences of androstenedione supplementation in men 35 to 65 years old participating in a high-intensity resistance training program. Arch Intern Med 2000;160: 3093–104.

[155] King DS, Sharp RL, Vukovich MD, et al. Effect of oral androstenedione on serum testosterone and adaptations to resistance training in young men: a randomized controlled trial. JAMA 1999;281:2020–8.

[156] Rasmussen BB, Volpi E, Gore DC, et al. Androstenedione does not stimulate muscle protein anabolism in young healthy men. J Clin Endocrinol Metab 2000;85:55–9.

[157] Beckham SG, Earnest CP. Four weeks of androstenedione supplementation diminishes the treatment response in middle aged men. Br J Sports Med 2003;37:212–8.

[158] Acacio BD, Stanczyk FZ, Mullin P, et al. Pharmacokinetics of dehydroepiandrosterone and its metabolites after long-term daily oral administration to healthy young men. Fertil Steril 2004;81:595–604.

[159] Buvat J. Androgen therapy with dehydroepiandrosterone. World J Urol 2003;21:346–55.

[160] Barnhart KT, Freeman E, Grisso JA, et al. The effect of dehydroepiandrosterone supplementation to symptomatic perimenopausal women on serum endocrine profiles, lipid parameters, and health-related quality of life. J Clin Endocrinol Metab 1999;84:3896–902.

[161] Genazzani AD, Stomati M, Bernardi F, et al. Long-term low-dose dehydroepiandrosterone oral supplementation in early and late postmenopausal women modulates endocrine parameters and synthesis of neuroactive steroids. Fertil Steril 2003;80:1495–501.

[162] Genazzani AD, Stomati M, Strucchi C, et al. Oral dehydroepiandrosterone supplementation modulates spontaneous and growth hormone-releasing hormone-induced growth hormone and insulin-like growth factor-1 secretion in early and late postmenopausal women. Fertil Steril 2001;76:241–8.

[163] Stomati M, Monteleone P, Casarosa E, et al. Six-month oral dehydroepiandrosterone supplementation in early and late postmenopause. Gynecol Endocrinol 2000;14:342–63.

[164] Kahn AJ, Halloran B, Wolkowitz O, et al. Dehydroepiandrosterone supplementation and bone turnover in middle-aged to elderly men. J Clin Endocrinol Metab 2002;87:1544–9.

[165] Kawano H, Yasue H, Kitagawa A, et al. Dehydroepiandrosterone supplementation improves endothelial function and insulin sensitivity in men. J Clin Endocrinol Metab 2003;88:3190–5.

[166] Wallace MB, Lim J, Cutler A, et al. Effects of dehydroepiandrosterone vs androstenedione supplementation in men. Med Sci Sports Exerc 1999;31:1788–92.

[167] Bohn AM, Khodaee M, Schwenk TL. Ephedrine and other stimulants as ergogenic aids. Curr Sports Med Rep 2003;2:220–5.

[168] Haller CA, Benowitz NL. Adverse cardiovascular and central nervous system events associated with dietary supplements containing ephedra alkaloids. N Engl J Med 2000;343:1833–8.

[169] Kockler DR, McCarthy MW, Lawson CL. Seizure activity and unresponsiveness after hydroxycut ingestion. Pharmacotherapy 2001;21:647–51.

[170] Morgenstern LB, Viscoli CM, Kernan WN, et al. Use of Ephedra-containing products and risk for hemorrhagic stroke. Neurology 2003;60:132–5.

[171] Pipe A. Efficacy and safety of ephedra and ephedrine for weight loss and athletic performance. Clin J Sport Med 2004;14:188–9.

[172] White LM, Gardner SF, Gurley BJ, et al. Pharmacokinetics and cardiovascular effects of ma-huang (Ephedra sinica) in normotensive adults. J Clin Pharmacol 1997;37:116–22.

[173] Dodd SL, Herb RA, Powers SK. Caffeine and exercise performance. An update. Sports Med 1993;15:14–23.

[174] Tarnopolsky MA. Caffeine and endurance performance. Sports Med 1994;18:109–25.

[175] Graham TE. Caffeine, coffee and ephedrine: impact on exercise performance and metabolism. Can J Appl Physiol 2001;26:S103–19.

[176] Doherty M, Smith PM, Davison RC, et al. Caffeine is ergogenic after supplementation of oral creatine monohydrate. Med Sci Sports Exerc 2002;34:1785–92.

ELSEVIER
SAUNDERS

EMERGENCY
MEDICINE
CLINICS OF
NORTH AMERICA

Emerg Med Clin N Am 23 (2005) 815–826

Anabolic Steroids: What Should the Emergency Physician Know?

James T. Brown, MD

OSF Saint Francis Medical Center, 530 N.E. Glen Oak, Peoria, IL 61637, USA

Common abuse of anabolic steroids among athletes, anabolic steroid use for chronic muscle wasting conditions, and conditions that are caused by anabolic steroid excess make knowledge of anabolic steroids important to the emergency medicine practitioner. Controlled scientific research is limited, but emerging, as the clinical application of anabolic steroids is increasing. Traditionally, if one was interested in learning about the use of anabolic steroids the gym would be the place to start their research. Many of the athletes abusing anabolic steroids have developed a "sophisticated" knowledge of steroid pharmacology based on subjective and anecdotal experiences. Unfortunately, these experiences are much more influential to an athlete than their physician's counseling. Publications about anabolic steroids are nearly absent in the emergency medicine literature, and frequently descriptive and poorly controlled in the sports medicine literature. This review will cover the epidemiology of anabolic steroid use and abuse, the physiologic effects, and their applications, both nonmedically and medically. Polycystic ovarian syndrome (PCOS) will be discussed briefly because of its association with excesses of anabolic steroid hormones.

Epidemiology of abuse

There have been estimates of more that 1 to 3 million current or former users in the United States [1]. The data on the actual prevalence of anabolic steroid abuse is limited, by the surveys that are used to describe this information. Surveys of the populations at risk may be influenced by a reluctance to admit the usage of a controlled substance. Recent reports have estimated that 4% to 12% of high school boys have used anabolic steroids at sometime in their life [2]. A survey conducted by Blue Cross and

---

E-mail address: JBrown5005@aol.com

Blue Shield Association [3] reported that anabolic steroids were the second most common substances know to be used for athletic performance among 12 to 17-year-old people, second only to creatine (31–57%, respectively). Considering the potential adverse effects on growth in this population, these statistics are quite alarming. Anabolic steroid use is reported in 1.1% of collegiate athletes [4], most commonly occurring in football players (29.3%) and male track and field athletes (20.6%) [5]. Traditionally, anabolic steroids were widely used and abused by body builders and recreational weight trainers, but are also reputedly used as training aids by endurance athletes to improve recovery from training loads [6].

Physiology

Testosterone is a steroid hormone that is synthesized in the Leydig cells of the testes in males; however, it is present in women, being produced in adrenal glands and the ovaries. Its synthesis is controlled by luteinizing hormone (LH), which is produced by the hypothalamus and secreted by the pituitary gland, which in turn targets the Leydig cells within the testes. This represents the pituitary–hypothalamic–gonadal negative feedback axis. The primary substrate for the production of testosterone is cholesterol.

The production of testosterone in males maintains plasma concentrations between 300 to 1000 ng/dL [6]. Approximately 44% of secreted testosterone is bound by plasma proteins (sex hormone binding globulin), and approximately 2% remains in the free form. The remaining 54% is bioavailable [7], and is loosely bound to albumin, which easily dissociates in the capillary beds [7]. In target tissues, skin, prostate, seminal vesicles, testosterone is acted on by the enzyme 5-alpha-reductase and converted to dihydrotestosterone, a much stronger androgen that testosterone. Fifty percent of the production of testosterone in females occurs extraglandularly. Androstenedione is produced by the adrenals and converted to testosterone. Subsequently, testosterone is acted on by aromatase in the adipose tissues and changed to estrogen. Plasma concentrations in females range from 15 to 65 ng/dL [6].

Testosterone is metabolized by the cytochrome P450 class of hepatic isoenzymes and in its pure form, is metabolized rapidly. Therapeutic preparations have changed the chemical structure enough to slow the metabolism in the liver, and increase their bioavailability. They are still metabolized in the liver, but at variable rates, with byproducts that are excreted in the urine and feces [7].

Specific organ effects

Muscle tissue

The exact mechanisms in which anabolic steroids produce muscle growth are not clearly delineated. Numerous proposed mechanisms of action related to athletic performance have been proposed. These include increased skeletal muscle protein synthesis and skeletal muscle hypertrophy [8,9], a decrease in the rate of protein breakdown [10], an increase in the number of mononuclei [11], activation of satellite cells [11], and an increase in the number of androgen receptors containing mononuclei [11].

At the cellular level, steroid hormones readily pass through the cell membrane of the target tissue, bind with the specific steroid receptors, and move to the nucleus where they attach to nuclear chromatin and stimulate specific messenger RNA by transcription. Ribosomal DNA then transforms into new proteins that mediate the hormone's function; the nature and quantities of proteins produced will vary depending on the type of tissue and its sensitivity to the hormone [12]. Well-known sites of action for anabolic steroids include muscle, bone, and hematopoietic tissue.

Effects of anabolic steroids on the muscles will be mediated by the interaction with the androgen receptor, and subsequent increase in protein synthesis, or by blocking the protein catabolic effects of endogenous glucocorticoids on the glucocorticoid receptor [13]. The primary mechanism for increases in muscle mass and performance are attributed to the anabolic effect on actin and myosin via somatomedin [14]. There is a trend toward a rise in myosin heavy chain, suggesting that testosterone enhances skeletal muscle mass by stimulating protein synthesis rather than decreasing muscle protein breakdown [15].

A common misconception among bodybuilders is that anabolic steroids increase the number of satellite cells or myocytes that do not mature into mature muscle cells (mononuclei). These satellite cells are recruited to repair myocytes injured during athletic activities. Kadi found that the anabolic steroids do not increase the number of satellite cells for recruitment, but the process of athletic training is responsible for the increase in satellite cells [11]. Bhasin et al [16] provided evidence that testosterone administration could increase muscle strength and size in males, but only in the presence of weight training. Consequently, the effects of anabolic steroids will not be demonstrated without adequate exercise and stress on the muscle.

Finally, the significance of androgens on the regulation of androgen receptors is not clearly delineated. Depending on the type of skeletal muscle, androgen receptors can either be upregulated or downregulated [11]. Strenuous exercise seems to be the way to increase the number of androgen receptor sites. The increase in androgen receptor sites consequently increases the effect of androgens at the cellular level, causing enlargement of the muscle unit [8].

Bone tissue

Androgen receptors have been found on osteoblasts, osteoclasts, mononuclear, and endothelial cells within the bone marrow. In vitro studies have demonstrated the stimulating effect of androgens on osteoblastic cell proliferation and differentiation by the inhibition of osteoclastic differentiation. Testosterone treatment in hypogonadal men rapidly increases 1,25-dihydroxy vitamin D levels and corrects calcium malabsorption, leading to an improvement in calcium balance and bone formation. In eugonadal men, testosterone treatment has demonstrated increase in spinal bone mass density by reducing the rate of bone resorption rather than increasing bone formation [17,18].

Hematopoiesis

Anabolic steroids cause an increase synthesis of erythropoietin. Subsequently, androgens will cause an increase in the hemoglobin and hematocrit, resulting in an increase oxygen carrying capacity [19]. Androgens were formerly used in the treatment of anemia, but with the advent of recombinant human erythropoietin, androgen use has fallen from favor [20]. This physiologic effect of androgens may result in erythrocytosis and sludging of the blood.

Efficacy of anabolic steroid use

Only limited evidence supports the use of anabolic steroids to enhance athletic performance [21]. Studies frequently have methodologic flaws in doses and administration strategies, limiting the applicability to current androgen use practices. Current practices among athletes include "stacking" of drugs. "Stacking" involves the combining of a number of different agents. In addition to "stacking," athletes will "cycle" (start and discontinue) androgens for periods of 7 to 14 weeks [22]. "Pyramiding" is the pattern of increasing a dose through a cycle [23]. Because of obvious ethical concerns, scientific studies have not examined these particular practices. Research has been conducted on single drug therapy, and much lower dosing than current practices.

Bhasin et al [16] demonstrated in a randomized, placebo controlled study, an increase in body weight (6.1 kg) in all groups receiving testosterone enanthate 600 mg/wk. There was also an increase in muscle size, as measured by the cross-sectional area of the triceps and quadriceps muscle. The testosterone group combined with the exercise group experienced the largest increase in muscle size and the only statistically significant increase in strength [16].

Additional studies have demonstrated the increased strength associated with the administration of metandienone and exercise [24]. Hervey et al [25] demonstrated that higher doses (25 mg/d) did not produce significant differences in strength over lower doses (10 mg/d) [25]. Anecdotal and case reports have documented much larger increases in bodyweight and strength. Obviously, these studies must be viewed with skepticism.

Adverse effects

Hepatic

There has been a documented, reversible association between anabolic steroid use and elevation of liver function tests [26]. The reversible course is the primary reason for athletes "cycling" drug use [27]. Dose-dependent jaundice and hepatic dysfunction are quite common with supraphysiologic androgen use for more than 2 months. Death from hepatotoxicity is rare [26]. Oral agents, C-17 alkylated, are more commonly associated with liver toxicity [26] (Table 1). Nonalkylated intramuscular agents, such as testosterone and nortestosteone, are less likely to produce liver problems [26]. Cases of carcinoma of the liver have been associated with high doses of anabolic steroid used, longer periods of administration, or in individual that had medical conditions predisposing to carcinoma.

Cardiovascular

Unpredictable changes may occur in the lipid profile of individuals using anabolic steroids [28]. Glazer conducted a meta-analysis in 1991 reporting a decrease in HDL of 39% to 70% (mean 52%). These changes usually occur within the first week, and will normalize within 3 to 5 weeks after discontinuation. Additionally, LDL elevations of 11% to 100% have been recorded (mean 36%) [29]. Long-term effect on morbidity or mortality associated with this adverse effect on the lipid panel is uncertain. All of the

Table 1
Anabolic steroids

Injectable agents	
Generic name	Trade name
Testosterone	
Propionate	Testex
Enanthate	Delatestryl, Everone, Durathate
Cypionate	Virilon, Depotest, Androcyp
Nandrolone decanoate	Deca-durabolin
Nandrolone phenpropionate	Durabolin
Topical Agents	
Testosterone	
Patches	Androderm, Testoderm
Gel	Androgel
Oral Agents (C-17 alkylated agents)	
Danazol	Danocrine
Fluoxymesterone	Halotestin
Methandrostenolone	Methandienone
Oxandrolone	Anavar, Oxandrin
Oxymetholone	Anadrol
Stanozolol	Winstrol

adverse effects have proven to be atherogenic in patient populations [30]. Blood pressure elevations have occurred with the use of anabolic steroids, most likely due to the elevation of blood volume [30]. Increases in heart rate have also been documented. This may contribute to cardiomegaly and its associated medical complications [30].

Reproductive/endocrine

In men, anabolic steroid use leads to hypogonadotropic hypogonadism, resulting from the suppression of LH and follicle stimulating hormone (FSH) mediated through the negative feedback loop of the hypothalamic–pituitary–gonadal axis [1]. Because LH and FSH are essential for spermatogenesis, the resulting physiologic effects of anabolic steroid use include decreased sperm density and sperm count, decreased sperm motility, abnormal sperm morphology, testicular atrophy, and no change in libido [1]. Increasing doses of anabolic steroids will lead to oligospermia and infertility [31]. Nomalization generally occurs within 1 year of cessation of the anabolic steroids [32,33]. Feminization in males can occur from the conversion of testosterone to estrogen metabolites (aromatization) [20]. The increased estrogens may result in increased voice pitch and gynecomastia.

In women, anabolic steroid use leads to hirsutism, acne, deepening of the voice, clitoral hypertrophy, decreased breast mass, decreased menstruation or amenorrhea, increased appetite, and male pattern baldness. Even after discontinuation of the causative agent, these effects are sometimes irreversible [34].

Psychiatric

There are few controlled studies associating anabolic steroid use to aggressive behavior in bodybuilders or weightlifters [1]. There are numerous case reports, animal studies, and controlled clinical trial that have linked the use of anabolic steroids with aggressive behavior and mood changes [35,36]. Controlled clinical trials have demonstrated little risk of mood changes or aggressive behavior with doses of less than 300 mg/wk [1]. The evaluation of the effects of anabolic steroids on aggression and mood changes is faced with the same problem that many of the other issues are. Studies are not done using multiple drugs, have different subject populations than the target population, and do not approach the high dosages that are used in the athletic community. There are data clearly suggesting that anabolic steroid abuse may be addictive. Interviewing anabolic steroid users demonstrates at least one DSM-III-R symptom of dependence in 94% of the sample. Three symptoms are required for the diagnosis of drug dependence. Copeland et al [37] found that 23% of their sample met the criteria in the DSM-IV for dependence, and 23% met the criteria for abuse.

Anabolic steroid abuse in adolescents

Athletic competition and the desire for success within athletics have increased dramatically over the last 20 years. Now, it is evident that only the biggest, strongest, and fastest have an opportunity to participate in athletics on an elite level. Athletes at all levels, with a desire to have that competitive edge, have been attracted to the use of anabolic steroids. It is no longer just the bodybuilders and the power lifters using anabolic steroids, but athletes on all levels and various age groups.

Anabolic steroid use in the adolescent population is commonplace. The 1997, Youth Risk and Behavior Surveillance System data showed that of 9th to 12th graders in public and private high schools in the United States; 4.1% of males, and 2.0% of females have used anabolic steroids at least once in their lives. These estimates translate into approximately 375,000 males and 175,000 females [38]. What are the risk factors associated with anabolic steroid use in the adolescent population? The most common characteristic would make an affluent, white, male, living with only one parent, and attending a larger school, in a metropolitan area, who is participating in muscular strength and size-dependent sports, such as football, wrestling, track and field, the highest risk candidate [39]. There were no specific personality or behavioral characteristics identified [40]. The hypothesis has been proposed that anabolic steroid users, because of their desire to improve their personal appearance, are less likely to abuse other illicit drugs. Unfortunately, it is quite the opposite; many of them are found to be polydrug abusers [39].

Preparations

Testosterone is rapidly absorbed and degraded causing researchers to search for a more stable chemical with a longer bioavailabilty. This search has resulted in three main classes of analogs of testosterone. Class A is made up of the analogs produced by the esterification of the 17(beta)-hydroxyl group with any of the several carboxylic acid groups. Longer carbon chain carboxylic acids yield chemicals which are more lipid soluble. Consequently, these chemicals, when suspended in oil, are perfect for injection [6]. Class B consists of those chemicals that have been alkylated at the 17(alpha) position, such as methyltestosterone. Class C medications are modifications of the Class A and B chemicals. Alkylated and modified ring structures are not metabolized by the liver as quickly as testosterone and are more appropriate for oral administration [41].

Anabolic steroid use in medical practice

Anabolic steroids have been used in medical practice rarely over the years. In the 1960s, before the development of growth hormone, oxandrolone, was used to treat the short stature of Turner syndrome [42]. Recently, the literature has reported on other uses for androgens. The most commonly cited uses for anabolic steroids in current medical practice include the treatment of severe muscle wasting illnesses, such as AIDs and chronic obstructive pulmonary disease (COPD). The use of anabolic steroids has also been examined in the setting of severe catabolic states, such as burns and wound healing.

AIDS

Weight loss greater than 10% from baseline body weight (HIV-associated wasting) in HIV-positive men is a strong predictor of mortality [43]. Because hypogonadism is common in this population, studies of testosterone replacement have taken place. Uncontrolled studies have demonstrated weight gains of 2.3 kg over 12 weeks [44]. Bhasin et al [16] completed a randomized, double blind, placebo-controlled 16 week trial of testosterone enanthate (100 mg/wk) and exercise (alone and in combination with testosterone administration) compared with placebo in HIV-infected males with hypogonadism and weight loss of 5%. The testosterone group experienced a total weight gain of 2.6 kg and a increase lean body mass of 2.3 kg. There was also an increase in muscle strength. The exercise alone group also demonstrated an increase in total body weight and lean body mass, whereas the placebo group lost weight. The testosterone and exercise group did not result in significantly greater gains than either intervention alone. In eugonadal men effected with HIV-associated weight loss Strawford et al [45] found that subjects receiving oxandrolone 20 mg/d combined with progressive resistance exercises had significantly greater weight gain and increased lean body mass than the placebo group. The effects were not altered in the group receiving protease inhibitors.

Chronic obstructive pulmonary disease

Similar to the HIV population, weight loss in the chronic lung population has been associated with an increased mortality [46]. Ferreira et al [14] found that administration of testosterone 250 mg at initiation, followed by administration of 12 mg/d of stanozolol for 27 weeks, resulted in improved body weight, body mass index, lean body mass, and muscle size compared with exercise alone patients. However, there were no improvements in maximum inspiratory pressures or measures of physical endurance.

Severe burns

There is a significant decrease in testosterone levels in patients with severe burn injuries [47]. Severe catabolism and loss of lean body mass are well recognized complications of major burns [48,49]. This catabolic state is thought to be mediated by increased levels of catabolic hormones (epinephrine and cortisol) and decreased levels of anabolic hormones (growth hormone and testosterone) [50–52]. In this hypermetabolic state 30% of the calories burned come from protein, primarily muscle proteins. Weight loss of 100 pounds per day has been well described [53]. Demling and DeSanti [54] found that the addition of oxandrolone 20 mg/d and a high protein diet resulted in significantly increased weight gain and improvement in the physical therapy index, over those patients treated with diet alone.

Polycystic ovarian syndrome

PCOS is a condition that will commonly be present in the emergency department patient population. Although their presentations will not be directly related to the elevated level of androgens, it is important to have a basic understanding of the condition, and its implications to the emergency department patient. PCOS is a heterogeneous disorder, of uncertain etiology, that will be present in 6% to 10% of females of reproductive age [55]. PCOS will present with clinical features of menstrual irregularity, anovulatory infertility and miscarriages, hirsutism, acne, and alopecia. The endocrine findings consist of elevated levels of androgens, LH, estrogen, and prolactin. Metabolic consequences of this syndrome include insulin resistance, obesity, lipid abnormalities, and increased risk for impaired glucose tolerance and type 2 diabetes mellitus [55].

The pathophysiology of PCOS is uncertain, despite its frequency. The association of glucose intolerance and hyperandrogenism was described as early as 1921 [56]. Mechanisms contributing to insulin resistance include peripheral target tissue resistance, decreased hepatic clearance, and increased pancreatic sensitivity [55]. Insulin resistance is found in all patients with PCOS, but is more pronounced in obese women. Studies have demonstrated the positive correlation between fasting insulin levels and androgen levels [57]. It is uncertain if hyperinsulinemia results from the hyperandrogenism state, or the other way around. Most of the current evidence supports the theory that hyperinsulinemia is the primary factor, although the exact mechanisms are unclear.

Some of the consequences of PCOS include glucose intolerance (diabetes mellitus type 2) and adverse effects on lipid profiles. Traditionally, both of these consequences are considered risk factors for cardiovascular disease. Long-term follow-up studies of 786 women by Pierpoint et al [58] reported no excess of coronary heart disease mortality or morbidity among middle-aged women with a history of PCOS, despite increased prevalence of several cardiovascular risk factors. However, the mortality and morbidity from diabetes and risk of nonfatal cerebrovascular disease were higher among women with PCOS.

Summary

Anabolic steroids have not currently made their way into the daily practice of emergency physicians. The patients that use and abuse them have. In addition, those patients that are suffering from the consequences of illnesses that have excess levels of androgens are commonly evaluated in the emergency department. Clinicians should familiarize themselves with the practices of anabolic steroid users, so they can provide more beneficial council to their patients. As research continues, the emergency physician may find uses for androgens within the emergency department.

References

[1] Kutscher EC, Lund BC, Perry PJ. Anabolic steroids: a review for the clinician. Sports Med 2002;32(5):285–96.

[2] Yates WR, Perry GJ, Anderson KH. Illicit anabolic steroid use: a controlled personality study. Acta Psychiatr Scand 1990;81:548–50.

[3] Blue Cross and Blue Shield Association. Health Competition Foundation National survey on performance enhancing drugs in sports. Blue Cross and Blue Shield Association. URL: http://www.bcbs.com. 2001; Jan 1.

[4] Green GA, Uryasz FD, Petr TA, et al. NCAA study of substance use and misuse habits of college student-athletes. Clin J Sport Med 2001;11:51–6.

[5] Yesalis CE, Buckley WE, Anderson WA, et al. Athletes' projections of anabolic steroid use. Clin Sports Med 1990;2:155–71.

[6] Basaria S, Wahlstrom JT, Dobs AS. Anabolic–androgenic steroid therapy in the treatment of chronic diseases. J Clin Endocrinol Metab 2001;86(11):5108–17.

[7] Pardridge WM. Serum bioavailability of sex steroid hormones. Clin Endocrinol Metab 1986; 15:259–87.

[8] Kadi F, Eriksson A, Holmer S, et al. Effects of anabolic steroids on the muscle cells of strength trained athletes. Med Sci Sports Exerc 1999;31:1528–34.

[9] Sheffield-Moore M. Androgens and the control of skeletal muscle protein synthesis. Ann Med 2000;32:181–6.

[10] Buckley WE, Yesalis CE, Bennell DL. A study of anabolic steroid use at the secondary school level: recommendations for prevention. In: Yesalis CE, editor. Anabolic steroids in sport and exercise. Champaign (IL): Human Kinetics Publishing; 1993. p. 71–86.

[11] Kadi F. Adaptation of human skeletal muscle to training and anabolic steroids. Acta Physiol Scand Suppl 2000;646:1–52.

[12] Sturmi JE, Kiorio DJ. Anabolic agents. Clin Sports Med 1998;17:261–82.

[13] Creutzberg E, Schols A. Anabolic steroids. Clin Nutr Metab 1999;2(3):243–53.

[14] Ferreira IM, Verreschi IT, Nery LE, et al. The influence of 6 months of oral anabolic steroids on body mass and respiratory muscles in undernourished COPD patients. Chest 1998;114: 19–28.

[15] Brodsky IF, Balagopal P, Nair KS. Effects of testosterone replacement on muscle mass and muscle protein synthesis in hypogonadal men—a clinical research center study. J Clin Endocrinol Metab 1996;81:3469–75.

[16] Bhasin S, Storer TW, Berman N, et al. The effects of supraphysiologic doses of testosterone on muscle size and strength in normal men. N Engl J Med 1996;335:1–7.

[17] Vanderschueren D, Boonen S. Androgen exposure and the maintenance of skeletal integrity in aging men. Aging Male 1998;1:180–7.

[18] Eastell R, Boyle IT, Compston J, Cooper C, et al. Management of male osteoporosis: report of the UK consensus Group. Q J Med 1998;91:71–92.

[19] Lamb DR. Anabolic steroids in athletics: how well do they work and how dangerous are they? Am J Sports Med 1984;12:31–8.

[20] Hickson RC, Ball KL, Falduto MT. Adverse effects of anabolic steroids. Med Toxicol Adverse Drug Exp 1989;4:254–71.

[21] Yesalis CE, Bahrke MS. Anabolic-androgenic steroids: current issues. Sports Med 1995;19: 326–40.

[22] Perry PJ, Anderson KH, Yates WR. Illicit anabolic steroid use in athletes: a case series analysis. Am J Sports Med 1990;18:422–8.

[23] American Academy of Pediatrics. Adolescents and anabolic steroids: a subject review. Pediatrics 1997;99(6):904–8.

[24] Crist DM, Stackpole PJ, Peale GT. Effects of androgenic-anabolic steroids on neuromuscular power and body composition. J Appl Physiol 1983;54:366–70.

[25] Hervey GR, Knibbs AV, Burkenshaw L, et al. Effects of methandienone on the performance and body compostion of men undergoing athletic training. Clin Sci 1981;60:457–61.

[26] Ishak KG, Zimmerman HJ. Hepatotoxic effects of the anabolic/androgenic steroids. Semin Liver Sis 1987;7:230–6.

[27] Blue JG, Lombardo JA. Steroids and steroid-like compounds. Clin Sports Med 1999;18: 667–89.

[28] Duchaine D. Underground steroid handbook II. Venice (CA): HLR Technical Books; 1989.

[29] Glazer G. Athrogenic effects of anabolic steroids on serum lipid levels. Arch Intern Med 1991;151:1925–33.

[30] Sullivan ML, Martinez CM, Gennis P, et al. The cardiac toxicity of anabolic steroids. Prog Cardiovasc Dis 1998;41:1–5.

[31] Turek PJ, Williams RH, Gilbauch JH, et al. The reversibility of anabolic steroid-induced azospermia. J Urol 1995;153:1628–30.

[32] Jarow JP, Lipshultz LI. Anabolic steroid-induced hypogonadotropic hypogonadism. Am J Sports Med 1990;18:429–31.

[33] MacIndoe JG, Perry PJ, Yates WR, et al. Testosterone suppression of the HPT axis. J Invest Med 1997;45:441–7.

[34] Straus RH, Liggett MT, Lanese RR. Anabolic steroid use and perceived effects in ten weight-trained women athletes. JAMA 1985;253:2871–3.

[35] Conacher GN, Workman DG. Violent crime possibly associated with anabolic steroid use. Am J Psychiatry 1989;146:679.

[36] Pope HG Jr, Katz DL. Affective and psychotic symptoms associated withanabloic sterod use. Am J Psychiatry 1988;145:487–90.

[37] Copeland J, Peters R, Dillon P. Anabolic-androgenic steroids use disorder among a sample of Australian competitive and recreational users. Drug Alcohol Depend 2000;60:91–6.

[38] Hewitt SM, Smith-Akin CK, Higgins MM, et al. Youth risk behavior surveillance: United States, 1997. MMWR CDC Surveill Summ 1998;47:61.

[39] Bahrke MS, Yesalis CE, Kopstein AN, et al. Risk factors associated with anabolic = androgenic steroid use among adolescents. Sports Med 2000;29(6):397–405.

[40] Chng CL, Moore A. A study of steroid use among athletes: knolwdge, attitude and use. Health Educ 1990;21(6):11–7.

[41] Griffin JE, Wilson JD. Disorders of the testes and the male reproductive tract. In: Wilson JD, Foster DW, Kronenberg HM, Larsen PR, editors. Williams textbook of endocrinology. 9th edition. Philadelphia: Saunders; 1998. p. 819–76.

[42] Dobs AS. Is there a role for androgenic anabolic steroids in medical practice? JAMA 1999; 281(14):1326–7.

[43] Suttmann U, Ockenga J, Selberg O, et al. Incidence and prognostic value of malnutrition and wasting in human immunodeficiency virus-infected outpatients. J Acquir Immune Defic Syndr Hum Retrovirol 1995;8:239–46.

[44] Wagner GJ, Babkin JG. Testosteron therapy for clinical symptoms of hypogonadism in eugonadal men with AIDS. Int J Stud AIDS 1998;9:1–4.

[45] Strawford A, Bargieri T, Van Loan M, et al. Resistance exercise and supraphysiologic androgen therapy in eugonadal men with HIV-related weight loss: a randomized controlled trial. JAMA 1999;28(14):1282–90.

[46] Schols AM, Slangen J, Volovics L, et al. Weight loss is a reversible factor in the prognosis of chronic obstructive pulmonary disease. Am J Respir Crit Care Med 1998;157:1791–7.

[47] Dolecek R, Dvoracek C, Jezek M, et al. Very low serum testosterone levels and severe impairment of spermatogenesis in burned male patients. Correlations with basal levels and levels of FSH, LF, and PRL after LHRH + TRH. Endocrinol Exp 1983;17:33–45.

[48] Moore FD. Response to starvation and stress. In: Moore FD, editor. Metabolic care of the surgical patient. Philadelphia (PA): W.B. Saunders; 1959. p. 202–75.

[49] Newsome T, Mason A, Pruitt B. Weight loss following thermal injury. Ann Sug 1973;178: 215–20.

[50] Watters JM, Bessey PQ, Dinarello CA, et al. Both inflammatrooy and endocrine mediators stimulate host response to sepsis. Arch Surg 1985;121:179–82.

[51] Wilmore DW, Long JM, Mason AD Jr, et al. Catecholamines: mediator of the hypermetabolidc response to thermal injury. Ann Surg 1974;180:653–8.

[52] Wilmore DW, Aulick LH, Mason AD, et al. Incluence of the burn wound on local and systemic responses to injury. Ann Surg 1974;180:653–7.

[53] Wilmore D, Aulick I. Metabolic changes in burned patients. Surg Clin North Am 1978;58: 1173–80.

[54] Demling R, DeSanti L. Oxandrolone, an anagolic steroid, significantly increases the rate of weight gain in the recovery phase after major burns. J Trauma 1997;43(1):47–51.

[55] Tsilchorozidou T, Overton C, Conway G. The pathophysiology of polycystic ovary syndrome. Clin Endocrinol 2004;60(1):1–17.

[56] Achard C, Thiers J. Le virilisme pilaire et son association a l'insuffisance glucolytique (diaberes des femmes a barb). Bull Acad Natl Med 1921;86:52–64.

[57] Burghen GA, Givens JR, Kitabchi AE. Correlation of hyperandrogenism with hyperinsulinism in polycystic ovarian disease. J Clin Endocrinol Metabol 1980;50:113–6.

[58] Pierpoint T, McKeigue PM, Isaacs AJ, et al. Mortality of women with polycystic ovary syndrome at long-term follow-up. J Clin Epidemiol 1998;51:582–6.

ELSEVIER
SAUNDERS

EMERGENCY
MEDICINE
CLINICS OF
NORTH AMERICA

Emerg Med Clin N Am 23 (2005) 827–841

External Causes of Metabolic Disorders

Mary Lynn Arvanitis, DO, FACOEP[a,b],
Julia L. Pasquale, MD[b,c],*

[a]*Emergency Medicine, Covenant HealthCare, 800 Cooper Avenue,
Saginaw, MI 48602, USA*
[b]*Emergency Medicine, Michigan State University College of Human Medicine,
East Lansing, MI 48823, USA*
[c]*Emergency Medicine, Synergy Medical Education Alliance, 1000 Houghton Avenue,
Saginaw, MI 48602, USA*

Common medical conditions, such as head trauma, malignancy, and pregnancy may be associated with rarely seen metabolic emergencies that require prompt recognition and therapy. This article focuses on three such emergencies: diabetes insipidus (DI), often associated with head injuries; the syndrome of inappropriate antidiuretic hormone (SIADH), associated with malignancies; and acquired postpartum hypopituitarism (Sheehan's syndrome). These clinical syndromes, although uncommon, are important to consider when evaluating patients, as prompt treatment may minimize their mortality and morbidity.

Diabetes insipidus

Diabetes insipidus is an abnormality in the synthesis, response, or degradation of vasopressin that affects about 3 out of every 100,000 people in the general population [1]. The most typical causes include intracranial trauma or tumor, genetic factors, medications, and some specific disease entities. DI can be either a temporary condition lasting a few days or a permanent condition. DI affects less than 1% of head injured patients [2], but it can occur abruptly in these patients. Therefore, recognition is important, and appropriate treatment should be initiated in the emergency department (ED).

* Corresponding author.
E-mail address: jpasquale@synergymedical.org (J.L. Pasquale).

0733-8627/05/$ - see front matter © 2005 Elsevier Inc. All rights reserved.
doi:10.1016/j.emc.2005.03.005
emed.theclinics.com

Emergency department presentation

The frequently cited descriptive presentation of DI is a patient with polyuria, polydipsia, findings of inappropriately low urine osmolality with a urine-specific gravity less than 1.005, and increased serum osmolality (greater than 300 mOsm/kg) [1,3]. Signs and symptoms of volume depletion may be seen if water loss is greater than water intake [4]. Patients incapable of compensating for the water loss may present with severe symptoms of dehydration, including hypotension and neurological changes that include headache, visual changes, seizures, coma, and encephalopathy [1,4].

One definition of polyuria is urinary output of more than 3 L per day or a 24-hour urine volume greater than necessary for the patient's circulating blood volume or serum sodium level [4]. The degree of polyuria depends on the amount of antidiuretic hormone (ADH) suppression, and this can vary from mild to severe (more than 15 L per day) [5]. Polydipsia is defined as free water intake by the patient in a 24-hour period greater than necessary for the effective sodium concentration or arterial blood volume [4]. The patient often craves very cold fluids as opposed to other types of fluid [1].

Emergency department patients presenting with this condition may be those with head injuries with direct insult to the hypopituitary system or indirect injuries that lead to acute blood loss or hypotension resulting in decreased intracranial pressure. Indirect injuries include infection and trauma to other parts of the anatomy, both out of hospital and post-operatively [2,3,6–10].

Multiple case reports of DI are found in the literature in patients with head injuries and in noninjured patients. Hadani described a 15-year-old boy with a small hemorrhagic brain contusion. He was discharged on the 14th day. Thirteen days later he presented with findings consistent with central DI (CDI) [11]. Kuwai et al described a 28-year-old man with a basilar skull fracture without brain injury who presented with DI 10 days after his injury [12].

Pathophysiology

The etiology of DI may be central, peripheral (nephrogenic), or physiologic. CDI is caused by either a failure to produce or a decrease in the secretion of vasopressin (also called ADH) from the hypopituitary system. Resistance of the renal collecting ducts to the adequately produced and circulating amount of vasopressin causes nephrogenic DI. Physiologic suppression of vasopressin may be the result of excessive intake of free water by the patient and is referred to as primary polydipsia [12].

Serum osmolality usually is maintained by the normal pituitary response and stays within a range of 285 to 295 mOsm/kg (mmol/kg). Osmolar receptors in the anterior pituitary gland sense an increase in serum osmolality when the patient starts to become dehydrated, signaling the release of ADH from the storage area in the posterior lobe of the pituitary gland. ADH then is bound to V2 receptors in the kidneys, resulting in an increased permeability and reabsorption of free water in the renal collecting ducts [1]. With normal ADH secretion and renal function, urine osmolality is normally between 100 and 1200 mOsm/kg (mmol/kg). This is based on the body's need to excrete or retain free water. In addition to ADH release, an increase in fluid intake is needed to maintain normal serum osmotic pressure. A healthy individual has a feeling of thirst and drinks fluids when the serum osmolality is greater than 290 mOsm/kg. In addition to osmolality, the release of ADH is sensitive to changes in volume. A decrease in blood volume greater than 10% will cause the release of ADH. Other factors that stimulate the release of ADH include nausea, decrease in serum glucose, and certain medications [1].

In the patient with a head injury or tumor resulting in CDI, there is a failure to produce ADH or a decrease in the secretion of the ADH from the hypopituitary system, leading to a water diuresis, dilute urine, and a hypertonic state with increased serum sodium. Most patients with an acute head injury recover from CDI in a few days, but some go through a three-phase response to their injury: diuresis, water retention, and then persistent or recurrent DI.

Differential diagnosis

The differential diagnosis for polyuria and polydipsia includes solute diuresis, psychogenic polydipsia, nephropathies, and medication effects. Solute diuresis may be caused by electrolyte or nonelectrolyte abnormalities, such as uncontrolled diabetes mellitus or diuretic use. Psychogenic polydipsia (often seen in psychiatric patients who drink up to 20 L of water daily) is notable for a patient with widely varying daily fluid intake. Resolving acute renal failure may lead to a diuresis. Medications that can cause polydipsia or polyuria include anticholinergics and antipsychotics. Simply stated, many of these medications may cause a dry mouth, and therefore the patient will increase water intake if he or she is capable of doing so [1,12].

Emergency department evaluation

In the patient with acute hyperosmolar coma, a suspicion of DI should be noted if the patient has an elevated serum sodium and serum osmolality. In these patients, initial stabilization measures of airway management and immediate intravenous fluid resuscitation are necessary before the full laboratory assessment. This may be followed by immediate administration of arginine vasopressin (AVP) or desmopressin (DDAVP). [4]. This is not only therapeutic but also diagnostic, because improvement in patient condition may confirm the suspected CDI [2,12].

In nonemergent, stable cases, the physician should begin evaluating the patient suspected of having DI with a 24-hour urine volume test to confirm polyuria before more expensive tests are ordered [4,12]. Other basic testing should include serum electrolytes, random plasma, and urine osmolality and renal function studies.

Although not practical in the ED, the water deprivation test confirms DI and differentiates between central and nephrogenic origin. Nephrogenic and central DI also can be distinguished by an aquaporin-2 level. Aquaporin-2 is made in the kidney and is excreted in response to vasopressin [12]. The details and interpretation of these tests are beyond the scope of acute ED management and this article.

Recently, MRI has been used to diagnose hypothalamic and pituitary lesions in nonfatal head injury, including those with a delayed presentation of DI up to several weeks after the original insult. Case studies discussing this technique suggest T1- or T2-weighted imaging is used to detect the absence of the usual hyperintense signal in affected areas [2,13,14].

Emergency department treatment

The goals are to correct any pre-existing water deficits and to decrease continued renal water losses. Therapy depends on clinical presentation. The patient with a more severe case of DI may present with volume depletion and hypotension. This may be life-threatening [4]. Despite hypernatremia, these patients may need normal saline 0.9% infusions to restore blood pressure to the appropriate level. Usually small amounts of this isotonic solution are all that is required, as the intravascular volume loss is only a small percentage of the total body water loss [4]. If the patient is alert with a normal thirst mechanism and adequate access to water, he or she may be asymptomatic except for polyuria and polydipsia. This patient will benefit from interventions to relieve the polyuria and polydipsia.

To correct the initial water deficit the physician may estimate the total body deficit with the following formula:

$$\text{Current water deficit} = 0.6 \times \text{premorbid lean body weight} \times [1 - (140/\text{serum Na (mEq/L)})].$$

To decrease the risk of central nervous system (CNS) damage from severe hypertonicity, plasma osmolality should be lowered quickly (1 to 2 mOsm/kg per hour) to approximately 330 mOsm/kg (serum sodium of 160 mmol/L). If the patient remains symptomatic (ie, seizures, or coma) at serum sodium of less than 160 mmol/L, continued aggressive treatment is recommended. Correction may continue at this rapid rate for symptomatic patients until the sodium reaches 147 to 149 mmol/L. After resolution of severe symptoms, or when the sodium is 147 to 149 mmol/L, decrease the serum sodium by 3 to 4 mmol/L every 1 to 2 hours. As hypertonicity resolves, and the initial treatment reverses symptoms, correct the serum sodium into a normal range slowly over a 48-hour period to avoid cerebral edema. Further details for calculations of rehydration are noted in the article by Lin et al in this issue. Chronic hypernatremia should be decreased more slowly than acute and symptomatic more quickly than asymptomatic [4].

The water deficit formula does not consider ongoing water loss. If this continues, frequent serum and urine electrolyte values should be obtained and replaced with oral water or intravenous dextrose in water 0.5% (D_5W), which is also isotonic with an osmolality of approximately 278 mmol/kg. Care should be taken with the use of D_5W for rehydration, because this can worsen hypokalemia, and very ill patients may be unable to metabolize this large a glucose load, leading to hyperglycemia, glycosuria, and more diuresis [4].

The choice of medication depends on acute versus chronic management. For acute emergent treatment of CDI that is diagnosed clearly, in addition to intravenous fluids, parenteral arginine vasopressin, 5 U subcutaneous or desmopressin 1 to 2 µg subcutaneous should be administered. This will decrease urinary output and might simplify fluid management [4,8,15]. Dosing frequency is determined by close observations of urine volume, urine electrolytes, and serum electrolytes. Management is based on desired urinary output (eg, when the hourly urine volume increases by 25%, another dose is indicated) [4].

For chronic therapy, three medications are recommended; the previously mentioned AVP and DDAVP, and lysine vasopressin. The dose of AVP for the initial phase of CDI is 5 to 10 U subcutaneously every 2 to 4 hours. Disadvantages include short half-life, frequent administration, and as the dose is increased, there is no increase in intensity, just duration. Because of its pressor effect if given intravenously, it may cause an increase in blood pressure and possibly induce coronary vasospasm [4].

Lysine vasopressin is a synthetic vasopressin available as a nasal spray with somewhat less, but not absent pressor activity. It has a rapid onset but short duration and has been replaced largely by DDAVP. It remains useful for partial CDI, because it is less expensive than the former, but this medication is available only on a compassionate-use basis from the manufacturer [4].

Desmopressin is the drug of choice for chronic CDI. It has a longer half-life and has very little pressor activity. It is available for intranasal administration, and the usual dose is 10 to 40 µg (0.1 to 0.4 mL) once or twice daily. Adverse effects are not common, and they are usually dose-related. DDAVP should be used carefully in at-risk patients, as it may cause coronary vasoconstriction [4].

Summary

Central DI may develop in a patient with head injury, either shortly after the injury or several days later. This is seen increasingly as patients survive the initial trauma (direct or ischemic) and are home or in a rehabilitation program. If CDI is suspected, intravenous fluids should be administered to correct instability from hypovolemia and hypertonicity. Initial laboratory work-up should include serum and urine electrolytes and osmolality in addition to renal function. The symptomatic hypertonic patient should be treated aggressively initially to halt seizures and other neurological changes; then a gradual decrease in serum sodium is required to prevent cerebral edema. To combat ongoing water loss, AVP or DDAVP is given with continued monitoring of urine volume and serum and urine electrolytes. In the severely hypertonic patient, vasopressin replacement is diagnostic and therapeutic. In more mild cases other testing is required, both to diagnose DI and distinguish between a central, nephrogenic, or physiologic event.

Syndrome of inappropriate antidiuretic hormone

Because the most common etiology of SIADH is a tumor, identification of this syndrome and investigation of its cause are imperative. This affliction has been identified since 1938, when there was an association made between lung cancer and hyponatremia. The first mention of the inappropriate secretion of an ADH-like substance causing dilutional hyponatremia in lung cancer was reported in 1957. By 1972, the biosynthesis of ADH by tumor cells of a patient was proven and shown to be almost identical to that made in the hypothalamus [16,17]. Although the production of ADH has been associated mostly with small cell lung cancer, more recent case studies have linked it with other tumors, including prostate [18], pancreatic, and pituitary tumors that metastasize to the brain or primary brain cancers [19]. In addition, it has been found that chemotherapeutic agents such as vincristine, cyclophosphamide, and cisplatin also may precipitate this syndrome [17,19].

Emergency department presentation

The hallmark findings of SIADH include a decrease in serum sodium associated with a low serum osmolality with increased extracellular fluid and persistent excretion of sodium. The patient must have a urine osmolality greater than expected compared with the serum osmolality when measured concurrently. The patient must be clinically euvolemic, because dehydration or other etiologies then would be suggestive as the cause of the hyponatremia and hypo-osmolality. In addition, the kidneys, thyroid, and adrenal glands must be functioning normally. The serum level of AVP is not included in the diagnostic criteria for SIADH [20].

The signs and symptoms of SIADH are the same as for hyponatremia, although many patients are asymptomatic and diagnosed through routine laboratory testing. The serum sodium concentration and rate of fall determine the severity of the symptoms, explaining why some patients are symptomatic at levels higher than others [21].

Even with very low serum sodium levels (less than 120 mmol/L), clinical symptoms are seen in only 27% to 44% of patients, likely because of prolonged time in which the hyponatremia developed [16]. Early and nonspecific symptoms may be present, including fatigue, anorexia, nausea, vomiting, diarrhea, headaches, myalgias, and increased thirst. With serum sodium levels less than 100 to 115 mmol/L, the patient may present with an altered mental status, confusion, lethargy, seizures, psychosis, coma, and occasionally death [17,19,20]. Additional signs can include pathological reflexes, papilledema, cerebral edema, and occasionally, focal neurological symptoms [20,22] Case reports of SIADH from malignancies and malignancy treatments are numerous, with many presenting complaints [23–25].

Pathophysiology

The inappropriate increased levels of serum arginine vasopressin or AVP-like substance result in excessive water reabsorption in the renal collecting ducts, leading to dilutional hyponatremia and weight gain without edema. The postulated mechanisms for excessive AVP release include:

- Secretion of AVP or AVP-like substances from the tumor cells
- Noncancerous lung tissue acquires the ability to make and release AVP, or a decrease in left atrial filling pressures caused by lung disease causes central AVP release.
- Central nervous system disease stimulates the release of AVP from the neurohypophysis without normal stimulation [17].
- The pituitary is possibly stimulated by chemotherapy to release AVP [19].

Studies indicate that a release of AVP alone is not sufficient to cause hyponatremia. Natriuresis only occurs after volume expansion, possibly because of the simultaneous release of a natriuretic factor such as atrial natriuretic peptide (ANP), among others [16]. As this is a newer finding, and there are many case reports without findings of increased ANP, this will not be addressed here.

Differential diagnosis

The differential diagnosis of SIADH includes other causes of hyponatremia and alternate diagnoses made from the physical exam. If the patient presents with an altered mental status and seizure, the diagnosis of bacterial meningoencephalitis initially should be considered. Up to 50% of children with bacterial meningoencephalitis have SIADH as part of their presentation. If a metabolic disease state is the source of the SIADH, the physical exam is frequently normal without signs of edema or hypertension [26]. The complete differential diagnosis of hyponatremia is found in the article by Lin et al elsewhere in this issue.

The other metabolic disease states also seen in oncologic patients that must be distinguished from SIADH is central and renal salt wasting syndromes. Central salt wasting is caused by renal salt loss mediated by ANP, leading to serum hyponatremia and hyperosmolality. Unlike SIADH, treatment includes fluid and sodium replacement. Renal salt wasting syndrome is characterized by an excessive urinary excretion of sodium, often secondary to or after chemotherapy. These patients present with dry skin and poor turgor. Laboratory data reveal hyponatremia, increased urinary sodium, and abnormal renal function, possibly caused by cisplatin related renal tubule damage. These patients may present with an increased level of ADH if they are dehydrated. Treatment is usually sodium re-placement [27].

Emergency department evaluation

Syndrome of inappropriate antidiuretic hormone is a diagnosis of exclusion and encompasses the classic triad of decreased serum osmolality (less than 270 mmol/L) with hyponatremia, urine osmolality inappropriately greater than serum osmolality, and an elevated urine sodium (less than 20 mEq/L) [26]. The patient must be clinically euvolemic to make the diagnosis.

Laboratory testing to establish the diagnosis of SIADH includes: sodium, glucose, serum urea nitrogen (BUN), uric acid, plasma osmolarity, urine osmolality, urine sodium, thyroid function, creatinine and morning cortisol. Solutes such as glucose can cause a relative decrease in sodium without a change in serum osmolality, so to avoid the misdiagnosis of SIADH, a direct measurement of serum osmolality or correcting for hyperglycemia is required.

A normal BUN is an important indicator of euvolemia in these patients. Another indicator of SIADH is the uric acid levels, which are low because of the enhanced extracellular volume clearance. The plasma osmolality may be calculated by the following formula: [26,28].

$$\text{Plasma osmolality} = [2 \times \text{Na (mEq/L)}] + \frac{\text{Glucose (mg/dL)}}{18} + \frac{\text{BUN (mg/dL)}}{2.8}$$

The urine osmolality must be increased inappropriately compared with serum to be consistent with SIADH. The urine osmolality must be greater than maximally dilute (eg, Uosm greater than 100 mOsm/kg water in the hypo-osmolar patient) [28].

Normally functioning kidneys and thyroid and adrenal glands are required to diagnose SIADH. Tests include serum creatinine, thyrotropin (TSH), free T4, and morning cortisol. Additional tests may include albumin and protein. Radiological studies that may aid in diagnosis include CT scan of the brain if seizures are part of the presentation and a CT or plain radiograph of the chest to look for malignancy. SIADH frequently is associated with small cell tumors of the lung and first may be diagnosed when the patient presents with SIADH.

Emergency department management

Emergency department management is aimed at correcting the hyponatremia. If the patient is symptomatic, or if the tumor eradication process is slow and the plasma sodium less than 130 mmol/L, fluid restrictions to 500 mL per day should increase the serum sodium [16,17,19,21]. If chemotherapy is required, careful monitoring and fluids of normal saline with a diuretic and electrolyte replacement are warranted.

Life-threatening hyponatremia with seizure or coma requires an initial bolus of 3% normal saline intravenously (300 to 500 cc over 3 to 4 hours) along with furosemide intravenously 1 mg/kg [17,20,21]. Normal saline increases serum sodium, while furosemide causes a negative fluid balance and prevents cardiac overload. The goal is to increase the sodium slowly, but no greater than 0.5 to 1 mEq/L per hour to prevent complications. Further details are found in the article by Lin et al elsewhere in this issue.

Monitoring should include hourly urinary outputs, urine sodium, serum sodium, and potassium, with replacement as needed. Central Venous Pressure monitoring is suggested in the elderly or patients with a cardiac history [17,19–21]. In patients with SIADH secondary to malignancy, approximately 7 to 10 days are required before improvement is noted. In those with a non-neoplastic cause, improvement within 3 days is expected [17].

Some patients are unresponsive to fluid restrictions or are unable to comply with the prescribed therapy because of antineoplastic treatment. This group can be treated with medications designed to interfere with the renal effects of AVP. These medications include diphenylhydantoin, dichlormethyl tetracycline, and lithium. Of these, dichlormethyl tetracycline is used most often. Diphenylhydantoin blocks the release of AVP at the neurohypophysis but has the disadvantage of being available for the intravenous route only. Lithium and dichlormethyl tetracycline act at the renal tubules directly inhibiting AVP-induced cAMP formation and block the effects of cAMP already made. This produces a nephrogenic DI that is dose-dependent, reversible, and consistently increases serum sodium levels without fluid restriction [17,20]. These medications are used if the underlying disorder is not eradicated and the patient needs long-term therapy [19–21,26].

Definitive treatment involves eradication of the tumor [16,17,19,20]. Chemotherapy of small cell cancer of the lung leads to resolution of SIADH in about 80% of patients treated, and the serum sodium returns to normal levels within 2 weeks in most [16,21]. If the SIADH is caused by a primary brain tumor or metastasis to the brain, radiation and corticosteroid treatment may be of benefit.

Disposition

When SIADH is diagnosed, treatment is based on the serum sodium level and extent of symptoms exhibited by the patient. These therapies vary from fluid restriction in mild cases to hypertonic saline and diuretic use in the more severely symptomatic. Eradication of the underlying cause of SIADH is the main goal of treatment, but if this is not feasible, long-term therapy with dichlormethyl tetracycline is available for those unable to tolerate fluid restriction. Disposition depends on the severity of the symptoms, laboratory evaluation, and ability to comply with therapy. The more symptomatic patients will be admitted. Those who may be discharged include patients with asymptomatic hyponatremia, serum sodium levels greater than 125 mmol/L, those without unstable comorbidities, and a known diagnosis of SIADH.

Sheehan's syndrome

Sheehan's syndrome, or postpartum pituitary necrosis, is a potentially devastating complication of pregnancy and delivery. It is a relatively rare acquired condition with diminished or decreased production of anterior pituitary hormones resulting in panhypopituitarism. Sheehan first described the syndrome in 1937 after autopsy study of patients who had died in the postpartum period [29]. It usually is associated with hemorrhage and shock in the postpartum period, but has been reported occasionally in patients who had no hemorrhage.

More recently, Molitch characterized Sheehan's syndrome into an acute form presenting within hours to days after delivery, and a chronic form presenting weeks to years later [30]. The acute presentation, which can be lethal, is dominated by symptoms and signs of adrenal insufficiency. The clinical presentation of the chronic form is more subtle; the degree of hormone deficiencies determines the clinical presentation.

The exact incidence of Sheehan's syndrome is unknown, although it appears to be more common in developing countries [31]. With prompt recognition and treatment, the morbidity and mortality should be minimized, because treatments for hypopituitarism exist.

Emergency department presentation

Sheehan's syndrome can occur with widely differing severity. It can be seen acutely in the puerperium with potentially lethal pituitary failure or may present years later with vague symptomatology. In the acute, potentially life-threatening form of the disease, the clinical presentation is one of an ill patient with symptoms and signs of adrenal insufficiency: hypotension, tachycardia, hypoglycemia, extreme fatigue, and nausea and vomiting. Also seen are failure to regrow shaved pubic hair, apathy, and failure to lactate [30]. One should consider this diagnosis in obstetrical patients with severe hemorrhage not responsive to blood replacement and prolonged hypotension. This disease may be seen by emergency physicians because of shorter postpartum hospitalizations.

In the chronic form, the clinical presentation may be seen from weeks to years after delivery. The degree of hormone deficiency determines the clinical presentation. The syndrome may be subclinical in some patients and manifest only if the patient is stressed. Signs and symptoms may be vague and nonspecific: lightheadedness, fatigue, failure to lactate, persistent amenorrhea, decreased body hair, dry skin, loss of libido, nausea and vomiting, and cold intolerance. DI has been reported in several cases of Sheehan's syndrome [8,38].

Pathophysiology

The pituitary gland lies in the sella turcica within the sphenoid bone [32]. The pituitary normally enlarges during pregnancy. The gland is comprised of an anterior and posterior lobe, which are anatomically distinct [33]. The blood supply to the anterior pituitary is through the internal carotid arteries and superior hypophyseal arteries. The inferior hypophyseal arteries supply the blood to the posterior pituitary. The anterior pituitary gland produces six major hormones: prolactin (PRL), growth hormone (GH), corticotropin (ACTH), luteinizing hormone (LH), follicle stimulating hormone (FSH), and thyroid stimulating hormone (TSH). The posterior pituitary gland produces ADH and oxytocin.

The pathogenesis of Sheehan's syndrome is not understood fully. During pregnancy, the normal pituitary enlarges, predominantly because of progressive lactotroph hyperplasia.

Based on extensive pathologic studies of patients, Sheehan proposed pituitary necrosis caused by occlusive spasm of the pituitary vessels. The size of the necrosis depends on the severity, duration, and distribution of the spasm. Massive or submassive ischemic necrosis of the pituitary gland should result in acute pituitary failure; however, delayed presentation of pituitary failure is common, with patients presenting years later with symptomatology. This slow clinical progression has led some authors to suggest a relationship between postpartum hemorrhage, pituitary antibodies, and the development of Sheehan's syndrome [34–36].

Differential diagnosis

Sheehan's syndrome should be considered in the patient with a recent obstetrical delivery with findings of shock. The differential diagnosis includes the long list of disease entities that may cause shock. Of special note, in the postpartum patient one must consider hypovolemia from ongoing blood loss or inadequate resuscitation, embolic disorders, and cardiac disorders associated with pregnancy. Unique conditions of the pregnant patient that may predispose one to hemorrhage include placenta previa, placenta abruption, uterine rupture, postpartum hemorrhage, puerperal hematoma, retained placenta, and uterine atony. Embolic disorders to consider in the postpartum patient with shock include amniotic fluid embolus, pulmonary thromboembolism, and venous air embolism. Cardiac conditions that may present with shock include peripartum cardiomyopathy, peripartum myocarditis, coronary artery dissection, atherosclerotic cardiovascular disease, and congenital heart disease. Life-threatening infection is an uncommon cause of maternal shock and death in the United States. Untreated infection, however, can lead to septic shock. Pituitary insufficiency as the etiology of shock may occur because of an autoimmune disorder such as lymphocytic hypophysitis [37].

The differential diagnosis of the chronic form of Sheehan's syndrome is extensive. The differential diagnosis of pituitary disease includes neoplasms (primary brain tumors and metastatic neoplasms), congenital deficiencies of each of the trophic hormones, vascular disorders, infectious causes (including tuberculosis, meningitis, and syphilis), sarcoidosis, and physical agents (radiation, surgery, and previous head trauma.)

Emergency department evaluation

In the acutely ill patient, evaluation and treatment must occur simultaneously. Attention to airway, ventilatory, and vascular support begins the resuscitation. Blood specimens should be obtained, and treatment should be initiated without waiting for results. Many of these test results are not likely to be available to the treating emergency clinician. The history may suggest a hypotensive period associated with delivery. The physical exam may exclude some entities in the long differential of shock.

Laboratory testing for Sheehan's syndrome includes baseline complete blood count, electrolyte panel, thyroid function studies, and assessment of the pituitary hormones (ACTH, PRL, GH, LH, FSH, and TSH). It would be expected to find low ACTH, cortisol, GH, PRL, and T3 levels. The T4 may be normal, as the levels may not yet be decreased because of the 7-day half-life of T4. Normally, one would see a 5- to 10-fold elevation in the PRL level in the puerperium, but in this scenario of pituitary failure, the PRL level is low.

The chronic form of Sheehan's syndrome may have an acute presentation. Months or years of vague symptoms may manifest with severe adrenal insufficiency when the patient is stressed. Laboratory testing should include baseline electrolyte panel, thyroid function studies, and assessment of pituitary hormones (ACTH, PRL, GH, LH, FSH, and TSH). All pituitary hormones may be low, consistent with hypopituitarism. Most of these laboratory studies will not be available to the physician initially evaluating the patient but will prove helpful to the clinician providing further care. Some patients may have normal baseline hormone levels but abnormal responses to stimulation. Stimulation testing may be necessary to confirm the diagnosis. This distinction is important for evaluating the subclinical patient who manifests with severe adrenal insufficiency when stressed. GH stimulation testing may be done by inducing hypoglycemia to reduce the blood glucose to 50% of the fasting level. This should increase the GH level to 6 to 8 ng/mL. Cortisol-stimulating tests are helpful in assessing the patient's ACTH activity.

Emergency department management

Acute treatment includes volume expansion, hydrocortisone 100 mg intravenously as a bolus followed by an additional 200 mg within the first 24 hours. Hospital admission, endocrinology consult, and further evaluation to assess the need for other hormone replacement are needed.

Treatment of the chronic form of Sheehan's syndrome is based on the patient's hormone deficiencies. Thyroid supplementation may be necessary with levothyroxine. Adrenal insufficiency is treated with oral prednisone. Hormone supplementation is necessary in times of stress, such as trauma or surgery. The disposition of the patient with chronic disease should be based on the clinical symptoms and findings with which she is presenting.

Summary

Sheehan's syndrome may present from hours to days after delivery, or may present with a long history of vague symptoms and acute decompensation in times of stress. The acute clinical picture is dramatic, a patient in shock. Initial treatment in the ED includes airway, ventilatory, and vascular support, followed by obtaining blood specimens for hormone testing. Initially, dexamethasone can be administered. Further hormone therapy is guided by results of laboratory testing.

References

[1] Adam P. Evaluation and management of diabetes insipidus. Am Fam Physician 1997;55(6): 2146–52.
[2] Kawai K, Aoki M, Nakayama H, et al. Posterior pituitary hematoma in a case of posttraumatic diabetes insipidus. J Neurosurg 1995;83:368–71.
[3] Alaca R, Bilge Y. Anterior hypopituitarism with unusual delayed onset of diabetes insipidus after penetrating head injury. Am J Phys Med Rehab 2002;81(10):788–91.
[4] Singer I, Oster J, Fishman L. The management of diabetes insipidus in adults. Arch Intern Med 1997;157(12):1293–301.

[5] Rose B. Urine output in diabetes insipidus. Available at: www.uptodate.com. Accessed August 5, 2004.

[6] Kuzeyli K, Cakr E, Baykal S, et al. Diabetes insipidus secondary to penetrating spinal cord trauma: case report and literature review. Spine 2001;26(21):E510–1.

[7] Edwards O, Clark J. Post-traumatic hypopituitarism. Six cases and a review of the literature. Medicine 1986;65(5):281–90.

[8] Kan A, Calligerous D. A case report of Sheehan's syndrome presenting with diabetes insipidus. N Z J Obstet Gynaecol 1998;38(2):224–6.

[9] Barzilay Z, Somekh E. Diabetes insipidus in severely brain-damaged children. J Med 1988; 19(1):47–64.

[10] Childers M, Rupright J, Jones P, et al. Assessment of neuroendocrine dysfunction following traumatic brain injury. Brain Inj 1998;12(6):517–23.

[11] Hadani M, Findler G, Shaked I, et al. Unusual delayed onset of diabetes insipidus following closed head trauma. J Neurosurg 1985;63:456–8.

[12] Maghnie M. Diabetes insipidus. Horm Res 2003;59(Suppl 1):42–54.

[13] Moses A, Thomas D, Canfield M, et al. Central diabetes insipidus due to cytomegalovirus infection of the hypothalamus in a patient with acquired immunodeficiency syndrome: a clinical, pathological, and immunohistochemical case study. J Clin Endocrinol Metab 2003;88(1):51–4.

[14] Maghnie M, Altobelli M, di Iorgi N, et al. Idiopathic central diabetes insipidus is associated with abnormal blood supply to the posterior pituitary gland caused by vascular impairment of the inferior hypophyseal artery system. J Clin Endocrinol Metab 2004;89(4):1891–6.

[15] Weimann E, Molenkamp G, Bohles H. Diabetes insipidus due to hypophysitis. Horm Res 1997;47:81–4.

[16] Mazzone P, Arroliga A. Endocrine paraneoplastic syndromes in lung cancer. Curr Opin Pulm Med 2003;9(4):313–20.

[17] Pimental L. Medical complications of oncologic disease. Med Clin North Am 1993;11(2): 407–19.

[18] Yalcin S, Erman M, Tekuzman G, et al. Syndrome of inappropriate antidiuretic hormone secretion (SIADH) associated with prostatic carcinoma. Am J Clin Oncol 2000;23(4):384–5.

[19] Tan S. Recognition and treatment of oncologic emergencies. J Infus Nurs 2002;25(3):182–8.

[20] Sorensen J, Anderson M, Hansen H. Syndrome of inappropriate secretion of antidiuretic hormone (SIADH) in malignant disease. J Int Med 1995;238:97–110.

[21] Markham M. Common complications and emergencies associated with cancer and its therapy. Cleve Clin J Med 1994;105–14.

[22] Advanced challenges in resuscitation. Section 1: life-threatening electrolyte abnormalities. [Guidelines 2000 for CPR and emergency cardiovascular care: International Consensus on Science]. Circulation 2000;102(8):I-217–22.

[23] Panayiotou H, Small S, Hunter J, et al. Sweet taste (dysgeusia): the first symptom of hyponatremia in small cell carcinoma of the lung. Arch Intern Med 1995;155(12):1325–8.

[24] Tzortzatou F, Dacou-Voutetakis C, Haidas S, et al. Electrolyte abnormalities in lympho-sarcoma after chemotherapy. Acta Paediatr Scand 1979;68(4):621–3.

[25] Galesic K, Krizanac S, Vrkljan M, et al. Syndrome of inappropriate secretion of antidiuretic hormone due to malignant thymoma. Nephron 2002;91(4):752–4.

[26] Vesely D. Inappropriate secretion of antidiuretic hormone. In: Schwartz G, Hanke B, Mayer T, et al, editors. Principles and practices of emergency medicine. 4th edition. Baltimore (MD): Williams & Wilkins; 1999. p. 969–72.

[27] Cao L, Joshi P, Sumoza D. Renal salt-wasting syndrome in a patient with cisplatin-induced hyponatremia. Case report. Am J Clin Oncol 2002;25(4):344–6.

[28] American College of Physicians. Syndrome of inappropriate antidiuretic hormone secretion (SIADH). Laboratory and other studies for hyponatremia. Available at: http://online. statref.com. Accessed August 25, 2004.

[29] Sheehan HL. Postpartum necrosis of the anterior pituitary. J Pathol Bacteriol 1937;45: 189–214.
[30] Molitch ME. Pituitary diseases in pregnancy. Semin Perinatol 1998;22:457–70.
[31] Sanuels MH. Sheehan's syndrome. Endocrinologist 2004;14:25–30.
[32] Melmed S, Braunstein G. Disorders of the hypothalamus and anterior pituitary. Available at: http://online.statref.com. Accessed September 5, 2004.
[33] Melmed S. Disorders of the anterior pituitary and hypothalamus. Available at: http:// online.statref.com. Accessed September 5, 2004.
[34] Goswami R, Kochupillai N, Crock P, et al. Pituitary autoimmunity in patients with Sheehan's syndrome. J Clin Endrocrinol Metab 2002;87(9):4137–41.
[35] Engelberth O, Jezkova Z. Autoantibodies in Sheehan's syndrome. Lancet 1965;1:1075.
[36] Pouplard A. Pituitary autoimmunity. Horm Res 1982;16:289–97.
[37] Prahlow J, Barnard J. Pregnancy-related maternal deaths. Am J Forensic Med Pathol 2004; 25(3):220–36.
[38] Barkan AL. Case report: pituitary atrophy in patients with Sheehan's syndrome. Am J Med Sci 1989;298(1):38–40.

ELSEVIER
SAUNDERS

EMERGENCY
MEDICINE
CLINICS OF
NORTH AMERICA

Emerg Med Clin N Am 23 (2005) 843–883

The Emergency Department Approach to Newborn and Childhood Metabolic Crisis

Ilene Claudius, MD, Colleen Fluharty, MD*,
Richard Boles, MD

*Department of Emergency and Transport Medicine,
Children's Hospital Los Angeles, 4650 Sunset Boulevard,
MS113, Los Angeles, CA 90027, USA*

For most emergency medicine physicians, the phrases "newborn workup" and "metabolic disease" are, at best, uncomfortable. This article, however, provides a simple approach to the recognition, evaluation, and treatment of infants with all manners of metabolic issues, including hypoglycemia, inborn errors of metabolism, jaundice, and electrolyte abnormalities. The disorders are grouped based on symptomatology, and have simple guidelines for work-up and management, with an emergency department practitioner perspective in mind.

The workup of a newborn with metabolic disease in the emergency department (ED) is a daunting endeavor for any physician. This article provides a simple approach to the recognition, evaluation, and treatment of infants with all manner of metabolic issues, including hypoglycemia, inborn errors of metabolism, jaundice, and electrolyte abnormalities.

Hypoglycemia

Definition

For years, the definition of hypoglycemia in neonates has varied widely, with some authors accepting a blood glucose of 30 mg/dL, while other sources change thresholds as an infant progresses through the first few days of life. More recently, neonatologists have accepted plasma glucose levels <45 mg/dL as a clear indication of hypoglycemia in any symptomatic

---

* Corresponding author.
  E-mail address: cfluharty@chla.usc.edu (C. Fluharty).

0733-8627/05/$ - see front matter © 2005 Elsevier Inc. All rights reserved.
doi:10.1016/j.emc.2005.03.010
emed.theclinics.com

neonate. In asymptomatic neonates, serum glucose ≤35 is considered an indication for treatment and close monitoring [1]. This change in thinking is predicated on several recent studies looking at neurologic outcomes of neonates with low glucose. Lucas [2] retrospectively showed poor intellectual performance in 18-month-old ex-premature babies who had been persistently below a serum glucose of 47 mg/dL as neonates. In 1999, Kinnala [3] observed abnormal cerebral magnetic resonance images and cranial ultrasounds at 2 months of age in 39% of otherwise well full-term neonates with blood glucose below 45 mg/dL versus 10% of euglycemic infants. Abnormal evoked potentials have also been measured in this population [4]. Because presentation to an ED selects for ill neonates, some of whom will have poor neurologic outcomes despite the most expeditious treatment, setting 45 mg/dL (2.5 mmol/L) as the threshold for hypoglycemia in all neonates is probably safest [5]. As reagent strips designed for rapid bedside glucose testing are widely variable in performance for this indication [6], the definition of hypoglycemia relies on confirmation by laboratory measurement of the serum glucose.

Physiology

Neonates are generally born with a serum glucose of 60% to 80% of maternal glucose. Within 2 to 4 hours, they stabilize and begin to regulate themselves. Maintenance of serum glucose requires the interplay of several systems. As the primary regulator, insulin stimulates the uptake of glucose by cells. Its counterregulatory hormones, specifically cortisol, glucagon, epinephrine, and growth hormone, are prevalent in times of starvation to encourage glycogenolysis and lipolysis. The liver both synthesizes glucose from amino acids, glycerol, and lactate, and coverts glycogen to glucose during fasting. When compared with adults, infants have decreased glycogen stores and poorly matured glycogenolysis [7]. In the normal well-nourished neonate, by 2 to 3 hours following a meal, insulin is suppressed and counterregulatory hormones are high. By 12 to 16 hours of fasting, the hepatic stores are depleted, and muscle and adipose begin to break down. Muscle can use its own glycogen stores during fasting, and although the glucose created is not released systemically, amino acids are released to the liver [8].

Emergency department presentation

Symptoms of hypoglycemia fall into two major categories: adrenergic and neuroglycopenic. Adults manifest high adrenergic tone as palpitations, anxiety, tremulousness, and diaphoresis, and neuroglycopenic symptoms as headache, fatigue, confusion, seizure, and unconsciousness. Neonates present similarly, but often translate the symptoms reported by adults into more subtle clues, such as jitteriness, tachycardia, apnea, cyanosis, tachypnea, hypotonia, temperature instability, lethargy, irritability, or an abnormal cry. Also, secondary hypoglycemia may be a concern for children presenting in extremis, regardless of etiology. In these children, signs of respiratory or cardiac failure may be attributed to the primary illness, leaving the hypoglycemia unrecognized. In one study, 9 of 49 children requiring resuscitative care for a medical condition exhibited hypoglycemia, suggesting glucose should be checked promptly on every patient requiring emergent resuscitation. The mortality in children with secondary hypoglycemia is higher than in nonhypoglycemia children with matched diagnoses [9].

Differential diagnosis

Primary hypoglycemia has an extensive differential, and the definitive underlying diagnosis is not the role of the emergency physician. However, low glucose may indicate another condition, like sepsis, requiring emergent diagnosis and attention. More commonly, the emergentologist has a unique opportunity to facilitate the workup of a hypoglycemic child. Insulin, cortisol, and growth hormone levels must be obtained while a child is hypoglycemic. If they are not drawn before treatment in the ED, a child will be subjected to the risks and discomfort of prolonged fasting in the hospital to replicate the hypoglycemia. Obviously, no reasonable physician would leave a seizing child untreated while an extensive workup is completed, but setting aside an additional red top tube before the administration of glucose may greatly assist the pediatrician or endocrinologist who assumes care.

Once the child is stabilized, a differential can be formed based on the presence of urinary ketones and the child's response to treatment. Ketones require lipolysis, which is suppressed by insulin and stimulated by the counterregulatory hormones. Therefore, diseases involving high levels of insulin production generally do not allow the formation of ketones. The quintessential disease in this category is hyperinsulinism from islet cell adenomas or overproduction, which can present either in the neonatal period or later in life. Although uncommon to see in a child returning to the ED after a hospital birth, infants of diabetic mothers have similar overproduction of insulin during the first 24 hours. Due to the lack of counterregulatory hormones, congenital panhypopituitarism may cause hypoglycemia, and is generally nonketotic (although individual hormone deficiencies may cause ketosis). Adrenal insufficiency, most commonly in the form of congenital adrenal hyperplasia (CAH), can cause a hyperinsulinism as well. Fatty acid oxidation deficiencies rarely present in the first month of life, but may cause a nonketotic hypoglycemia [10]. Finally, a rare condition known as Beckwith-Wiedemann can cause hyperinsulinism, and is usually recognized by hemihypertrophy of the patient's body and internal organs. Most of the nonketotic forms of hypoglycemia involve an inability of the body to produce glucose and other forms of energy despite appropriate glycogen storage. Therefore, glucagon has an important diagnostic and therapeutic role. If it is effective in normalizing serum glucose, this confirms that hepatic energy stores are present, suggesting one of these diagnoses.

On the other hand, children with ketotic hypoglycemia often lack the glycogen stores to respond to glucagon [11]. Children who are thin, when subjected to prolonged fasting or gastroenteritis, can easily become hypoglycemic. In fact, simple ketotic hypoglycemia from fasting is the most common etiology in a nondiabetic child. One study showed this to account for 24.4% of episodes of hypoglycemia presenting to the ED in nondiabetic children over 6 months [12]. Of course, there are more serious etiologies for a ketotic hypoglycemia, and metabolic diseases such as galactosemia, hereditary fructose intolerance, and glycogen storage disease type 1 should be considered in a neonate who appears ill or has abnormal physical findings like hepatomegaly [13].

Common secondary reasons for hypoglycemia include ingestions (ethanol, insulin, oral hypoglycemia, salicylates, and propranolol), liver failure [14], and sepsis. One study of septic neonates demonstrated hypoglycemia in 20 of 56 babies, suggesting prompt diagnosis and treatment of hypoglycemia is warranted in this population [15].

Infants born in the department

Early discharge of neonates has been a convenient and cost-effective measure, but increases the likelihood of a 1- to 2-day-old hypoglycemia infant presenting, undiagnosed, to the ED. Even without this consideration, many of us have witnessed the "virginal" teen with abdominal pain give birth in the department, and the risk factors for hypoglycemia in these children must be discussed. Of paramount importance is to recognize the symptoms of hypoglycemia. The unexpected birth of a child in the department can cause significant stress, particularly if the baby is not doing well. Any concern of respiratory difficulty, vital sign instability, or neurologic findings should prompt performance of a bedside glucose.

Infants of diabetic mothers have a significant risk of early hypoglycemia—most sources quote 25% [17], but in one study 47% of infants of diabetic mothers developed hypoglycemia in the first 2 hours of life [18]. The glucose crossing the placental barrier causes hypertrophy of the islet cells, which continues for 24 hours following birth [17]. Large-for-gestational-age babies, even without maternal diabetes, may have sufficient hyperinsulinism to become hypoglycemic [7]. On the opposite end of the spectrum, premature or small-for-gestational-age babies can lack the stores to maintain their glucose. Transient hyperinsulinism without predisposing factors is rare, but has been reported [19]. Maternal factors, such as use of sympathomimetic medications, may also cause low blood sugar in the neonate [16]. If proper incubators and warming lights are not used, the cold stress alone can cause the glucose to plummet. Many of these children will not become hypoglycemic until 2 to 4 hours after birth. Therefore, if awaiting a bed or a transfer requires a high-risk neonate to remain in the ED for several hours, a repeat assessment and bedside glucose is warranted, even in the absence of symptoms, and certainly immediately if symptoms develop.

Emergency department evaluation

As previously stated, hypoglycemia is a symptom, rather than a diagnosis. The hypoglycemia may be suggested on a bedside glucose, and confirmed by a laboratory run serum glucose, but additional labs can confirm the etiology. A minimum workup includes serum glucose, growth hormone, insulin level, cortisol, and ketones obtained while the patient is hypoglycemia. A urinalysis can give an early indication regarding the presence of ketones, as the serum ketones may take hours to run. Electrolytes are indicated, although mild acidosis is often associated with hypoglycemia and will correct without intervention. A more significant acidosis may be due to ketosis or may indicate the presence of lactic acid from sepsis or metabolic diseases [11]. Second tier tests that may be ordered from the ED or later include lactate, free fatty acids, ammonia, acylcarnitine, organic acid profiles.

Emergency department management

Significant alterations in mental status may resolve slowly, even after the child has been given adequate glucose [8]. For children in whom intravenous (IV) access cannot be obtained, oral or nasogastric glucose is an option, as is intramuscular glucagon. Once IV access is obtained, a small bolus 0.25 to 0.5 g/kg of dextrose should be administered. Neonatologists would suggest administering this as 2 to 4 mL/kg of D_{10}, but D_{25} is likely also safe if the IV is secure in a large vein at a dose of 1 to 2 mL/kg. The bolus should be followed by a infusion, and generally a D_{10} with 0.2NS drip at 1.5 times maintenance [8] will provide 6 to 8 mg/kg/min, which is a physiologic glucose delivery rate. Clearly, hyperinsulinemic or ill neonates may require a higher glucose delivery rate. If a concentration above $D_{12.5}$ is required to maintain the blood glucose, central access should be obtained. If the hypoglycemia is refractory to glucose administration, glucagon, a pancreatic polypeptide hormone [20], may be administered, and may be followed 1 hour later by hydrocortisone. However, these modalities require substrate and, therefore, are unlikely to work in a patient with ketotic hypoglycemia, or in the absence of simultaneous IV glucose. If a patient responds to glucagon transiently, an IV glucagon drip has been proven effective in the glucagon-responsive neonate [21,22]. Diazoxide or an octreotide drip may also work for hyperinsulinism-induced hypoglycemia [14]. Clearly, if an underlying disease is suspected, it should be treated as well, with attention to antibiotics if sepsis is suspected, and to hormone replacement if panhypopituitarism or CAH are possible. These treatments are summarized in Table 1.

Table 1
Treatment for hypoglycemia

Medication	Indication	Route	Dose	Maximum (adult) dose
Dextrose	Hypoglycemia	IV	0.25–0.5 g/kg given as 1–2 cc/kg D_{25} or 2–4 cc/kg D_{10}	25 g (1 amp)
Glucagon	Nonketotic hypoglycemia	IV or IM	0.03 mg/kg	1 mg
Hydrocortisone	Suspected hormone deficiency without shock	IV or IM	1–2 mg/kg (shock dose is higher)	100 mg
Diazoxide	Hyperinsulinemia	PO	5 mg/kg/dose	150 mg
Octreotide	Hyperinsulinemia	SC or IV	1 µg/kg bolus followed by 1 µg/kg/h infusion	100 µg

From Refs. [23,24]. Taketomo C, (ed.) Childrens Hospital Los Angeles pediatric dosing handbook and formulary. Ohio: Lexicomp; 2003. p. 269, 390, 408, 564; Tarascon Pocket Pharmacoepia. Loma Linda: Tarascon Publishing; 2001. p. 43, 56.

Goals of treatment are markedly different than definitions of hypoglycemia. For an otherwise well baby requiring treatment, a level of >45 mg/dL is acceptable [1]. For a child with other incurrent medical issues, prematurity, or suspected hyperinsulinism, maintenance of glucose between 72 to 90 mg/dL is prudent [6].

Disposition

Clearly, most patients with hypoglycemia will require admission, either to the floor, or to a more monitored setting if frequent neurologic checks or bedside glucose checks are required. In a healthy older child with ketotic hypoglycemia, disposition home is acceptable once the hypoglycemia resolves and the child is taking food well [14]. In a neonate, however, admission for further workup and observation is indicated.

Long term

As previously mentioned, hypoglycemia in the early neonatal period can have devastating long-term neurologic consequences, particularly when symptomatic, prolonged, or early in onset. Hyperinsulinism as a cause of hypoglycemia may also be a risk factor for poor neurologic outcome. In one study, 52% of patients requiring subtotal pancreatectomy for hyperinsulinemia suffered mental retardation [25]. Meissner also demonstrated a poorer outcome in the hyperinsulinemic children with neonatal onset of hypoglycemia than in those with an onset later in childhood [26]. In Menni's study of 90 patients with persistent hyperinsulinemic hypoglycemia, seven patients had severe mental retardation, 12 patients had intermediate delay, and 16 had epilepsy. Early onset of neonatal hypoglycemia was highly correlated with these outcomes [27].

Inborn errors of metabolism

Whether due to the large variety of diseases or the intricacy of the biochemical pathways, studying inborn errors of metabolism is daunting. Yet despite their seeming complexity, an emergency physician or pediatrician can easily care for these children by remembering several basic underlying principals. The hundreds of specific diseases involved generally cause symptoms by three major mechanisms of illness: (1) the acute accumulation of toxic small molecules, (2) energy deficiency, or (3) the chronic accumulation of large molecules. These are summarized in Table 2. With some overlapping and exceptions, these different mechanisms lead to three different categories of presenting signs, abnormalities on diagnostic testing, and treatment modalities. All these disorders have in common that each is caused by a genetic mutation that disables a protein, resulting in a blocked metabolic pathway. The defective proteins are generally enzymes, although increasingly defects in proteins involved in crossmembrane transport, assembly, and cofactor maintenance are being identified as the cause of various metabolic disorders. Inborn errors of metabolism can present in older children, but this article will address the inborn errors of metabolism that commonly present in the neonatal period.

Emergency department presentation

Defects in enzymes/proteins involved in small molecule catabolism generally cause disease due to a toxic intermediate that accumulates at high concentration because of the metabolic block. Pathology does not begin until after birth because the placenta easily removes these small molecules. When enzymatic function is absent or minimal, these toxic intermediates can accumulate rapidly, and reach concentrations sufficient to cause disease generally between the second and fifth postnatal days [28]. Many, but not all, of these disorders involve the catabolic pathway of one or more amino acids ("aminoacidemias/urias" or "organicacidemias/urias"), and the accumulating toxic intermediates are acids. Thus, severe metabolic acidosis is a feature common to many of these disorders. Hyperpnea/tachypnea can be secondary to metabolic acidosis or hyperammonemia, which is also commonly present. Many, but not all, of these toxic intermediates cause acute neurologic dysfunction, and thus altered mental status (irritability or lethargy) and vomiting are frequently the presenting signs of early illness. Altered mental status and vomiting interfere with feeding, leading to

Table 2
Metabolic disorders in early infancy

Mechanism	Classes of disorder	Examples	Signs	Labs	Treatment
Toxic small molecules	Organic and amino acidemias	Methylmalonic acidemia, propionic acidemia, maple syrup urine disease	Altered mental status (irritability, lethargy, coma), poor feeding, vomiting, neurologic symptoms, hyperpnea/tachypnea, Frequently present at age 2–5 days	Anion gap acidosis, ketonuria, increased ammonia, uric acid, and lactate, low glucose (rare)	NPO IV glucose L-carnitine Insulin HD Liver transplantation
	Urea cycle disorders	Citrullinemia, ornithine transcarbamoylase deficiency		Elevated ammonia, respiratory alkalosis	NPO IV glucose L-arginine (some disorders) Na benzoate, Na phenylacetate and/or Na phenylbutyrate[a] Insulin HD Liver transplantation
	Sugar intolerances	Galactosemia	Liver failure with jaundice hemorrhage, ascites, and edema	Elevated transaminases and bilirubin, low glucose, coagulopathy	NPO IV glucose, Antibiotics

Exceptions (amino acidemias with distinct presentations)	Nonketotic hyperglycinemia	Lethargy, apnea, Hypoventilation, and seizures in the first week	Elevated CSF to peripheral glycine ratio	None effective
	Tyrosinemia Type 1	Liver failure at 2 months hepatomegaly at 3 weeks	Liver failure	NTBC
Energy deficiency	Mitochondrial disorders Electron transport chain and related disorders	Neurological dysfunction, seizures, hepatomegaly cardiomyopathy, birth defects	Metabolic acidosis, elevated lactate, LFTs may be abnormal	IV glucose L-carnitine
Storage disorders	Lysosomal disorders Gaucher disease Hurler syndrome	Progressive neurologic disease, hepatosplenomegaly, coarse facies, Skeletal dysplasia	Specific enzymatic tests for disease, biopsy, urine mucopoly and oligosaccrides	Increasingly enzyme replacement, bone marrow transplantation
	Peroxisomal disorders Zellweger syndrome		Very long chain fatty acids	None effective

Abbreviations: NPO, non per os; NTBC, 2-nitro-4-trifluromethylbenzoyl-1, 3 cyclohexanedione.
a Are often used for the hyperammonemia of organic and aminoacidemias as well, but are not approved for that indication.
From Refs. [28,31,32,35,36].

a fasting-induced catabolic state. The resultant release of endogenous amino acids, which also cannot be metabolized, creates a cycle of acidosis and neurologic dysfunction that rapidly leads to coma, multisystem failure, and death in the absence of appropriate treatment.

It is not uncommon for these same disorders to present later in life. Milder degrees of enzymatic dysfunction may not present until prolonged fasting results in a sufficient degree of catabolism. Although these "late-onset" disorders can present at any time from the second month through adulthood, the most common presentation is in toddlers with common viral illnesses, especially gastroenteritis. The clinical signs and laboratory features are identical to the early-onset varieties, except that the patient is older and there are generally signs and symptoms of a viral infection with associated fasting. As intravenous glucose-containing fluids are both part of routine emergency management and the mainstay of therapy for these disorders, a child may be successfully treated without the presence of the metabolic disorder being revealed. These children sometimes suffer many such episodes of acute encephalopathy associated with subsequent viral infections.

There are exceptions in which, toxic small molecules accumulate rapidly after birth, yet they cause damage only slowly over months and years. Thus, these disorders generally present at some point after the neonatal period. A classic example is phenylketonuria, in which the accumulating metabolite, phenylalanine, is neurotoxic, resulting in mental retardation. In another example caused by a block further down in the same metabolic pathway, several hepatotoxic intermediates accumulate in tyrosinemia type 1, resulting in liver failure that occurs at about age 2 months in the early-onset variety, or at any age thereafter in the later onset varieties.

High-energy phosphates such as adenosine triphosphate cannot cross membranes, and thus fetuses with disorders of energy metabolism ("mitochondrial disorders") are not protected by the placenta and can present prenatally (eg, birth defects, dysmorphic facies, Intrauterine growth retardation) or immediately after birth without a symptom-free period. Although mitochondrial disorders are highly complex in terms of their genetics, treatment, prognosis, diagnosis, and pathophysiology, those individuals presenting as neonates generally have autosomal recessive inheritance, an ultimately fatal prognosis, and are characterized by severe lactic acidosis and multisystem failure. Seizures, cardiomyopathy, and hepatocellular disease are common hallmarks.

Finally, the chronic accumulation of large molecules ("lysosomal storage disorders") results in a progressive disease burden related to the volume of stored material. Clinical manifestations depend on what tissues preferentially accumulate the stored material, and how quickly this material is stored. Again, as large molecules cannot cross membranes, storage begins prenatally and disease may be apparent at birth or soon thereafter [29]. Storage predominately in connective tissues results in some combination of coarse facial features, joint contractures, cardiac valvular disease, and cataracts. Storage predominately in the brain often results in the failure to achieve or a loss in acquired milestones, or leukodystrophy noted by magnetic resonance imaging. The lysosomal storage disorders rarely present emergently; therefore, the remaining sections concentrate on disorders in the other two previously mentioned categories.

Common to many specific diseases in all three metabolic disorder categories are neurologic signs such as seizures, apnea, hyperventilation, opisthotonus [30], stroke (often of the basal ganglia with resultant dysatonia), and abnormal tone (frequently central hypotonia possibly with peripheral spasticity). Abnormal odors, from that of maple syrup to smelly socks, have also been associated with some of the metabolic disorders of small molecule and energy metabolism [30]. Abnormal odor can be very helpful when present, but is an infrequent occurrence. Almost all of the metabolic disorders are autosomal recessive; thus, a history of consanguinity or affected siblings (including unexplained early death) certainly helps support the suspicion of a metabolic disorder. However, most children with metabolic disease have a completely noncontributory family history.

Differential diagnosis

Most metabolic disorders are initially misdiagnosed as sepsis [31], as the presentations can be difficult to distinguish. Vital sign abnormalities are similar, with metabolic patients often demonstrating a low core temperature [32,33], an elevated heart rate (due to dehydration), and a rapid respiratory rate (due to acidosis or hyperammonemia). In a metabolic disorder, however, the alteration in mental status far outweighs other signs early on, and a child is more likely to present comatose, but with a preserved blood pressure. Previous episodes of culture negative "rule-out sepsis" may provide an additional clue to an inborn error of metabolism. Certainly, the coexistence of sepsis and a metabolic disorder is not a rare phenomenon: in many metabolic disorders clinical disease is triggered by either a viral or a bacterial infection, and certain disorders, quintessentially galactosemia, are frequently associated with sepsis [8]. Therefore, ill-appearing neonates should be fully cultured and given antibiotics, even in light of a suspected metabolic disorder [30]. Many of these children present with hyperventilation or apnea; thus, pneumonia and other respiratory conditions must be considered. Additionally, hypoxia, hypoglycemia, child abuse with intracranial hemorrhage, electrolyte disturbances, CAH, seizure disorders, gastrointestinal catastrophe (eg, malrotation), and congenital cardiac disease should all be considered in the acutely ill neonate.

Emergency department evaluation

Each disorder has specific associated laboratory abnormalities, and these are listed in Table 3. In the ED, when metabolic disease is suspected, or

Table 3
Metabolic disorders and associated laboratory abnormalities

Disorder	Causes of decompensation	Signs and symptoms	Labs	Treatment following stabilization with glucose
Type 1 Glycogen Storage Disorder	Period of brief fasting	Growth failure, hepatomegaly	Lactic acidosis Hyperuricemia	Frequent feedings, cornstarch
Galactosemia	Often postprandial hypoglycemia (from galactose-containing foods)	Jaundice, vomiting, hepatomegaly, Gram-negative sepsis, cataracts	Positive urine for reducing substances	Stop formula or breast feeding
Hereditary fructose intolerance	Often postprandial hypoglycemia (from fructose-containing foods)	Vomiting, poor feeding, hepatomegaly, jaundice	Nongap acidosis, proteinuria	Avoidance of fructose or sucrose in diet
Disorders of fatty chain metabolism	Rarely symptomatic before 6 months unless prolonged fasting or infection	Reye-like syndrome Sudden death (SIDS) AMS ± Hepatomegaly, heart failure	Rarely ketotic Send organic acids and acylcarnitines	Carnitine Avoid fasting
Ketotic hypoglycemia	Often in thin child with incurrent illness; usually in ages 1–5 years	Evidence of gastroenteritis or upper respiratory infection with po intolerance (or water only)	Positive urine and serum ketones	po or IV glucose, depending on mental status and ability to take pos

Hyperinsulinism (B-cell regulatory defect)	Postprandial	May be familial (AR)	No ketones Elevated insulin level	Glucagon, Hydrocortisone, diazoxide or octreotide, Surgery
Congenital hypopituitarism (component hormone deficiency)	Lack of counterregulatory hormones following insulin release	Microphallus, midline facial defects, mixed hyperbilirubinemia	±ketones	Glucagon, steroids; hormone replacement
CAH	Hypoglycemia is due to cortisol deficiency	Females may be virilized, vomiting	May be hyponatremic, hyperkalemic ±ketones	Steroids, treat electrolyte disturbances, Hydration
Hypothyroidism	Unless central, should be noted on newborn screen	Prolonged jaundice	±ketones Low T4	Levothyroxine

Abbreviations: AR, autosomal recessive; AMS, altered mental status; CAH, congenital adrenal hyperplasia; SIDS, sudden infant death syndrome.
From Refs. [10,11,16].

when it is only one of many conditions on a differential diagnosis, the following widely available and relatively inexpensive laboratory tests can serve as a reasonable screening battery: electrolytes, urea nitrogen, creatinine, glucose, blood gas (can be venous), complete blood count (CBC), ammonia and possibly lactate, and urine dip stick for ketones and specific gravity. In some cases, alanine aminotranserase (ALT), bilirubin, albumin, or prothrombin time are helpful to evaluate liver function. A creatinine kinase (CK) can confirm a clinical suspicion of myopathy. If infection is in the differential, add a routine urinalysis and blood and urine cultures. Ammonia and lactate must be collected as free flowing blood without prolonged tourniquet time, and immediately placed on ice and run within 90 minutes by the laboratory [34]. Capillary blood is not acceptable [35]. Specific disorders associated with laboratory abnormalities are listed in Table 4.

The most sensitive and specific single sign of metabolic crisis due to an organic acidemia is an increase in the serum anion gap. Although mild to moderate degrees of dehydration may result in an anion gap of 16 to 17, possibly as high as 20, an anion gap above 20 is highly abnormal, with shock, diabetic ketoacidosis, renal failure, poisoning, and metabolic disease being the principal causes. Shock can be of any variety (hypovolemic, cardiogenic, septic, and so on), and shock resulting in a highly elevated anion gap should be clinically obvious. Most of the other conditions in the differential can be generally excluded by history, and blood glucose and creatinine determination, leaving only metabolic disease and cryptic poisoning as serious contenders.

An elevated ammonia (generally at least three to five times the upper range of normal, or > 150–200 micromolar) is the hallmark of an inborn error of the urea cycle. The most common presentation is a 2- to 5-day-old male who did well for the first few days of life, then developed the poor feeding, vomiting, and neurologic signs seen with significant hyperammonemia. Males are primarily affected by the X-linked disorder ornithine transcarbamylase deficiency, but both genders are affected equally by each of the other urea cycle defects. However, as acidosis from any cause results in a nonspecific downregulation of the urea cycle, hyperammonemia is frequently present in many organic acidemias as well, and can be just as severe.

Much as been written about "inappropriate ketosis" being a sign of a metabolic disorder. Although this is complicated and there are exceptions, large ketones in the first 12 hours of fasting is not normal, and is suggestive of an organic acidemia, while the absence of ketosis with frank hypoglycemia is suggestive of a fatty acid oxidation disorder. The latter group of disorders is not covered in this article, as presentation in the neonatal period is rare. Although hypoglycemia can be seen in many metabolic disorders, particularly late in the course, normoglycemia is more common, and the absence of hypoglycemia should never be used to exclude the presence of metabolic disease.

Table 4
Laboratory abnormalities and associated metabolic disorders

Laboratory	Likely metabolic disorder	Other considerations	Notes
Anion gap acidosis	Organic/amino acidemia, Fatty acid oxidation disorder, mitochondrial disease	Shock (extreme dehydration, bleeding, cardiac failure, hypoxia, sepsis, etc.), poisoning, DKA, renal failure	Tissue hypoxia without metabolic disease produces acidosis without urinary ketones. However, ketones may be present simply as an effect of fasting
Urinary ketones	Organic/amino acidemia, mitochondrial disease	Starvation DKA poisoning	Trace ketones in neonate who has not eaten for hours can be normal
Elevated ammonia (μg/mol)	Urea cycle disorder, organic acidemia, fatty acid oxidation deficiency	Primary liver disease, shock of any cause, Inappropriate collection, transient hyperammonemia of the neonate	Lab dependent, but often: normal <50 concerning >80 Ill or asphyxiated neonate up to 180 likely metabolic disease >200 (early presentations may be lower)
Liver failure /dysfunction	Tyrosinemia type 1, galactosemia, hereditary fructose intolerance, glycogen storage disease, Hemochromatosis, Zellweger, rare mitochondrial disorders	Primary liver disease, sepsis	Nonglucose reducing substances in carbohydrate disorders
Respiratory alkalosis	Urea cycle defect	Agitated neonate Aspirin overdose	
Neutropenia and/or thrombocytopenia	Methylmalonic and proprionic acidemia, glycogen storage disorder 1b, some mitochondrial disorders		May become neutropenic only during times of crisis
Elevated CK	Glycogen storage disorders, fatty acid oxidation disorders, mitochondrial disorders		Is evidence of myopathy, aldolase may also be affected

Abbreviation: DKA, diabetic ketoacidosis.

In the absence of an associated infection, the CBC is frequently normal, but certain disorders can have an associated neutropenia or thrombocytopenia [32]. Tests of liver function frequently are mildly abnormal in the acute phase of many different metabolic disorders. Hepatocellular dysfunction can also be the result of a metabolic disorder. Of course, primary liver disease of any cause can result in hyperammonemia. Elevated muscle enzymes such as CK or aldolase can confirm myopathy.

Although confirmation of the specific metabolic diagnosis is not the role of the emergency physician, there are advantages to collecting specimens in the emergency departmemt. Not only is early diagnosis helpful [35,37], but occasionally the definitive diagnostic test (ie, urine organic acids) is only positive when the child is acutely decompensated. Therefore, at a minimum it is recommended that urine and plasma be collected in the ED and frozen for potential future testing. Whole blood should not be frozen.

Emergency department management

Early treatment involves the withdrawal of potentially toxic substances, typically meaning stopping breast milk or formula, and the administration of intravenous dextrose. As the mainstay of therapy, dextrose infusions provide energy as well as result in an endogenous insulin excretion that combats catabolism. A standard intravenous order that is applicable to most metabolic disorders and clinical conditions is 10% dextrose in 0.2 normal saline to run at 1.5 times maintenance. If the patient is clearly dehydrated or in hypovolemic shock, a normal saline bolus can be run concurrently through a "Y" connector or a second line. Do not stop the dextrose infusion to give a normal saline bolus. Another option is to give 10 cc/kg of D_5NS over 30 to 60 minutes, which provides volume as well as a moderate dextrose infusion. However, unless shock is present, the bulk of rehydration should be done slowly, over 48 hours, to prevent cerebral edema. Cerebral edema is frequently present even before treatment, and care must be taken not to overwhelm the infant with fluid or sodium. Highly concentrated dextrose solutions given through central access is a strategy often successfully employed to provide large quantities or dextrose without resulting in cerebral or pulmonary edema. Because many of the adjunctive treatments involve large doses of sodium containing medicines, a lower concentration of sodium is often preferred in the rehydration fluid (0.2 normal saline). Bicarbonate, if required, should be used sparingly to prevent cerebral edema and hemorrhage [30]. Some patients may need additional stabilizing care, such as intubation for apnea, or correction of hypoglycemia (2–4 cc/kg of 10% dextrose) as well.

In critical patients, simultaneous insulin and dextrose drips may be beneficial in terminating catabolism rapidly and reversing metabolic acidosis and hyperammonemia. Clinical experience suggests starting at 0.05 units/kg/h of insulin and 10 mg/kg/min of glucose, and titrate both upwards, frequently obtaining rapid blood glucose measurements, until the patient is on 0.1 to 0.2 units/kg/h of insulin, and about 8 to 12 mg/kg/min of glucose. In the converse of the logic employed in the treatment of diabetic ketoacidosis, in critical metabolic decompensation the glucose infusion is titrated to maintain the desired insulin dosage. The goal is to achieve a serum glucose between 120 to 170 mg/dL [33]. If protein-containing feedings have been not tolerated or withheld for greater than about 48 to 72 hours, essential amino acid deficiency can result in a catabolic state regardless of the dextrose infusion, yet will respond to about 0.5 to 0.7 g/kg/d of amino acids delivered in hyperalimentation.

Toxic metabolites, specifically ammonia, can generally be removed pharmacologically with sodium benzoate, sodium phenylacetate, or sodium phenylbutyrate. The intravenous form of these medications are only approved for urea cycle defects, but acutely should be administered in the presence of severe hyperammonemia until the etiology is determined. Symptoms of hyperammonemia generally occur at a level three to five times normal, and this is also a reasonable threshold for hospitalization and directed treatment [37]. If pharmacologic treatment fails and the patient's ammonia remains greater then 10 times normal, hemodialysis should be considered. Peritoneal dialysis, although much easier in this age group, is less effective [32].

Administration of cofactors may be helpful, and should be done under the guidance of a consulting metabolic specialist, particularly if the specific metabolic disorder is not yet known. If a metabolic specialist is not available, L-carnitine may be beneficial [3], and is highly unlikely to cause harm. Until infection is excluded, antibiotics, generally ampicillin and either cefotaxime or gentamicin, should be administered. Indications and dosing of common medications are listed in Table 5.

Treatment of children with a known metabolic disorder

For several disorders, special synthetic formulas are used to restrict the precursors of the defective enzyme to the minimal intake needed to promote normal growth. The resultant diets are highly unpalatable, and noncompliance by ingesting either too little or too much can result in metabolic decompensation and substantial morbidity. In particular, children with inborn errors of metabolism are highly dependent on maintaining their caloric intake, and any intercurrent illness that causes the refusal or the inability to eat can precipitate a crisis [31]. During viral illnesses, patients are commonly instructed to take a sick-day regimen of protein free juices at home for 24 to 48 hours [38], and to monitor their mental status and urinary ketones by dipsticks. Altered mental status, vomiting, or other feeding intolerance, or "large" ketones (80 or greater) are indications for evaluation by a physician. If the child presents to the ED, several hours of 1.5 times maintenance with 10% dextrose in 0.2 normal saline may avert the crisis and return the patient's anion gap and

Table 5
Treatments commonly employed in neonates with metabolic disorders

Condition	Medication	Route	Dose	Caution
Most conditions	L-carnitine	IV/PO	100 mg/kg/d	
Hyperammonemia	Sodium benzoate /sodium phenylacetate /sodium phenylbutyrate	IV	IV: 0.25 g/kg bolus over 2–4 h, then infusion of 0.25 g/kg over 24 h	Hypernatremia, hypokalemia, acidosis, transient hyperammonemia, confusion, cerebral edema, hypotension
Citrulinemia, Argininosuccinate lyase deficiency	L-arginine	IV	0.2–0.6 g/kg then infusion of 0.25 g/kg over 24 h	Acidosis, extravasation, can be harmful in some urea cycle disorders
Biotinidase deficiency, multiple carboxylase deficiency	Biotin	PO	10 g/d	

From Summar M. Current strategies for the management of neonatal urea cycle disorders. J Pediatr 2001;138:S30–9; Batshaw ML, MacArthur RB, Tuchman M. Alternative pathway therapy for urea cycle disorders: twenty years later. J Pediatr 2001;138:S46–55.

urine ketones to normal; hyperammonemia corrects slowly over multiple hours. Antiemetics, especially phenothiazines, which may alter mental status should be used with caution, but the administration of ondansetron may allow a patient to tolerate oral intake. However, if the patient has acute neurologic signs or laboratory abnormalities that persist or worsen, or the child remains unable to take the appropriate formula, he/she will require hospitalization [39]. Patients with methylmalonic acidemia, propionic acidemia, glycogen storage disease type 1b, and certain mitochondrial disorders require a complete blood count and differential, as they are prone to neutropenia or thrombocytopenia during periods of acute illness. Certain medications, such as valproic acid, haloperidol, or steroids can precipitate hyperammonemia in some children with metabolic disorders and should be used with caution.

Death

Some of these disorders have a mortality as high as 50% with their initial presentation, so it is not uncommon to encounter a patient with a suspected metabolic disorder who dies in the ED or is dead upon arrival [40]. Generally, the cause of death is cardiovascular compromise, arrhythmia, hypoglycemia, pulmonary hemorrhage, or cerebral edema. Some sudden infant death syndrome deaths are thought to be attributable to metabolic disorders [28]. An autopsy later may be diagnostic, but often body fluids are not available or reliable by the time an autopsy is performed. It is recommended to collect blood and urine for the tests listed in the "workup" section above, plasma amino acids (2 cc, green top heparin sulfate tube), an additional tube of heparinized plasma for freezing, urine organic acids, and additional urine for freezing. In addition, facilitating that an autopsy be performed on the recently deceased infant may allow the family to obtain appropriate genetic counseling and possibly prevent a similar death in a future (or possibly a current) sibling.

Outlook

Prognosis varies widely in terms of morbidity, mortality, and cognitive abilities, depending on the specific metabolic defect and the care given. Infants presenting with severe hyperammonemia (generally > 1000 micromolar) or prolonged coma (generally > 3 days) have a poor long-term neurologic prognosis. Neonatal screening by tandem mass spectroscopy is performed in many states and foreign nations, and despite many false positives and false negatives, can identify a substantial proportion of affected infants with several different metabolic disorders, in some cases before symptom onset, improving outcomes. Liver or bone marrow transplantation has been employed to provide a long-term cure for some metabolic disorders [41]. Enzyme replacement is increasingly being made available for the treatment of lysosomal storage disorders. Gene therapy has not yet been successfully applied toward metabolic disease treatment, but is a future possibility.

Jaundice

Hyperbilirubinemia is a very common finding in the newborn, with 60% of newborns having some degree of jaundice [42]. Therefore, ED physicians must be very comfortable with diagnosis and management of newborn hyperbilirubinemia.

Emergency department presentation

Most infants will present with parental concerns regarding a change in skin color, but jaundice may be noted first by the physician in the course of treating a dehydrated or ill neonate.

Pathophysiology

Bilirubin is produced, via the intermediary metabolite biliverdin in the breakdown of hemoglobin. Initially, bilirubin is soluble in lipids, but not water. In the blood stream, it is albumin bound, and any substrate competing for binding sites, such as organic acids or drugs, can increase the amount of free bilirubin available. In this unconjugated state, bilirubin is difficult to excrete, and can pass easily into the central nervous system, causing the toxicity known as kernicterus. Bilirubin is then conjugated in the liver, converting it to a water-soluble compound that can be excreted via the biliary or renal tract. Decreased enzyme activity in the liver and low amounts of binding substrate in neonates predispose them to the development of jaundice.

The first step in the evaluation of newborn jaundice is to determine whether the hyperbilirubinemia is unconjugated or conjugated by measurement of the fractionated serum bilirubin. As the further workup, differential diagnosis, and management depends completely upon whether an infant has a pure unconjugated hyperbilirubinemia, or a component of conjugated hyperbilirubinemia, these abnormalities will be discussed independently.

Unconjugated hyperbilirubinemia

Differential diagnosis

Physiologic jaundice refers to the normal bilirubin released by the breakdown of red cells and exacerbated by the immature conjugation ability of the liver. Levels generally peak at a level of 12 mg/dL when a term infant is 72 hours old, but may climb as high as 17 mg/dL in breast-fed infants [43]. This higher peak with breast feeding is likely due to mild dehydration, and should be differentiated from "breast milk jaundice," which occurs in babies at 1 to 2 weeks of age due to a poorly understood property of breast milk that interferes with the conjugation of bilirubin. Studies show that preterm infants mount higher bilirubin levels, with nearly any degree of prematurity [44], and peak a few days later [43]. Although physiologic jaundice is quite common, it remains a diagnosis of exclusion, and pathologic causes must be excluded. Indicators for pathologic jaundice in patients with unconjugated hyperbilerubinemia include jaundice in the first 24 hours of life, a rapid rate of rise of the bilirubin level (0.5 mg/dL/h or 5 mg/dL/d), or in the presence of anemia or hepatosplenomegaly [43,45,46].

In any neonate who is significantly compromised from any illness, jaundice may be a secondary finding. It is particularly common in the infant suffering from dehydration, infection, and inborn errors of metabolism. Some of the inborn errors of metabolism, such as hereditary fructose intolerance and tyrosinemia, can cause liver failure, and jaundice may be the most notable sign of that. Significant hemolysis may be also be responsible for hyperbilirubinemia, either from a disease inherent to the infant itself, like hereditary spherocytosis, or due to an incompatibility with the maternal Rh or ABO blood type. Breakdown of extravascular blood, like cephalohematomas or swallowed maternal blood, may also increase bilirubin if the quantity is sufficient. Rarer causes include an upper gastrointestinal obstruction like pyloric stenosis, or duodenal atresia, congenital hyperthyroidism, Crigler-Najjar syndrome, Lucey-Driscoll syndrome, Down's syndrome, or maternal diabetes [45].

Emergency department evaluation

Clearly, the workup must be guided by the appearance of the infant. However, in a well-appearing, afebrile infant, fractionated bilirubin and hemoglobin are a reasonable place to begin. If the hyperbilirubinemia is indeed unconjugated and the hemoglobin normal, no further tests are required. It has recently been shown that physiologic jaundice is associated with asymptomatic urinary tract infections, and some practitioners would also check a urinalysis and culture [47]. If, on the other hand, anemia is present, a CBC with peripheral smear, Coomb's test, and maternal and fetal blood types should be analyzed. If there is a positive coombs test, ABO or Rh incompatibility is a likely cause for the jaundice. Most other causes of hemolysis will be Coombs negative [48]. Most recently, it is recommended that glucose-6-phospate dehydrogenase level be checked for any infant receiving phototherapy with an appropriate genetic or geographic background or for any infant who does not respond well to phototherapy.

Emergency department management and disposition

Clearly, if a serious illness is identified, priority must be given to its treatment. For the majority of children with physiologic jaundice, the goal of management is prevention of kernicterus. The likelihood of kernicterus depends not only on the bilirubin level, but also on the age of the child and their comorbidities. Age-appropriate criteria for treatment of jaundice are included in Table 6. It is important to remember that certain factors increase the risk of kernicterus, and many practitioners reduce these thresholds slightly in patients with evidence of hemolysis or dehydration.

If initiated, treatment requires correction of dehydration with normal saline boluses and initiation of phototherapy. This is generally done as an inpatient, but home bili-blankets and home nursing services make outpatient treatment an option as well. After correction of dehydration, oral feeds should be reinstituted, as frequent feeds and frequent stooling help excrete bilirubin. Discontinuation of breast feeding is not recommended. Continuation of breast feeding with close monitoring, supplementation with formula, or a brief interruption of breast feeding and substitution of formula are all accepted strategies, each done with or without adjuvant phototherapy, depending on the degree of hyperbilirubinemia [45]. In the event that bilirubin levels are dangerously high, exchange transfusion in an intensive care setting should be considered.

In cases of breast milk jaundice, many practitioners would encourage temporary cessation of breast milk with reintroduction after the bilirubin has fallen to a safe level.

Table 6
Management of hyperbilirubinemia in the healthy term newborn[a]

| Age, hours | TSB Level, mg/dL (pmol/L) | | | |
	Consider Phototherapy[b]	Phototherapy	Exchange Transfusion if Intensive Photo therapy Fails[c]	Exchange Transfusion and Intensive Phototherapy
≤24[d]	—	—	—	—
25–48	≥12 (210)	≥15 (260)	≥20 (340)	≥25 (430)
49–72	≥15 (260)	≥18 (310)	≥25 (430)	≥30 (510)
>72	≥17 (290)	≥20 (340)	≥25 (430)	≥30 (510)

[a] TSB mdicates total serum bilirubin.

[b] Phototherapy at these TSB levels is a clinical option, meaning that the intervention is available and may be used on the basis of individual clinical judgment. For a more detailed description of phototherapy (see the Appendix).

[c] Intensive phototherapy (Appendix) should produce a decline of TSB of 1 to 2 mg/dL within 4 to 6 h and the TSB level should continue to fall and remain below the threshold level for exchange transfusion. If this does not occur, it is considered a failure of phototherapy.

[d] Term infants who are clinically jaundiced at <=24 h old.

From Subcommittee on Hyperbilirubinemia. Management of hyperbilirubinemia in the newborn infant 35 or more weeks of gestation. Pediatrics 2004;114(1):297–316.

Conjugated hyperbilirubinemia

As mentioned above, conjugated bilirubin lacks the toxicity potential of unconjugated bilirubin, but is a marker for a serious underlying disease of either hepatocellular damage or cholestasis [43]. Other findings associated with conjugated hyperbilirubinemia are pale, acholic stools, and dark urine, although these are not always present in a newborn. Most cases will present with clinical jaundice in the first 4 weeks of life. The differential diagnosis can be seen in Table 7.

Emergency department evaluation

Appropriate evaluation of patients with conjugated hyperbilirubinemia is directed at identifying the underlying condition. Infection is not only a common cause for conjugated hyperbilirubinemia, but one that requires prompt identification and treatment. A complete septic workup, including a CBC, blood and urine cultures, as well as cerebral spinal fluid and stool studies when appropriate, should be sent on any ill-appearing infant, and jaundice itself should be included as a risk factor for neonatal sepsis. Keep in mind that the presence of sepsis, however, does not exclude an associated serious underlying disease [46]. Most of the TORCH infections are associated with jaundice and a TORCH panel as well as hepatitis B virus serology, and urine for cytomegalovirus should be sent. Inborn errors of metabolism may present with jaundice and should be worked up as outlined previously. Alpha 1-antitrypsin deficiency, cystic fibrosis, and Wilson's

Table 7
Differential diagnosis of conjugated hyperbilirubinemia

Common causes:	Sepsis
(Infectious)	CMV (Cytomegalovirus)
	Other TORCH infections
	(Congenital Toxoplasmosis, Rubella,
	CMV, Herpes, and Syphilis)
Infrequent causes:	Biliary atresia
(anatomic)	choledochal cyst
Infrequent causes:	Inborn errors of metabolism
(other)	Cystic fibrosis
	Alpha 1-antitrypsin deficiency
	Neonatal iron storage diseases
	Alagille syndrome
	(arteriohepatic dysplasia)
	Hepatic infarction
	Byler disease

From Behrman RE, Kliegman RM. Fetal and neonatal medicine. In: Nelson, Essentials of pediatrics. 4th edition. Philadelphia: W.B. Saunders; 2002. p. 179–249, 682–8.

disease may also cause liver damage, resulting in a conjugated hyperbilirubinemia and, as with the inborn errors of metabolism, may have an insidious onset heralded by inconstant jaundice and failure to thrive. Complete liver function studies including aspartate aminotransferase, ALT, and gamma-glutamyltranspeptidase, ammonia, albumin, total protein, alkaline phosphatase, and coagulation studies should also be ordered. Electrolytes, blood urea nitrogen (BUN), creatinine, and blood glucose are recommended as well. Urine for reducing substances, alpha 1-antitrypsin, sweat chloride, and red blood cell galactose-1-phosphate uridyltransferase activity may be useful for the ultimate diagnosis. Finally, it is crucial to identify those cases of biliary atresia or obstruction early, as they require surgical intervention, and if missed, may have poor surgical outcomes. Due to their healthy appearance, patients with biliary atresia may be initially be missed. Infants with complete obstruction should have a history of clay-colored stools, but obstruction can be intermittent and stools may remain pigmented for a few weeks. Abdominal ultrasonography and hepatobiliary scintigraphy should identify cases of biliary atresia and cholydocal cyst, mandating surgical intervention.

Emergency department management and disposition

The treatment of conjugated hyperbilirubinemia is aimed at treating the underlying pathology. For sepsis or infectious causes, appropriate antimicrobials are indicated. For suspected inborn errors of metabolism, withholding galalactose and fructose from the diet may be prudent until definitive diagnosis is made. Other treatment, again, depends on the underlying cause: infants should be admitted to the hospital for further workup and definitive therapy [49].

Electrolyte disturbances

As with many of the inborn errors of metabolism, infants presenting to the ED with electrolyte disturbances may have a myriad of nonspecific symptoms. With the atypical presentations seen in this age group, and the likelihood of coexisting abnormalities, it is difficult to present electrolyte disturbances in a truly symptom-based manner. However, some of the more common disturbances tend to be associated with jitteriness and seizures, while tend to manifest as weakness and vomiting, or as cardiovascular embarrassment. Therefore, they are grouped here by characteristic presenting symptoms.

Electrolyte abnormalities associated with seizures

Although much attention has been given to the judicious use of electrolyte testing in pediatric and adult patients with new onset seizures [50–52], studies support metabolic screening the newborn population [53–55]. In a newborn or infant, seizure activity may be less obvious than in adult or older pediatric patients. Neonatal seizures may be subtle, and frequently are not recognized as seizure activity by caretakers or medical personnel. Subtle symptoms of neonatal seizures include sucking or chewing motions, lip smacking, bicycling of the legs, apnea, eyelid fluttering, eye deviation, laughter, or tonic posturing. This group of neonatal seizures, in particular, is often not associated with EEG findings. Tonic, clonic, and myoclonic neonatal seizures may be either focal or generalized and are more commonly associated with EEG abnormalities [56].

Overall, there are relatively few medical conditions that account for the majority of neonatal seizures [57], and metabolic causes are common, in particular sodium abnormalities and hypocalcemia. The complete differential diagnosis must include hypoxic–ischemic encephalopathy, metabolic abnormalities (including electrolyte disorders, hypoglycemia, pyridoxine deficiency, and inborn errors of metabolism), intracranial hemorrhage, infections, cerebral dysgenesis, drug withdrawal, toxins (ie, lidocaine), and familial epilepsy [57]. Some maternal and birth conditions will predispose an infant to electrolyte abnormalities and subsequently seizure activity. Therefore, it is imperative that the ED physician, as with any infant patient, obtain a thorough history of the pregnancy, delivery, and resuscitation, as well as a detailed description of the presenting complaint.

Hyponatremia

In a well infant with seizures and without fever, hyponatremia, defined as serum sodium levels less than 130 mEq/L [58], should be foremost on the differential [59,60]. Hyponatremia is second only to febrile seizure as a cause for first-time seizure in an infant [61]. For those patients presenting to the ED, water intoxication and gastrointestinal losses are the most frequent causes, with water intoxication more likely in infancy [58]. Neonates lack the ability to appropriately concentrate their urine to accommodate for serum sodium shifts. Therefore, a parent who gives their young infant free water, or inappropriately dilutes the formula to make it last longer, may induce hyponatremia in their child. This phenomenon is often associated with poverty, and may be increasing in the United States [62–64].

Emergency department presentation

Symptomatolgy in hyponatremia is more reflective of the rate of fall of the serum sodium than on the absolute value. Significant symptoms generally begin to appear with serum sodium values less than 120 mEq/L, but may be observed with a rapid fall of the sodium levels into the normal range [43,58]. Symptoms such as anorexia, agitation, disorientation, and apathy may be difficult to appreciate in an infant. More pronounced symptoms include lethargy, muscle cramping or decreased deep tendon reflexes (DTRs), vomiting, acute respiratory failure, and seizures [57]. When seizures occur in these patients, they tend to be refractory to standard anticonvulsant therapy and often require high enough doses of medication to necessitate ventilatory support, unless the hyponatremia is recognized and corrected promptly [59,65,66] Hyponatremic children frequently have a cocumbenent hypothermia and hyperglycemia [59,60,62,63,66].

As with adults, pediatric hyponatremia is classified based on total body water content into hypervolemic, hypovolemic, and euvolemic hyponatremia.

Differential diagnosis

Most cases of hyponatremia in infants are associated with either dietary causes or gastrointestinal illness. Euvolemic hyponatremia is most likely due to water intoxication in healthy infants. This can occur as a result of inappropriate dilution of formula or with the addition of solute-poor fluids to the diet [60,62–64]. A change in diet is often due to recent gastrointestinal illness or summer weather dehydration, and so careful interviewing may reveal this history. Most hyponatremic infants studies were formula fed, so this may be another risk factor [62–64,66]. Moreover, patients with a history of vomiting, diarrhea, and dehydration are likely to have hypovolemic hyponatremia due to gastrointestinal losses, another common cause for pediatric hyponatremia. This is more likely when replacement fluid is solute poor. Other causes to consider include syndrome of inappropriate secretion of antidiuretic hormone (SIADH), in light of a history of underlying neurologic or pulmonary disease, CAH if the hyponatremia is associated with hyperkalemia and hypoglycemia, or in edema-forming states such as congestive heart failure, cirrhosis, and nephrosis. Other renal disorders may result in excessive renal excretion. Finally, hyperglycemia or hyperlipidemia may be the cause for pseudo or factitious hyponatremia, respectively [67].

Emergency department evaluation

The immediate workup of hyponatremia should include complete serum electrolytes, BUN, creatinine, and glucose and urinanalysis with specific gravity. As most cases are due to dietary or gastrointestinal causes, this will likely suffice for the ED evaluation. If the history, physical examination, and initial laboratory studies do readily suggest a cause, there is probably a more serious underlying condition, and the infant should be admitted for additional workup. The constellation of hyponatremia, hypoglycemia, hyperkalemia, and acidosis may indicate CAH. Serum and urine omolality should be tested, as urine osmolality greater than serum osmolality suggests SIADH. Liver function testing may be necessary if there is evidence of cirrhosis, nephrosis, or hypoalbuminemia in association with edema. Additionally, urine sodium, and creatinine should be tested [58].

Emergency department management and disposition

Any infant with severe symptoms of hyponatremia should be treated immediately with IV administration of 3% NaCl at a dose of 10 to 12 mL/kg over 1 hour. Another method is to calculate the volume required to raise serum sodium by 10 mEq/L using the following formula: volume of 3% NaCl to give = 10 mEq/L × body weight (kg) × 0.6 (extracellular fluid space). For less symptomatic patients, treatment is based on the cause. For water intoxication, restriction of daily free water by 25% to 50% is the treatment of choice. For hyponatremia associated with dehydration and gastrointestinal losses, serum sodium should correct with rehydration with isotonic saline over approximately 24 hours. SIADH will require fluid restriction as well, and in edema-forming states diuretics may be appropriate. Most hyponatremic patients will require admission, and certainly symptomatic hyponatremia without obvious cause mandates hospital admission [58].

Hypernatremia

Emergency department presentation

Hypernatremia may also be a cause for seizures and altered mental status in the newborn period [58,67]. Other signs and symptoms may include increased DTRs, tetany and tonic spasm, and tremulousness, rigidity, fever, and high-pitched cry [67].

Differential diagnosis

Hypernatremia is defined as serum sodium greater than 145 mEq/L, and is also divided based on total body sodium and water content [58]. Insensible free water losses leading to hypovolemic hypernatremia account for most cases of hypernatremia likely to be seen in the ED, with diarrhea(especially if fluid replacement has a high sodium relative to water content) the most common cause overall in pediatric ED patients [58]. As with hyponatremia, improper diet (boiled milk) or formula preparation can be a cause of hypernatremia. Furthermore, hypernatremia has been found in breast fed infants, due to poor oral intake [68–70]. Other causes include vomiting, insensible skin or respiratory losses, diuretic use, hypertonic sodium-containing enemas, or diabetes insipidus (more likely with a history of cental nervous system pathology). Euvolemic hypernatremia may be essential, iatrogenic, or due to formula errors. Hypervolemic hypernatremia is very rare, and can result from hyperaldosteronism, although it is usually iatrogenic in origin [67].

Emergency department evaluation

Evalution of hypernatremia is much the same as hyponatremia: initial laboratory studies should include complete chemistries, BUN, creatinine, and glucose, and a urinalysis in the ED. Additional workup will likely be done on an in-patient basis and will include liver enzyme analysis, serum, and urine osmolality and serum electrolyte testing.

Emergency department management and disposition

The treatment of hypernatremia depends on the underlying cause and the relative total body water content. In patients with underlying disease, such as a premature neonatal intensive care unit (NICU) graduate or a history of anoxic ishcemic event, diabetes insipidus is much more likely, and treatment for this is slow correction with free water replacement, along with initiation of ddAVP. Without a history of underlying medical disease, a history of improper formula preparation should be sought. In this case, the rate of correction of sodium should reflect the rate of sodium rise. Without a history of salt poisoning, one should search for any signs or symptoms or history consistent with dehydration. Treatment for hypertonic dehydration depends on degree of dehydration. Emergently, severely dehydrated infants with signs of shock require volume expansion with isotonic saline. Water and sodium losses may be replaced with hypotonic electrolyte solutions over 48 hours. It is recommended that for every 1 mEq/L of serum Na greater than 145 mEq/L, a free-water deficit of 4 mL/kg should be replaced over 48 to 72 hours [57]. As free water should not be given IV, it may either be given by mouth, or calculated out so that a child gets an appropriate volume of 0.45 or 0.2 normal saline. For mildly dehydrated infants, 10 to 20 cc/kg normal saline bolus is appropriate, and may be repeated as needed. Finally, without stigmata or findings of dehydration, hyperaldosteronsim, obstructive uropathy, osmotic diuretic use, and essential hypernatremia remain in the differential. These are rare in infants and will mandate further workup with treatment reflective of the underlying condition.

Hypocalcemia

Emergency department presentation

Hypocalcemia is one of the most common electrolyte abnormalities encountered in the newborn period, and often presents with jitteriness or seizures. It is important for the ED physician to recognize hypocalcemia as a cause of newborn seizures, as patients are frequently treated without assessment of serum calcium [71]. Other symptoms of hypocalcemia may include lethargy, poor feeding, irritability, and vomiting. As with adult patients, the QT interval on ECG may be increased and infants are at risk for myocardial depression and sudden cardiac death. Unlike older patients Chvostek and Trousseau signs will likely not be present in this age group [72].

Hypocalcemia is defined as a level <6 mg/dL in preterm newborn, <7 mg/dL in a term newborn, and <8 mg/dL in a term infant over 1 week of age [73], and is divided into early-onset hypocalcemia, delayed hypocalcemia, and childhood hypocalcemia thereafter [73].

Differential diagnosis

All infants have a slight decline in serum calcium levels just after birth with the nadir at approximately 24 to 48 hours of age. Generally, this is asymptomatic and resolves without therapy by the fifth day of life. Symptomatic hypocalcemia is much more common in infants of diabetic mothers, preterm infants, and infants with a history of anoxic encephalopathy, and may be an exaggeration of the normal fall in serum calcium after birth [72,74]. With the trend toward 24- and 48-hour newborn discharge, ED physicians may see more of this early neonatal population. Up to 80% of infants with symptomatic early neonatal hypocalcemia have concomitant hypomagnesemia and will not respond to calcium therapy without correction of the hypomagnesemia [72].

Delayed neonatal hypocalcemia is a disease of term-healthy infants, presenting at 5 to 10 days of age, and is associated with hyperphosphatemia [72]. Classically, this was the result of a diet of unmodified cow's milk formula, which has a very high phosphate-to-calcium ratio. Similar cases have been described with phosphorus overload, such as with administration of a phosphate containing enema [75].

Any form of vitamin D deficiency or resistance may lead to hypocalcemia associated with rickets. Congenital rickets, although now a rare condition

[74], is the result of severe maternal vitamin D deficiency. It should be noted that rickets can occur secondary to hypophospatemia due to renal wasting or dietary insufficiency as well [71]. Rickets of prematurity is secondary to birth before sufficient in utero skeletal calcification and subsequent dietary phosphorous deficiency.

Findings of arrhythmia, congenital heart disease, or heart murmur on examination, dysmorphology, and a history or seizures or jitteriness should prompt a workup for hypocalcemia secondary to DiGeorge syndrome. Familial hypocalcemia with hypercalciuria is a dominantly inherited condition associated with hypocalcemia, severe hypercalciuria, and nephrolithiasis.

Other less common causes of late hypocalcemia include pseudohypoparathyroidism (insensitivity at the parathyroid hormone receptor), maternal hypocalcemia with downregulation of parathyroid production, and secondary to citrate chelation associated with blood transfusions.

Emergency department evaluation

In an infant presenting with hypocalcemic seizures or tetany, obtaining a serum calcium level is critical, preferably ionized serum calcium [71], as treatment needs to be initiated immediately. Magnesium and phosphorus abnormalities should also be identified and treated in the ED. Ideally, before treatment is started, intact PTH and vitamin D metabolites should be drawn (an extra red top placed on ice or frozen), as these will help the consultant to identify the specific cause for the hypocalcemia [73]. Spot urine for calcium, phosphate, and creatinine should be collected within a few hours of the hypocalcemic event if possible, to assist the primary physician in a specific diagnosis. Additional workup will include renal and liver function testing may also aid in definitive diagnosis [73]. If indicated, radiographs of the skull and long bones may be useful in rickets [71].

Emergency department management and disposition

Treatment for hypocalcemia is much as with adult patients. Severely symptomatic patients, such as patients with seizures or myocardial dysfunction, need immediate IV calcium replacement. Ten percent calcium gluconate should be given, starting with 0.5 to 1.0 cc/kg up to 2 cc/kg, given over slow continuous infusion. As with adults, calcium infusions must be given very carefully, with close monitoring for cardiac arrhythmias, IV infiltration, and levels should be followed closely [58,74]. The infusion should be stopped for any signs of bradycardia and once symptoms have resolved [58]. Continuous replacement can then be started with 20 to 100 mg/kg of elemental calcium added to IV fluids [58,74], or by oral supplementation. Again, hypomagnesemia frequently accompanies hypocalcemia and must also be corrected. Generally, mild asymptomatic hypocalcemia does not need therapy, but levels less than 7.0 to 7.5 mg/dL in neonates warrant treatment to prevent tetany [74].

Hypomagnesemia

Emergency department presentation

As mentioned above, hypomagnesemia should be suspected in any infant with evidence of hypocalcemia, and can be associated with tetany and seizures. In fact, most of the symptoms of hypomagnesemia parallel those of hypocalcemia: lethargy, nausea, muscle cramping, parasethesias, fasciculations, and irritability [76]. There may be similar ECG changes as well.

Differential diagnosis

Causes for hypomagnesemia in children include gastrointestinal losses or malabosorption, renal losses due to renal insufficiency, or medications, as with the pseudo-Bartters syndrome (described later), or due to underlying metabolic conditions, such as primary hypomagnesemia. For the newborn, it is imperative to keep in mind that infants of diabetic mothers and infants with a history of anoxia are at increased risk of hypomagnesemia [77].

Emergency department evaluation

The evaluation of hypomagnesemia should, thus, be much the same as that of hypocalcemia with complete electrolyte testing, assessment of renal and liver function, urine electrolytes, and ECG testing. Recent studies have recommended ionized magnesium as a more accurate measurement [78], but this may be impractical in the ED.

Emergency department management and disposition

Any symptomatic patient with hypomagnesemia needs treatment. IV replacement is recommended, although it can be given intramuscularly. An IV dose of 25 to 50 mg/kg can be given as a 10% solution (100 mg/mL) or as a 50% solution (500 mg/mL) every 4 to 6 hours as needed [58].

Electrolyte abnormalities associated with weakness and vomiting

Infants who present with poor tone, vomiting, lethargy, or alterations in consciousness need prompt evaluation for common causes, such as sepsis or dehydration, but also should be evaluated for electrolyte abnormalities. In particular, hypercalcemia and hypokalemia can cause this clinical picture.

Hypercalcemia

Emergency department presentation

Hypercalcemia is very rare in infancy [79], but can have serious sequelae. Patients may present with poor feeding, vomiting, and constipation with associated failure to thrive and dehydration. They may have poor tone, weakness, and irritability as well [72]. Hypercalciuria will lead to polyuria and dehydration, exacerbating the potential for nephrocalcinosis and renal insufficiency. Patients are often hypertensive, and may even present with seizures [79].

Hypercalcemia is defined by ionized serum calcium levels greater than 5.4 mg/dL with or without the total serum calcium greater than 10.8 mg/dL [79]. Other diagnostic findings include bradycardia, a narrow QT interval, and, as mentioned above, hypertension. On renal function analysis, patients frequently have elevated creatinine with evidence of hematuria and pyuria due to urine calcium exretion [79].

Differential diagnosis

Although individually rare, the causes of infantile hypercalcemia are many. Overall, iatrogeic exposure is the most common etiology, but in ED patients the most common cause is idiopathic infantile hypercalcemia (IIH) [79]. IIH is divided into mild and severe forms. Mild IIH, otherwise know as Lightwood variant IIH, has been associated with elevated vitamin D metabolites or increased sensitivity to vitamin D with increased gut absorption of calcium. It is generally self-limited, resolving by 12 months of age, and treated with diet. Severe IIH is now recognized as Williams syndrome. A history of small-for-gestational age, hypotonia, feeding difficulties, and cardiac murmur on exam should tip the ED physician to screen for hypercalcemia associated with Williams syndrome. The hallmark "elfin facies," loquaciousness, and mental retardation may not become evident until later in life. As with mild IIH, the hypercalcemia of William's syndrome patients may have increased sensitivity to vitamin D metabolites, and the hypercalcemia generally resolves spontaneously by 1 year of age. It should be recognized that although an astute ED physician could make this diagnosis with a careful history and physical and a high index of suspicion, the marked hypercalcemia is often not recognized until many weeks of age, and is not a cause for the mental retardation [74].

Hypercalcemia due to severe neonatal hyperparathyroidism, while very rare, is an absolute medical emergency. This is the result of homozygous mutations in a calcium-sensing receptor. These patients will have critically high calcium levels and require immediate correction. It is imperative to recognize these patients, as they will require surgical treatment with parathyroidectomy. Heterozygousity for this leads to only modest asymptomatic hypercalcemia, so parents do not need medical intervention, but should have genetic counseling [79].

Infants may also have secondary neonatal hyperparathyroidism due to exposure to maternal calcium hypocalcemia. This is a self-limited, transient disorder requiring only symptomatic treatment of the hypercalcemia [79].

One other cause for infantile hypercalcemia is vitamin D intoxication. This can be exogenous, due to inappropriate choice of formulas, or due to over production. Extensive neonatal fat necrosis can cause excess vitamin D synthesis. In any infant with symptoms of hypercalcemia and a history of large-for-gestational age or traumatic delivery, the examination should focus on signs of fat necrosis, and this diagnosis should be entertained [72,79].

Emergency department evaluation

ED workup of hypercalcemia should include a complete set of electro-lytes, BUN, and creatinine to assess degree of dehydration and to look for renal insufficiency and other associated electrolyte abnormalities. If at all possible, measurement of an intact serum PTH level at the time of hypercalcemia is crucial. High levels of PTH in the face of markedly elevated calcium suggest neonatal hyperparathyroidism requiring surgical manage-ment, and thus will affect management, consultation, and disposition. Low levels of PTH will mandate futher calcitrophic hormone testing [79].

Emergency department management and disposition

Asymptomatic hypercalcemia does not need treatment emergently. Mild hypercalcemia can be managed with a low calcium diet and close follow-up [79]. This is best done by the primary care provider given the risk of calcium and phosphate depletion in a growing child [74]. For more significant hypercalcemia, intervention is warranted. The goals of treatment for hypercalcemia are: rehydration, increasing calcium excretion, decreasing gut absorption, and treatment of the underlying disorder. Intravenous normal saline should be used to expand the extracellular fluid compartment at approximately 1.5 to 2.5 times maintenance therapy [79]. This will also enhance calcium excretion by inducing a calciuresis [72]. Furthermore, furosemide at 0.5 to 1.0 mg/kg IV every 6 hours will enhance this calciuresis [79]. These steps are simple and familiar to the ED physician, and are effective for all causes of hypercalcemia [79].

In severe cases, additional therapy can include calcitonin subcutaneously at 4 IU/kg every 6 hours. Glucocorticoids, while ineffective in hyperparathy-roidism, may be helpful in cases of hypervitaminosis D as a short-term measure [74,80]. Bisphosphonates have not been tested well in infants, but may have a future role for PTH-mediated hypercalcemia and vitamin D toxicity [81]. Ultimately, dialysis may be required if these methods are unsuccessful.

Hypokalemia

Emergency department presentation

Hypokalemia is an uncommonly described electrolyte disturbance in infants, and is defined as a serum potassium level below 3.5 mEq/L [58]. Symptoms range from muscle weakness, polyuria, ileus, tetany, areflexia, and paralysis [58]. Disturbances in cardiac conduction can be seen as well including ST depression, T-wave reduction, and the hallmark finding of U waves on ECG. Patients with severe hypokalemia can progress to acute respiratory failure, and can develop myoglobinuria from muscle paralysis leading to acute renal failure [58].

Differential diagnosis

In previously healthy patients gastrointestinal losses can cause hypokalemia. Gastric potassium loss from vomiting can cause hypokalemia. Metabolic alkalosis from vomiting can exacerbate this by inducing renal potassium wasting and shifting potassium intracellularly. This, coupled with diarrhea, can frequently be the cause for hypokalemia in an otherwise well child [58] Hypokalemia may be an associated finding in an infant with pyloric stenosis as well [58].

Bartter syndrome, although rare, may present in infancy with polyuria, salt craving, muscle weakness, constipation, tetany, and failure to thrive [82]. It is characterized by hypokalemia and hypochloremia associated with metabolic alkylosis without hypertension. Patients may also have hyponatremia, hypercalcemia, hypomagnesemia, and hyperuricemia [82]. Although Bartter syndrome is a very rare disease, it should be noted that there have been reported cases of transient Bartter syndrome associated with gentamycin therapy continuing weeks to months after discontinuation of the drug [83,84]. Hence, the index of suspicion for hypokalemia should be heightened in infants with a history of gentamycin therapy in the NICU.

Many underlying disease are associated with hypokalemia. Renal tubular acidosis is another cause of hypokalemia. In contrast to Bartter syndrome, this causes a nonanion gap metabolic acidosis with hyperchloremia and an alkaline urine pH [58]. Another underlying condition that leads to hypokalemia is cystic fibrosis. Diabetic ketoacidosis is well recognized as a cause of hypokalemia in older pediatric patients, but is extremely uncommon in the newborn period. Pediatric hypokalemia, in association with normal acid-base status, is generally reflective of unusual diets, Cushing's syndrome, or hyperaldosteronism [58].

Emergency department evaluation

The immediate workup of hypokalemia should start with the serum electrolytes, BUN, creatinine, glucose, and urinalysis. In addition, an arterial blood gas should be obtained to ascertain acid-base balance. Additionally, an ECG should be done for any suspicion of conduction abnormalities and an ultrasound or upper gastrointestinal series to rule out pyloric stenosis when appropriate [58]. If a cause is not identified, additional evalution with urine Na, K, Cl, pH, and osmolality may be helpful, but may be done in conjunction with hospital admission or consultation.

Emergency department management and disposition

The treatment of hypokalemia in infants does not differ from that in adult patients. Treatment can generally be slow oral or intravenous potassium supplementation, and will be dependent somewhat on the cause of the hypokalemia. In alkalosis with associated intracellular potassium shifts, treatment of the underlying alkalosis is appropriate. For familial periodic hypokalemic paralysis judicious oral potassium supplementation is recommended with close monitoring. Any patient with life-threatening symptoms from hypokalemia requires immediate IV potassium replacement. Intravenous potassium should be given at 0.5 to 1 mEq/kg per hour with continuous cardiac monitoring. For patients with associated alkalosis, potassium chloride should be used, and for patients with acidosis, potassium bicarbonate can be used. In addition, infants with evidence of dehydration will also need volume replacement to prevent further renal losses. Most infants with a serum potassium less than 3.0 mEq/L require admission, and certainly those who are symptomatic and requiring correction [58].

Cardiovascular or respiratory compromise

A subset of electrolyte disorders may present with signs of cardiac or respiratory failure. Hyperkalemia can cause conduction abnormalities in addition to skeletal muscle weakness. Hypermagnesemia is associated with respiratory depression and can progress to apnea. Finally, CAH, causing a constellation of electrolye abnormalities, can present with profound hypotension and shock.

Hyperkalemia

Emergency department presentation

Symptomatic hyperkalemia, as with adult patients, is a true medical emergency. The clinical findings of hyperkalemia can range from weakness and paralysis to significant cardiac conduction abnormalities, arrhythmia, and cardiac arrest. ECG changes tend to parallel the degrees of hyperkalemia if it has occurred acutely. As in adults, the earliest finding is peaking of the T-wave, then widening of the PR interval, followed by first degree heart block, loss of the P wave, ventricular arrhythmia, and ultimately, asystole.

Hyperkalemia is defined as serum potassium levels greater than 5/5 mEq/L. It is relatively common to find elevated potassium levels on laboratory serum analysis due to hemolysis and this should be considered in the face of significantly potassium elevation without peaking of the T-wave on ECG.

Differential diagnosis

Extracellular shift of potassium due to acidosis may also result in an elevated serum potassium value, although the true total body potassium may be normal or decreased. Significant burn or crush injury can release extracellular potassium from damaged cells, and these patients should be screened for hyperkalemia, even in the absence of symptoms. Finally, potassium levels can rise with decreased renal excretion, and this is nearly always the case with life-threatening hyperkalemia [58]. As with older patients, acute renal failure, especially with oliguria, can result in hyperkalemia. In the infant age group, acute adrenal insufficiency due to CAH must be ruled out.

Emergency department evaluation

In the ED, it is imperative to assess renal function: measurement of the BUN and creatinine is mandate. Neonates have such little muscle mass that a creatinine level that is acceptable in adults may be abnormal in neonates, and values should be compared with age-appropriate normals. Complete electrolytes and glucose should also be obtained to screen for other electrolyte abnormalities and evidence of CAH. An ABG is recommended to establish if acidosis is present and serum creatinine phosphokinase should be included to exclude rhabdomyolysis as a cause for hyperkalemia. ECG testing should be done in any patient with abnormalities in serum potassium, especially in the face of hyperkalemia [58]. As with other electrolye abnormalities, urinalysis, urine electrolytes (Na, K, Cl), urine pH, and osmolality will help the pediatrician evaluate more esoteric causes such as renal tubular acidosis, but need not be done emergently. Finally, for patients with elevated laboratory values and normal ECG or no history compatible with hyperkalemia, repeating the test is prudent.

Emergency department management and disposition

The treatment of hyperkalemia in newborns and infants is exactly the same as with adult patients. Any patient with evidence of arrhythmia or serum potassium level above 8.0 mEq/L needs immediate treatment. Calcium is given to restore the membrane potential at a dose of 0.5 mL/kg of 10% calcium gluconate over 2 to 5 minutes. This must be followed with a reduction in serum potassium. The most expeditious way to achieve this is to force potassium out of the extracellular component and into the intracellular space. This is can be achieved by the use of IV bicarbonate therapy (Na bicarbonate 7.5% 2–3 mL/kg over 30–60 minutes), and a combination of IV glucose and insulin (1 unit of insulin for every 5–6 g of glucose given) [57]. Patients with only minimal elevation of serum potassium can be treated with Kayexalate (sodium polystyrene sulfate) at a dose of 1 g/kg. This is appropriate for longterm treatment, but should be considered in more acute patients in addition to symptomatic treatment, as the above measures are only temporizing. Diuresis with furosemide will also enhance renal potassium excretion. For asymptomatic patients with mildly elevated K+ levels (<6.5 mEq/L) and a normal or near normal (peaked T-waves only) ECG, no specific treatment is needed other than correction of acidosis if present and withdrawal of supplemental potassium. However, if the hyperkalemia is the result of acute renal failure or rhabdomyolysis, more active treatment is indicated, as levels may climb rapidly. In these patients, dialysis should be considered if the underlying condition cannot be quickly reversed. Admission to the hospital is warranted for patients with potassium levels greater than 6.5 mEq/L or if symptomatic [58].

Hypermagnesemia

Emergency department presentation

Hypermagnesemia, although rare, can be seen in the newborn period. Symptoms associated with hypermagnesemia correlate well with serum levels. Decreased DTRs are noted first, with magnesium levels of 4 to 5 mEq/L. ECG changes (increased P-R, QRS, and QT intervals) and a drop in blood pressure can be seen with levels above 5 mEq/L. At levels of 8 to 10 mEq/L, decreased respirations and apnea ensue, and at levels greater than 15 mEq/L, heart block can occur [58].

Differential diagnosis

Hypermagnesemia is seen in the NICU in infants of mothers who received magnesium therapy for hypertension and seizure prophylaxis. Hypoxic ischemic encepholopathy has been described in association with hypermagnesemia [77], as well as hypomagnesemia. Infants have also presented with hypermagnesemia when inappropriately given such medications as magnesium hydroxide [85].

Emergency department evaluation

Serum magnesium levels should be ordered, in addition to complete serum electrolytes for any suspicion of hypermagnesemia. BUN, creatinine, and urinalysis should also be checked.

Emergency department management and disposition

Treatment for mild hypermagnesemia includes hydration and diuresis. For any severe signs or symptoms, IV calcium gluconate can be given at a dose of 0.5 mL/kg of 10% Ca gluconate, with careful monitoring as described earlier. For any patient with evidence of renal failure, dialysis is indicated.

Congenital adrenal hyperplasia

Finally, CAH should be mentioned, as it is associated with many of the described electrolyte abnormalities and can cause severe symptoms related to corticosteroid insufficieny and salt wasting.

Emergency department presentation

The symptomatology of CAH is twofold. There can be virilization or ambiguous genitalia present at birth. Other affected infants who have symptoms of acute salt-wasting crisis generally present in the second week of life and may initially have nonspecific symptoms of poor feeding or weight gain, lethargy, irritability, and vomiting. Symptoms progress to profound shock and death if not recognized and treated [86].

Differential diagnosis

CAH is often misdiagnosed with a delay in treatment [86]. Symptoms may suggest gastroenteritis, formula, or feeding intolerance, or a number of the diseases already described. Careful physical examination will alert the astute ED physician to this disorder. Appreciation of an enlarged clitoris, fusion of the labial folds, or testes palpable in the labia in females or a micropenis, hypospadias, or palpable gonads in the inguinal canal or labioscrotal folds is highly suggest of CAH and electrolyte abnormalities should be sought.

Emergency department evaluation

The first priority for workup of these infants includes serum electrolytes and glucose. Most commonly the infant will be found to have hyperkalemia and hyponatremia, often associated with hypoglycemia and acidosis. As mentioned before, an adrenal steroid profile, including 17-hydroxyproges-terone, dehydroepiandrosterone, and testosterone should be obtained before treatment with hydrocortisone [86]. That said, if the clinical suspicion is high and the patient unstable, these studies should not delay treatment.

Emergency department management and disposition

For these patients, as with any infant with shock, fluid rehydration will be the first step in resuscitation. An IV bolus of 20 mL/kg on normal saline should be initiated immediately and repeated as needed to correct the volume deficit. IV hydrocortisone should be given in the ED at a dose of 25 mg, followed by hydrocortisone 50 mg/m^2 over 24 hours continuous infusion. If IV access cannot be established, intramuscular cortisone acetate at a dose of 25 mg may be life saving. The hydrocortisone should provide some mineralocorticoid activity, but some patients will require fludrocortisone for long-term management. Electrolyte correction may occur with volume and glucorticoid replacement [86]. For any significant symptoms secondary to the electrolyte abnormalities, treatment is as outlined earlier in the article. Infants diagnosed with CAH should be admitted, and consultation with an endocrinologist is recommended.

References

[1] Cornblath M, Hawdon JM, Williams AF, et al. Controversies regarding the definition of neonatal hypoglycemia: suggested operational thresholds. Pediatrics 2000;101(5):1141–5.

[2] Lucas A, Morley R, Cole JJ. Adverse neurodevelopmental outcome of moderate neonatal hypoglycemia. BMJ 1988;297:1304–8.

[3] Kinnala A, Rikalainen H, Lapinleimu H, et al. Cerebral magnetic resonance imaging and ultrasonography findings after neonatal hypoglycemia. Pediatrics 1999;103(4):724–9.

[4] Koh TH, Aynsley-Green A, Tarbit M, et al. Neural dysfunction during hypoglycemia. Arch Dis Child 1988;63:1353–8.

[5] Marcus C. How to measure and interpret glucose in neonates. Acta Paediatr 2001;90(9): 963–4.

[6] Kalhan S, Peter-Wohl S. Hypoglycemia: what is in it for the neonate? Am J Perinatol 2000; 17(1):11–8.

[7] Schwartz RP. Hypoglycemia in infancy and childhood. Indian J Pediatr 1997;64(1):43–55.

[8] Yu dkoff M. Metabolic Emergencies (Inborn Errors of Metabolism). In: Fleisher GR, Ludwig S, editors. Textbook of pediatric emergency medicine. 4th edition. Philidelphia: Lippencott, Williams, and Wilkins; 2000. p. 1117–27.

[9] Losek JD. Hypoglycemia and the ABC's (sugar) of pediatric resuscitation. Ann Emerg Med 2000;35(1):43–6.

[10] Sunehag AL, Haymond MW. Glucose extremes in newborn infants. Clin Perinatol 2002; 29(2):245–60.

[11] Louis C, Weizimer SA. A 12-day-old infant with hypoglycemia. Curr Opin Pedriatr 2003; 15(3):333–7.

[12] Daly LP, Osterhoudt KC, Weizimer SA. Presenting features of idiopathic ketotic hypoglycemia. J Emerg Med 2003;25(1):39–43.

[13] Gomella TL, editor. Neonatology management, procedures, on-call problems, diseases, and drugs. 3rd edition. Norwalk (CT): Appelton & Lange; 1994. p. 217–20.

[14] Crain EF, Gershel JC, editors. Clinical manuel of emergency pediatrics. New York: McGraw-Hill; 1997. p. 157–9.

[15] Yeung CY. Hypoglycemia in neonatal sepsis. J Pediatr 1970;77(5):812–7.

[16] Cowett RM, Loughead JL. Neonatal glucose metabolism: a differential diagnosis, evaluation, and treatment of hypoglycemia. Neonatal Netw 2002;21(4):9–19.

[17] Jones CW. Gestational diabetes and its impact on the neonate. Neonatal Netw 2001;20(6): 17–22.

[18] Agrawal RK, Lui K, Gupta JM. Neonatal hypoglycemia in infants of diabetic mothers. J Paediatr Child Health 2000;36(4):354–6.

[19] Yap F, Hogler W, Vora A, et al. Sevre transient hyperinsulinaemic hypoglycaemia: two neonates without predisposing factors and a review of the literature. Eur J Pediatr 2004; 163(1):38–41.

[20] Pollack CV. Utility of glucagons in the emergency department. J Emerg Med 1993;11(2): 195–205.

[21] Charsha DS, McKinley PS, Whitfield JM. Glucagon infusion for the treatment of hypoglycemia: efficacy and safety in sick, preterm infants. Pediatrics 2003;111(1):220–1.

[22] Miralles RE, Lodha A, Perlman M, et al. Experience with intravenous glucagons infusions as a treatment in resistant neonatal hypoglycemia. Arch Pediatr Adolesc Med 2002;156(10): 999–1004.

[23] Taketomo C, editor. Childrens Hospital Los Angeles pediatric dosing handbook and formulary. Ohio: Lexicomp; 2003. p. 269, 390, 408, 564.

[24] Tarascon Pocket Pharmacoepia. Loma Linda: Tarascon Publishing; 2001. p. 43, 56.

[25] Thomas CG, Cuenca RE, Azizkhan RG, et al. Changing concepts of islet cell displasia in neonatal and infantile hyperinsulin. World J Surg 1988;12:598–609.

[26] Meissner T, Wendel U, Burgard P, et al. Long term follow-up of 114 patients with congenital hyperinsulinism. Eur J Endocrinol 2003;149(1):43–51.

[27] Menni F, de Lonlay P, Sevin C, et al. Neurologic outcomes of 90 neonates and iinfants with persistent hyperinsulinemic hypoglycemia. Pediatrics 2001;107(3):476–9.

[28] Seashore MR, Rinaldo P. Metabolic disease of the neonate and young infant. Semin Perinatol 1993;17(5):318–29.

[29] Saudubray JM, Nassogne MC, deLonlay P, et al. Clinical approach to inherited metabolic disease in neonates: an overview. Semin Neonatol 2002;7:3–15.

[30] Burlina AB, Bonafe L, Zacchello F. Clinical and biochemical approach to the neonate with a suspected error of amino acid and organic acid metabolism. Semin Perinatol 1999;23(2): 162–73.

[31] Leonard JV, Morris AAM. Urea cycle disorders. Semin Neonatol 2002;7:27–35.

[32] de Baulny HO. Management and emergency treatment of neonates with a suspicion of inborn errors of metabolism. Semin Neonatol 2002;7:17–26.

[33] Summar M. Current strategies for the management of neonatal urea cycle disorders. J Pediatr 2001;138:S30–9.

[34] Steiner RD, Cedarbaum SD. Laboratory evaluation of urea cycle disorders. J Pediatr 2001; 138:S2–29.

[35] Consensus statement from a conference for the management of patients with urea cycle disorders. J Pediatr 2001;138(1):S1–5.

[36] Burton BK. Inborn errors of metabolism in infancy: a guide to diagnosis. Pediatrics 1998; 102(6):E69.

[37] Batshaw ML, MacArthur RB, Tuchman M. Alternative pathway therapy for urea cycle disorders: twenty years later. J Pediatr 2001;138:S46–55.

[38] Berry GT, Steiner RD. Long-term management of patients with urea cycle disorders. J Pediatr 2001;138:S56–61.

[39] Dixon MA, Leonard JV. Intercurrent illness in inborn errors of intermediary metabolism. Arch Dis Child 1992;67(11):1387–91.

[40] Summar M, Tuchman M. Proceedings of a consensus conference for the management of patients with urea cycle disorders. J Pediatr 2001;138:S6–10.

[41] Lee B, Goss J. Long-term correction of urea cycle disorders. J Pediatr 2001;138:S62–71.

[42] American Academy of Pediatrics. Provisional Committee for Quality Improvement and Subcommittee on Hyperbilirubinemia. Practice parameter: management of hyperbilirubi-nemia in the healthy term newborn. Pediatrics 1994;94:558–65.

[43] Behrman RE, Kliegman RM. Fetal and neonatal medicine. In: Nelson, Essentials of pediatrics. 4th edition. Philadelphia: W.B. Saunders; 2002. p. 179–249, 682–8.

[44] Sarici SU, Serdar MA, Korkmaz A, et al. Incidence, course, and prediction of hyper-bilirubinemia in near-term and term newborns. Pediatrics 2004;113(4):775–80.

[45] Mandal KD. Jaundice—unconjugated hyperbilirubinemia. In: Fleisher GR, Ludwig S, editors. Textbook of pediatric emergency medicine. 4th edition. Philadelphia: Lippincott Williams & Wilkins; 2000. p. 355–61.

[46] Mowat AP. Disorders of the liver and biliary system. Part II. In: Roberton NRC, editor. Textbook of neonatalolgy. 2nd edition. Edinburgh: Churchill Livingstone; 1992. p. 619–31.

[47] Garcia FJ, Nager AL. Jaundice as an early diagnostic sign of urinary tract infection in infancy. Pediatrics 2002;109(5):846–51.

[48] Herschel M, Karrison T, Wen M, et al. Isoimmunization is unlikely to be the cause of hemolysis in ABO-incompatible but birect antiglobulin test-negative neonates. Pediatrics 2002;110(1):127–30.

[49] Singer JI. Jaundice—Conjugated Hyperbilirubinemia. In: Fleisher GR, Ludwig S, editors. Textbook of pediatric emergency medicine. 4th edition. Philadelphia: Lippincott Williams & Wilkins; 2000. p. 363–74.

[50] Lowe RA, Wood AB, Burney RE, et al. Rational ordering of serum electrolytes: development of clinical criteria. Ann Emerg Med 1987;16(3):260–9.

[51] Npaver MM, Reynolds SL, Tanz RR, et al. Emergency department laboratory evaluation of children with seizures: dogma or dilemma? Pediatr Emerg Care 1992;8(1):13–6.

[52] Turnbull TL, Vanden Hoek TL, Howes DS, et al. Utility of laboratory studies in the emergency department patient with a new-onset seizure. Ann Emerg Med 1990;19(4): 373–7.

[53] Bui TT, Delgado CA, Simon HK. Infant seizures not so infantile: first-time seizures in children under six months of age presenting to the ED. Am J Emerg Med 2002;20(6): 518–20.

[54] Scarfone RJ, Pond K, Thompson K, et al. Utility of laboratory testing for infants with seizures. Pediatr Emerg Care 2000;16(5):309–12.

[55] Valencia I, Sklar E, Blanco F, et al. The role of routine serum laboratory tests in children presenting to the emergency department with unprovoked seizures. Clin Pediatr 2003;42: 511–7.

[56] Grover G, Silverman BK. Problems of the very early neonate. In: Fleisher GR, Ludwig S, editors. Textbook of pediatric emergency medicine. 4th edition. Philadelphia: Lippincott Williams & Wilkins; 2000. p. 1241–4.

[57] Hill A, Volpe JJ. Neonatal seizures Part II. In: Roberton NRC, editor. Textbook of neonatalolgy. 2nd edition. Edinburgh: Churchill Livingstone; 1992. p. 1043–7.

[58] Cronan K, Norman ME. Renal and electrolyte emergencies. In: Fleisher GR, Ludwig S, editors. Textbook of pediatric emergency medicine. 4th edition. Philadelphia: Lippincott Williams & Wilkins; 2000. p. 811–28.

[59] Farrar HC, Chande VT, Fitzpatrick DF, et al. Hyponatremia as the cause of seizures in infants: a retrospective analysis of incidence, severity, and clinical predictors. Ann Emerg Med 1995;26:42–8.

[60] Medani CR. Seizures and hypothermia due to dietary water intoxication in infants. South Med J 1987;80:421–5.

[61] Cornelli HM, Gormley CJ, Baker RC. Hyponstremia and seizures presenting in the first two years of life. Pediatr Emerg Care 1985;1:190–3.

[62] David R, Ellis D, Gartner JC. Water intoxiacation in nornal infants: role of antidiuretic hormone in pathogenesis. Pediatrics 1981;68(3):349–53.

[63] Keating JP, Schears GJ, Dodge PR. Oral water intoxication in infants. An American epidemic. ADJC 1991;145:985–90.

[64] Vanapruks V, Prapaitrakul K. Water intoxication and hyponatremic convulsions in neonates. Arch Dis Child 1989;64:734–5.

[65] Sarnaik AP, Meert K, Hackbarth R, et al. Management of hyponatremic seizures in children with hypertonic saline: a safe and effective strategy. Crit Care Med 1991;19(6):758–62.

[66] Sharf RE. Seizure from hyponatremia in infants. Early recognition and treatment. Arch Fam Med 1993;2:647–52.

[67] Gruskin AB, Baluarte HJ, Prebis JW, et al. Serum sodium abnormalities in children. Pediatr Clin North Am 1982;29(4):907–32.

[68] Laing IA, Wong CM. Hypernatremia in the first few days: is the incidence rising? Arch Dis Child Fetal Neonatal Ed 2002;87:F158–62.

[69] Macdonald PD, Grant L, Ross SRM. Hypernatremia in the first few days: a tragic case. Arch Dis Child Fetal Neonatal 2003;88(4):F350–1.

[70] Oddie S, Richmond S, Coulthard M. Hypernatremic dehydration and breast feeding: a population study. Arch Dis Child 2001;85:318–20.

[71] Singh J, Moghal N, Pearce SHS, et al. The investigation of hypocalcemia and rickets. Arch Dis Child 2003;88:403–7.

[72] Barnes ND. Endocrine disorders. In: Robert NRC, editor. Textbook of neonatology. 2nd edition. Edinburgh: Churchill Livingstone; 1992.

[73] Umpaichitra V, Bastian W, Castells S. Hypocalcemia in children: pathogenesis and management. Clin Pediatr 2001;40:305–12.

[74] Gerner JM. Mineral metabolism in the newborn. In: McMillan JA, DeAngelis CD, Feigin RD, Warshaw JB, editors. Oski's pediatrics: principles and practice. Philadelphia: Lippincott Williams & Wilkins; 1999.

[75] Walton DM, Thomas DC, Aly HZ, et al. Morbid hypocalcemia associated with phosphate enema in a six-week-old infant. Pediatrics 2000;106(3):e37.

[76] Rudolph CD. Disorders of magnesium metabolsim. In: Miller WM, associate editor. Rudolph's pediatrics. 21st edition. New York: McGraw-Hill Publishing Division; 2002.

[77] Ilves P, Kiisk M, Soopold T, et al. Serum total magnesium and ionized calcium concentrations in asphyxiated term newborn infants with hypoxic–ischaemic encephalopathy. Acta Paediatr 2000;89:680–5.

[78] Marcus JC, Valencia GB, Altura BT, et al. Serum ionized magnesium in premature and term infants. Pediatr Neurol 1998;18:311–4.

[79] Rodd C, Goodyer P. Hypercalcemia of the newborn: etiology, evaluation, and management. Pediatr Nephrol 1999;13:542–7.

[80] Root AW. Disorders of calcium and phosphorous metabolsim. In: Miller WM, associate editor. Rudolph's pediatrics. 21st edition. New York: McGraw-Hill Publishing Division; 2002.

[81] Lteif AN, Zimmerman D. Bisphosphonates for treatment of childhood hypercalcemia. Pediatrics 1998;102(4):990–3.

[82] Boineau FG, Lewy JE. Disorders of the kidneys and urinary tract, Part I. In: Roberton NRC, editor. Textbook of neonatalolgy. 2nd edition. Edinburgh: Churchill Livingstone; 1992. p. 839–51.

[83] Landau D, Kher KK. Gentamicin-induced Bartter-like syndrome. Pediatr Nephrol 1997;11: 737–40.

[84] Shetty AK, Rogers NL, Mannick EE, et al. Syndrome of hypokalemic metabolic alkalosis and hypomagnesemia associated with gentamicin therapy. Case reports. Clin Pediatr 2000; 39:529–33.

[85] Sullivan JE, Berman BW. Hypermangesmia with lethargy and hypotonia due to administration of magnesium hydroxide to a 4-week-old infant. Arch Pediatr Adolesc Med 2000;154:1272–4.

[86] Hale DE. Endocrine emergencies. In: Fleisher GR, Ludwig S, editors. Textbook of pediatric emergency medicine. 4th edition. Philadelphia: Lippincott Williams & Wilkins; 2000. p. 1101–4.

ELSEVIER
SAUNDERS

EMERGENCY
MEDICINE
CLINICS OF
NORTH AMERICA

Emerg Med Clin N Am 23 (2005) 885–899

The Porphyrias

Teague A. Dombeck, MD,
Robert C. Satonik, MD, FACEP*

*Department of Emergency Medicine, Synergy Medical Education Alliance,
1000 Houghton Avenue, Saginaw, MI 48602, USA*

A 19-year-old female presents to the emergency department (ED) complaining of chronic, intermittent, crampy abdominal pain, which is associated with nausea and vomiting. She also reports that she has muscle pain and weakness. Her past medical history is positive for depression and fibromyalgia.

Although the differential diagnosis of the patient describe above is certainly extensive, it is important to consider that this is a classic presentation of porphyria. There are several forms of porphyria, each caused by separate defects in the heme synthesis metabolic pathway. This pathway, although complex, is responsible for producing the precursors for oxygen transport, cytochromes, and various other biologic functions. It is certainly not essential for the ED physician to master these metabolic pathways; however, with a prevalence roughly the same as acromegaly or autoimmune hemolytic anemia, porphyria is a disease that can be encountered and even diagnosed in the ED.

Among the different porphyrias, porphyria cutania tarda is by far the most common and has a reported prevalence of about 1to 2/100,000 world wide [1]. Porphyria appears to be less prevalent in the United States. Despite the rare occurrence of this disease, the cardinal signs and symptoms are certainly recognizable in the correct clinical setting. Patients presenting with a long history of undiagnosed abdominal pain, somatic and autonomic neural complaints, and psychiatric conditions deserve to have porphyria in their differential diagnosis.

The porphyrias collectively are caused by particular enzymatic defects in the biosynthesis of heme [2]. There are seven major entities described in the literature, and each has its own associated enzyme defect. Each of

---

* Corresponding author.

E-mail address: rsatonik@synergymedical.org (R.C. Satonik).

0733-8627/05/$ - see front matter © 2005 Elsevier Inc. All rights reserved.
doi:10.1016/j.emc.2005.03.014   *emed.theclinics.com*

these entities displays neurovisceral symptoms, photocutaneous symptoms, or both. The neurovisceral symptoms arise from an accumulation of porphyria precursors, namely aminolevulinic acid and porphobilinogen. Although the exact mechanism of neurotoxicity has yet to be elicited, aminolevulinic acid is analogous to gamma-aminobutyric acid (GABA), and this may interact with GABA receptors [3]. Another theory is that the precursors aminolevulinic acid and porphobilinogen are directly neurotoxic [4–6]. Photocutaneous symptoms occur in connection with the accumulation of porphyrins. These porphyrins are activated by long-wave ultraviolet light, and subsequently generate oxygen radicals that damage the skin [7].

The porphyrias may be classified according to their specific site of expression of the enzymatic defect, or on the basis of their clinical characteristics. Sites of enzymatic defects can generally be categorized as either acute hepatic or erythropoietic. The acute hepatic porphyrias include acute intermittent porphyria (AIP), variegate porphyria (VP), hereditary coproporphyria, and delta-aminolevulinate dehydratase (ALAD)- deficiency porphyria. Erythropoetic porphyrias include congenital erythropoietic porphyria and erythropoietic protoporphyria (EPP) [3]. Differentiation of the porphyrias on the basis neurovisceral vs. photosensitivity is outlined in Fig. 1.

The following review of the porphyrias is intended to be an overview of the most current information regarding this disease entity. Each of the seven forms of porphyria is discussed in order of their respective prevalence. Each type of porphyria is discussed with respect to its pathophysiology, precipitating factors, clinical features, diagnosis, and treatment.

Porphyria cutanea tarda

Porphyria cutanea tarda (PCT) is the most common of the porphyrias in both the United States and Europe. It is caused by a deficiency in the enzyme uroporphyrinogen decarboxylase (UROD). Manifestations are primarily cutaneous, with iron overload playing a key role in the pathogenesis of the disease. PCT can be inherited; however, it is more commonly an acquired porphyria [8].

Pathophysiology

UROD is an enzyme in the heme synthesis pathway that catalyzes the removal of four carboxyl groups from uroporphyrinogen to form coproporphyrinogen. There are three types of PCT, and each has different degrees of UROD deficiency. The most common (80-90%) of these is type I, which is an acquired form characterized by decreased hepatic UROD deficiency but normal erythrocyte UROD activity. Although this acquired form can be

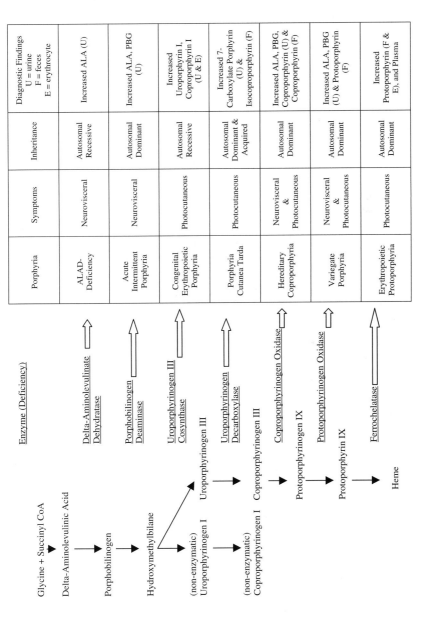

Fig. 1. Heme synthesis pathway with major enzyme deficiencies. Associated porphyrias with major symptomatology, inheritance pattern, and accumulation products.

spontaneous, more commonly it is precipitated by the use of alcohol, estrogen, iron overload, and certain drugs. Alcoholism is associated with roughly 70% of PCT; however, the extent of liver disease is usually mild. Iron overload is universally present, and is an important factor in the pathogenesis of PCT. Other precipitating factors appear to be estrogen containing compounds. These become clinically apparent usually when women begin taking birth control pills or males are placed on estrogen therapy for prostate cancer. Other entities that have been reported to precipitate PCT include chlorinated hydrocarbons, autoimmune disorders, and viral hepatitis. Skin photosensitivity results from absorption of light in the 400 nm to 410 nm range. This excites the porphyrins and causes direct damage as well as free radical production. These free radicals disrupt cell membranes and lysosomes in the dermis and epidermis [9].

Signs and symptoms

The most distinguishing feature of PCT is the formation of vesicles on the sun exposed areas of skin. Most commonly this includes the hands, face, and extremities. The vesicles become crusted, scarred, and residually pigmented. The skin of these individuals is very fragile and minor trauma may cause blistering eruptions. These individuals develop severe chronic changes of the skin and typically have hyperpigmentation of the malar and periorbital regions. Almost half of individuals with PCT will develop hypertrichosis of the cheeks and lateral eyebrows [9].

Diagnosis

Although clinical features tend to distinguish this type of porphyria from others, a definitive diagnosis may be obtained by measuring porphyrin levels in the urine and feces. Patients will typically have increased levels of urine uroporphyrin and coproporphyrin in a five-to-one respective ratio. This ratio distinguishes PCT from the variegate form of porphyria, as both will have elevated levels of the two precursors. Elevated isocoproporphyrin levels in the serum, as well as feces, are diagnostic of PCT. It should be noted that a rare form of cutaneous porphyria, hepatoerythropoietic porphyria (HEP), will display childhood onset of similar clinical symptoms and have identical diagnostic labs.

Treatment

Although avoidance of precipitating factors including sunlight, alcohol, and estrogens is a necessity, the primary therapy for PCT involves the reduction of total body iron stores. This is obtained by repeated phlebotomy of 1 unit of blood twice a month for a total of 5 to 10 liters. Other treatments include subcutaneous desferrioxamine infusion and chloroquine therapy [10].

Acute intermittent porphyria

AIP is caused by a deficiency in the enzyme porphinobillinogen (PBG) deaminase. The defect results in the inability to convert PBG to uroporphyrinogen I. AIP is inherited in an autosomal dominant fashion, and typically, individuals have a 50% decrease in enzyme activity [8]. AIP has its highest incidence in people of Swedish descent. The incidence is reportedly 1.5/100,000 in the United States Swedish population and 1/1,000 in Lapland Sweden [11]. AIP is primarily associated with neurovisceral symptoms, with abdominal pain being the most frequent complaint.

Pathophysiology

The mutations of porphobilinogen deaminase can be divided into three subtypes and account for three variants of AIP. Functional and non-functional enzymes can be distinguished by crossreactions with antibodies specific to the normal enzymatic protein. These antibodies are termed crossreacting immunologic material [3]. Clinically, patients with AIP and ALAD deficiency porphyria typically become symptomatic when a precipitating factor induces aminolevulinic acid (ALA) synthetase, which in turn, promotes heme synthesis.

Precipitating factors

There are four general categories of precipitating factors that can induce or worsen symptoms of AIP. Drugs, starvation, infection, and hormonal factors all play key roles in instigating attacks. Most patients with porphyria do not experience significant symptoms unless one or more of these factors are present.

Several drugs have been clearly implicated in inducing porphyria. These include the barbiturates, sulfonamides, griesofulvin, sulfonylureas, phenytoin, and many others (see Box 1). Experimentally, there are a number of medications that pose a theoretical risk, as their ability to induce porphyria has been demonstrated in laboratory animals. Some of these include ciprofloxacin, cimetidine, erythromycin, furosimide, and metocloprimide [2,3]. Although the exact mechanism by which different medications can induce an attack of porphyria is not clear, many experts agree that the induction of cytochromes is a likely mechanism. As the upregulation of cytochromes is activated, total body heme stores become depleted leading to an induction of aminolevulinic acid synthetase.

Hormones have been shown to play a key role in the induction and severity of AIP. Experimentally, porphyrin precursor production is increased in diseased individuals who are taking estrogens. One study from Sweden reported that oral contraceptives precipitated acute attacks in 24% of individuals studied [12]. AIP is generally more common in females,

Box 1. Safe and unsafe drugs in acute porphyria

Drugs safe in acute porphyria
  Acetaminophen
  Acetazolamide
  Acyclovir
  Allopurinol
  Amiloride
  Aminoglycosides*
  Asprin
  Atropine
  Beta-blockers
  Bromides*
  Bumetanide
  Bupivicaine*
  Buprenorphine
  Chlorpromazine
  Codiene
  Corticosteroids*
  Deferoxamine
  Demerol
  Diazoxide*
  Digitalis
  Epinephrine
  Fentanyl
  FSH
  Fenoprophen*
  Gabapentin
  Gentamicin
  Glipizide
  Haloperidol
  Hepzrin
  Ibuprophen*
  Indomethacin
  Insulin
  Labetolol
  Lithium salts
  Metformin
  Metoprolol
  Morphine
  Nadolol
  Nitrouos oxide
  Oxytocin
  Pencillin
  Procaine
  Prochlorperazine*
  Propofol
  Propoxyphene
  Quinine
  Ranitidine*
  Salbutamol
  Senna
  Sulindac
  Temazepam
  Thyroxine*
  Warfarin

Drugs unsafe in acute porphyria
  Alpha-methyldopa[+]
  Barbiturates[+]
  Captopril
  Carbamazepine
  Cimetidine
  Chloramphenicol[+]
  Chlorpropamide
  Diazepam
  Diliazem
  Dimenhydrinate
  Doxycycline
  Ergot compounds[+]
  Erythromycin
  Estrogen
  Tehanol[+]
  Furosemide
  Griesofulvin[+]
  Hydralazine
  Hydrochlorothiazide
  Imipramine[+]
  Lidocaine
  Metoclopramide
  Metronidazole
  Nifedipine
  Oral contraceptives
  Orphenadrine[+]
  Oxycodone
  Pentazocine[+]
  Phenobarbital
  Phenytoin[+]

---

  * Denotes medications that are likely to be safe.
  [+] Denotes medications that are known to cause acute attacks.

and demonstrates a temporal coincidence with the onset menses in 10% to 20% of women [13,14]. Rarely does AIP occur before puberty, and pregnancy typically worsens the disease or brings about an acute attack. Therefore, it is highly recommended that endogenous sex hormones be restricted in those who have AIP.

Another precipitating factor of AIP appears to be the induction of the synthesis of ALA synthetase associated with starvation. Decreased caloric intake of carbohydrates in particular seems to desuppress the activity of ALA synthetase.

Finally, infections and surgeries have been shown to exacerbate or precipitate AIP. The exact mechanism is not known; however, it appears to be related to the release of endogenous steroids and the presence of a starvation state. Infections both viral and bacterial may produce oxidative stressors that induce heme oxygenase-1 [3]. This, in turn, leads to heme catabolism and the lifting of suppression of ALA synthetase. The induction of ALA synthetase initiates the heme production pathway, which becomes interrupted by PBG deaminase deficiency (the enzyme deficient in AIP). This inability to convert PBG to hydroxymethylbilane (HMB) slows the heme production cascade, thereby increasing the amount of PBG and ALA in the cells which are hypothesized to be neurotoxic.

Signs and symptoms

The most common initial symptom in AIP is abdominal pain, which is present in roughly 90% of patients. Other common symptoms include nausea/vomiting (43%), extremity pain/parasthesias (50%), and constipation (48%) [4]. Gastrointestinal symptoms include the above as well as diarrhea, abdominal distention, and ileus. AIP can easily be mistaken for an acute surgical abdomen, as often times patients will have a tender abdomen with dilated loops of bowel on plain radiographs. Typically however, patients will not have rebound tenderness or guarding. These finding are likely due to a visceral neuropathy and complicate the clinical picture when combined with the accompanying leukocytosis and low-grade fever that can be present. Tachycardia occurs due to autonomic dysfunction in approximately 80% of patients. Other autonomic signs include urinary retention, incontinence, hypertension, and postural hypotension.

Commonly, AIP will manifest with neurologic symptoms, including mental status changes and hallucinations. The motor neuropathy associated with acute attacks tends to manifest itself as muscle weakness. This weakness tends to involve the proximal muscles of the extremities including the hips and shoulders, and is usually symmetric. Patients present with cramping, weakness, and often a noticeable muscle wasting. Deep tendon reflexes may be lost; however, fasiculations are typically absent. Although the weakness and wasting will usually spontaneously resolve with the resolution of an acute attack, there have been reports of foot drop and wasting of the intrinsic muscles of the hand. Rarely, the motor neuropathy involves the cranial nerves and can resemble Guillain Barre' syndrome [15]. These complications can arise from patients receiving medication that exacerbate AIP and can progress to respiratory paralysis.

Approximately 15% of patients experiencing an acute attack of porphyria will present with seizures [4]. These tend to be generalized, and are more common in patients who are hyponatremic. Low sodium states in AIP arise from vomiting, syndrome of inappropriate antidiuretic hormone (SIADH), and inappropriate fluid replacement. Other electrolyte disturbances include hypokalemia, hypomagnesemia, hypochloremia, and azotemia [16]. Last, many psychologic manifestations of AIP have been described. These include anxiety, depression, confusion, and psychotic episodes. An obvious distinguishing feature of AIP is the lack of cutaneous symptoms.

Diagnosis

Classically, AIP has been crudely diagnosed by exposing a patient's urine to sunlight and open air. This exposure converts the PBG in the urine to porphobilin, which is a reddish-brown porphyrin-like compound and essentially turns the urine a port-wine color. A Woods lamp may also be used to detect PBG in the urine. Upon exposure, urine containing this precursor will give off a red or pink fluorescence. Patients with AIP will have increased amounts of ALA and PBG in their urine during acute attacks. This can be confusing, however, as patients with AIP may also display these precursors in their urine between attacks. Therefore, it is necessary to quantitatively determine the presence of ALA and PBG, as well as identify the disease furthermore on a molecular-genetic basis.

Screening for urine PBG can be obtained by using the Watson-Schwartz or the Hoesch test. Both these methods provide quantitative data and use the Ehrlich reagent to detect a chromogen. These methods do require 24-hour urine collection [2,3].

Due to the fact that other porphyrias may exhibit increased levels of ALA, PBG, or both, it is necessary to perform further assays to differentiate between them. An erythrocyte PBG deaminase assay is available to detect decreased PBG deaminase activity in red blood cells. This will correctly identify AIP types I and III. Further identification of the specific genetic mutations is beyond the scope of this article; however, it must be remembered that identification of the molecular-genetic aspects of AIP is not alone sufficient to diagnose an acute attack of porphyria. The symptoms must also be accompanied by elevated ALA and PBG in the urine.

Treatment

Treatment is essentially the same for the other hepatic porphyrias (VP, hereditary coproporphyria, and ALAD deficiency) as AIP. Therapy is generally three pronged, and is aimed at alleviating the inciting event, symptomatic relief, and reversing ALA synthase activity.

Patients who present with medications as precipitating factors should have the medication discontinued, and other current medications should be scrutinized for their potential to exacerbate their condition. Patients who have decreased oral intake or are in starvation states need aggressive fluid hydration with glucose containing solutions. Careful examination for underlying infections must be undertaken, and treatment for them must be initiated with mediations "safe" for patients with porphyria (see list).

Symptomatic treatment can become complex, and again, care needs to be used to avoid exacerbating medications. The gastrointestinal symptoms of AIP respond well to chlorpromazine as well as other phenothiazines. The use of these medications, however, can give false positives for urine PBG. This coincidence is unfortunate given the usefulness of ganglionic blockade the phenothiazines have to treat the autonomic neuropathy particular of AIP. Pain control can be maintained by morphine or by consulting the list of safe medications in porphyria. Propanolol is useful, and has been shown to be safe in treating hypertension as well as tachycardia. Patients presenting with an acute attack and having seizure activity can be safely treated with diazepam. Chronic management of seizures can be treated by valproate, clonazepam, or magnesium sulfate. The management of seizures can be a potential source of iatrogenicity as phenytoin, carbamazepine, ethosuximide, and barbituates; all can induce acute attacks of porphyria [17–19].

ALA synthetase is the primary enzyme whose activity is the cause of acute attacks. Reversal of this activity is essential in the management of AIP as well as the other hepatic porphyrias. Initial treatment consists of high glucose intake of at least 400 g/d [20]. This may be via oral or parenteral, and directly acts to suppress the activity of ALA synthetase. An infusion of $D_{10}W$ at 166 cc/h or eating 12 Snickers bars/24 h (both would give 400 g/d) is unreasonable. Therefore, combination therapy using oral and intravenous glucose therapy is likely the best method. Hematin infusions at a rate of 4 mg/kg every 12 hours are also very effective in inhibiting the activity of ALA synthetase. Derived from outdated HbsAg-negative blood, hematin directly inhibits ALA synthetase due to its high heme content [21]. Infusions are continued until signs and symptoms are improved. Patients receiving hematin can have elevations of the prothrombin time and the partial thromboplastin time, and may have bleeding diathesis [22]. Other rare complications include transient renal insufficiency and chemical phlebitis [23]. Once an acute attack is adequately treated, prevention consists of adequate carbohydrate diets, avoidance of exacerbating drugs, and prompt treatment of any infection. With the increasing popularity of low-carbohydrate diets, it will be interesting to see if the clinical presentations of the porphyrias will also increase.

Erythropoietic protoporphyria

EPP is one of the more common forms of porphyria. Patients with EPP have roughly a 75% to 90% reduction in the activity of the enzyme ferrochelatase. This enzyme is essentially the last step in the heme synthesis pathway, and reduction of its activity results in massive accumulations of protoporphyrin in the plasma, feces, and in erythrocytes [2,3]. EPP displays an autosomal dominant inheritance pattern. However, due to different types of mutations of the allele, family members of patients with EPP may show a 50% reduction in enzyme activity and still be essentially asymptomatic [8]. Sun exposure is the major precipitating factor in EPP, and the photo-cutaneous lesions produced tend to be characteristically distinct from both congenital erythropoetic porphyria (CEP) and PCT.

Signs and symptoms

Clinical diagnosis of EPP may be adequate to distinguish EPP from the other forms of porphyria. The skin lesions formed by sun exposure tend to have a predictable time course and a characteristic appearance. Typically, within 1 hour after sun exposure, patients with EPP experience burning or stinging pains in the skin. These symptoms can appear within minutes and are usually pruritic. This acute phototoxic reaction is followed by the development of edema, erythema, and burning pain in the sun exposed areas. Eventually these areas develop petechiae, vesicles, and rarely purpura. Finally, these lesions will crust over and severe chronic skin changes typically follow. Chronic changes include "velvet knuckles," which are marked by thick, hyperkeratotic skin, with deep skin markings over the dorsum of the hands, which can also be seen on the bridge of the nose [24,25]. Other skin changes such as lichenification, pigmentation, and premature aging are common.

Diagnosis

Biochemical diagnosis of EPP hinges upon the presence of increased amounts of protoporphyrin in erythrocytes, plasma, bile, and feces. Protoporphyrin levels are not increased in the urine of these patients as it is poorly water soluble.

Treatment

Treatment of EPP involves avoidance of sun exposure and use of topical sunscreens. Oral beta-carotene is recommended as an adjuvant to increase systemic photo protection. Benefits are not seen typically until a few months after therapy is initiated. and dosages of up to 180 mg/d is recommended. The mechanism of beta-carotene likely involves the quenching of activated oxygen radicals [5].

Variegate porphyria

Also known as South African porphyria, VP is a very rare form of porphyria. In the South African population, however, it has an estimated incidence of 3/1000 individuals [26]. Interestingly, this high incidence is traced back to two Dutch settlers whose union in 1688 appears to be the source of nearly all of the South African cases of VP [27,28]. As the name implies, VP can present with photosensitivity, neurovisceral symptoms, or both.

Pathophysiology

VP is caused by a decrease in the activity of the enzyme protoporphyrinogen oxidase (PPO). This enzyme is responsible for the oxidation of protoporphyrinogen to protoporhyrin. Patients with VP are almost universally heterozygous, and will display a 50% reduction in enzyme activity. Rarely, there have been reported cases of homozygous individuals with VP; however, the particular PPO mutations appear to be less severe in these patients, and the enzyme has been shown in these patients to have residual activity. Cases have been documented of individuals with essentially no PPO activity, and these patients have severe growth and mental retardation, as well as marked photosensitivity and neurologic abnormalities. Precipitating factors that can bring about acute attacks of VP are nearly identical to that of the other hepatic porphyrias (hereditary coproporphyria [HCP] and ALAD).

Signs and symptoms

The neurovisceral symptoms in VP are essentially indistinguishable form that of the other hepatic porphyrias. Abdominal pain, peripheral neuropathy, weakness, and gastrointestinal symptoms predominate. Photosensitivity, however, tends to be more chronic than the symptoms of hereditary coproporphyria. Blisters, as well as superficial ulcers, typically present in various stages of healing and scarring. Sites of bony protuberances tend to be areas of high fragility, and severe chronic scarring is common.

Diagnosis

Because VP shares portions of its major symptoms with AIP, ALAD, HCP, and PCT, the definitive diagnosis can be made demonstrating an elevated concentration of protoporphyrin IX in the plasma and feces. This finding is the hallmark of VP, and the plasma will typically fluoresce when exposed to ultraviolet light.

Treatment

Treatment of the neurovisceral symptoms of VP is identical to the three-pronged approach used to treat both AIP and ALAD. Avoidance of precipitating factors, symptomatic treatment, and reversing the activity of ALA synthetase are the cornerstones of therapy. The photosensitivity in VP tends to be grossly undertreated, and patients essentially need to avoid any contact with sunlight. Patients need to use sunscreen, protective clothing, and even wide-brimmed hats to minimize exposure [29].

Hereditary coproporphyria

HCP is a rare form of porphyria, which is clinically similar to AIP; however, it is typically much milder. It is caused by a reduction in the activity of the enzyme coproporphyrinogen. Although neurovisceral symptoms predominate in patients with HCP, it has been associated with photocutaneous exacerbations.

Signs and symptoms

The symptoms of HCP are essentially identical to that of the other hepatic porphyrias. Abdominal pain, nausea, vomiting, neurologic, and psychologic symptoms predominate. Roughly 30% of patients will have photosensitivity. Acute attacks are triggered by essentially the same precipitating factors as AIP (eg, medications, hormones, starvation).

Diagnosis

Definitive diagnosis of the disease involves detection of coproporphyrin in the urine and feces. Similar to AIP, ALA and PBG will be elevated in the urine; however, it typically does not stay elevated between attacks [2,3].

Treatment

Treatment of HCP is essentially identical to that of AIP. Both precipitating factors and preventative measures are also the same as those in AIP.

Congenital erythropoietic porphyria

This form of porphyria manifests with both neurovisceral and photosensitive symptoms. It is one of the rarest forms of the disease, and reported cases number between 100 and 200, some of which were not confirmed on a molecular level. The defective enzyme uroporphyrinogen cosynthetase (UCS) is inherited as an autosomal recessive trait. CEP is also referred to as Gunther disease, and has no clear gender or racial predilection [8].

Pathophysiology

UCS is responsible for the conversion of HMB to uroporphyrinogen III. In patients with the defective UCS, HMB is shunted down the pathway to be nonenzymatically converted to uroporphyrin I. Uropoyphyrin I is subsequently catalyzed to coproporphyrin I. This isomer of coproporphyrin is the porphyrin that causes erythrodontia or red staining of the teeth.

Signs and symptoms

Erythrodontia presents early in infancy and is accompanied by staining of the bones, hemolysis, dark urine, and photosensitiviy. Interestingly, these particular features may be the fodder from which vampire folklore was contrived [30]. The cutaneous symptoms of CEP are like those of the other porphyrias. However, the skin changes tend to become chronic with repeated sun exposure, and can lead to disfiguring hyper- and hypopigmented lesions. Hypertrichosis, alopecia, and disfigurement of the hands, extremities, and face are not uncommon. Systemic symptoms include hemolytic anemia, splenomegaly, porphyrin containing gallstones, and fragile bones. Bone density suffers as a result of erythroid hyperplasia of the marrow, and is typified by pathologic fractures, vertebral compression fractures, and short stature.

Diagnosis

CEP is typically diagnosed early in infancy, with children having characteristically pink-stained diapers and severe photosensitivity. Diagnosis is further obtained by demonstrating increased levels of urinary, fecal, and erythrocyte porphyrins, along with elevated type I isomers of uroporphyrin and coproporphyrin. Elevated erythrocyte porphyrins will cause nucleated erythrocytes to fluoresce.

Treatment

Treatment of CEP begins primarily with avoiding damage to the skin. Avoiding sunlight, and minimizing trauma or infections of the skin is paramount. Sunscreens are essential, and oral beta-carotene can be used to diminish photosensitivity. Splenectomy is useful in reducing red blood cell destruction and transfusions of packed red blood cells can decrease hemolysis and suppress bone marrow erythropoesis, thereby decreasing porphyrin excretion. Recently, cases of severe CEP have been cured by bone marrow transplantation [31].

Delta-aminolevulinate dehydratase deficiency porphyria

ALAD deficiency porphyria is the rarest of the porphyrias. Aptly named, it is characterized by the inability to catalyze the conversion of delta-aminolevulinic acid to porphobilinogen. It is inherited as an autosomal recessive disorder, and predominantly manifested as neurologic symptoms. Although it is well described in the porphyria literature, there have been only four molecularly confirmed cases reported [3].

Pathophysiology

ALAD enzyme activity is less than 2% normal in both erythrocytes and nonerythroid cells of individuals with this disorder. Parents of these individuals have enzyme activity of roughly half that of normal individuals, but are largely asymptomatic [3]. In the heme synthesis pathway ALAD adjoins two molecules of aminolevulinic acid (ALA) to form PBG. Two molecules of water are lost in the reaction. The active form of ALAD requires zinc as a cofactor. Individuals with ALAD deficiency porphyria have lead displacing zinc in their altered form of the enzyme [32].

Diagnosis

Diagnosis of ALAD deficiency porphyria is confirmed by the presence of increased levels of ALA in the urine in conjunction with the absence of accumulated urine PBG. This lack of PBG distinguishes ALAD deficiency porphyria from AIP. Although this distinction is obvious on a molecular basis, the symptomatology and treatment are nearly identical to patients with AIP.

Summary

In summary, the porphyrias are a group of disorders involving enzymatic defects in heme synthesis. The signs and symptoms characteristic of porphyria are primarily neurovisceral and photocutaneous. Although encounters with these patients are rare, emergency physicians should simply consider porphyria in their differential diagnosis in particular patients to avoid unnecessary morbidity and mortality. These particularities include patients with longstanding histories of undiagnosed abdominal pain, autonomic dysfunction, musculoskeletal complaints, and photosensitivity.

References

[1] Elder GH. Porphyria cutanea tarda. Semin Liver Dis 1998;18(1):67–75.
[2] Sassa S, Kappas A. The porphyrias. 2003;9:1–9 [Available from WebMD Inc., Accessed May 1, 2004].
[3] Werman H. The porphyrias. Emerg Clin North Am 1989;7(4):927–42.
[4] Bonkowsky HL, Schady W. Neurologic manifestations of acute porphyria. Semin Liver Dis 1982;2:108–24.
[5] Shanley BC, Neethling AC, Percy VA, et al. Neurochemical aspects of porphyria: studies on the possible neurotoxicity of delta-aminolevulinic acid. S Afr J Med 1975;49:576–80.
[6] Shanley BC, Percy VA, Neethling AC. Neurochemistry to acute porphyria: experimental studies on delta-aminolevulinic acid and porphobilinogen. In: Doss M, editor. Porphyrins in human disease. Basel: S Karger; 1976.
[7] Spikes JD. Porphyrins and related compounds as photodynamic sensitizers. Ann N Y Acad Sci 1975;244:496–508.

[8] Kappas A, Sassa S, Galbraith RA, et al. The porphyrias. In: Scriver CR, Beaudet AL, Sly WS, et al, editors. The metabolic and molecular basis of inherited disease. New York: McGraw-Hill; 1995. p. 2103–59.

[9] Poh-Fitzpatrick MB. Pathogenesis and treatment of photocutaneous manifestations of the porphyrins. Semin Liver Dis 1982;2:164–76.

[10] Gilbertini P, Rocchi E, Cassanelli A, et al. Advances in the treatment of porphyria cutanea tarda: effectiveness of slow subcutaneous desferrioxamine infusion. Liver 1984;4:280–4.

[11] Goldberg A, Rimingron C. Diseases of porphyrin metabolism. Springfield (IL): Charles C. Thomas; 1962.

[12] Andersson C, Innala E, Backstrom T. Acute intermittent porphyria in women: clinical expression, use and experience of exogenous sex hormones: a population-based study in northern Sweden. J Intern Med 2003;254:176–83.

[13] Zimmerman TS, McMillin JM, Watson CJ. Onset of manifestations of hepatic porphyria in relation to the influence of female sex hormones. Arch Intern Med 1966;118:229–40.

[14] Welland FH, Hellman ES, Collins A, et al. Factors affecting the excretion of porphyrin precursors by a patient with acute intermittent porphyria: II. The effect of ethinyl estradiol. Metabolism 1964;13:251–8.

[15] Elder GH, Hift RT, Neissner PN. The acute porphyrias. Lancet 1997;349:82–3.

[16] Disler PB, Eales L. The acute attack of porphyria. S Afr Med J 1982;61:82–3.

[17] Bonkowsky HL, Sinclair PR, Emery S, et al. Seizure management in acute hepatic porhyria: risks of valproate and clonazepam. Neurology 1980;30:588–92.

[18] Larson AW, Wasserstrom WR, Felsher BF, et al. Post-traumatic epilepsy and acute intermittent porphyria: effects of phenytoin, carbamazepine, and clonazepam. Neurology 1978;28:824–8.

[19] Magnessen CR, Doherty JM, Hess RA, et al. Grand mal seizures and acute intermittent porphyria. Neurology 1975;25:1121–5.

[20] Sassa S. Diagnosis and therapy of acute intermittent porphyria. Blood Rev 1966;10:53–8.

[21] Mustajoki P, Tenhunen R, Pierach C, et al. Heme in the treatment of porphyrias and hematological disorders. Semin Hematol 1989;26:1–9.

[22] Pierach CA. Hematin therapy for the porphyric attack. Semin Liver Dis 1982;2:125–31.

[23] Lamon JM, Frykholm BC, Hess RA, et al. Hematin therapy for acute porphyria. Medicine 1979;58:252–69.

[24] DeLeo BA, Poh-Fitzpatrick MB, Matthews-Roth M, et al. Erythropoietic protoporphyria, 10 years experience. Am J Med 1976;60:8–22.

[25] Poh-Fitzpatrick MB. Erythropoietic protoporphyria. Int J Dermatol 1978;17:359–69.

[26] Eales L, Day RS, Blekkenhorst GH. The clinical and biochemical features of variegate porphyria: an analysis of 300 cases studies at Groote Schuur Hospital, Cape Town. Int J Biochem 1980;12:837–53.

[27] Meissner PN, Dailey TA, Hift RJ, et al. A R59W mutation in human protoporphyrinogen oxidase results in decreased enzyme activity and is prevalent in South Africans with variegate porphyria. Nature 1996;13:95–7.

[28] Dean G. The porphyrias: a study of inheritance and environment. London: Pitman Medical; 1971.

[29] Muhlbauer JE, Pathak MA, Tishler PV, et al. Variegate porphyria in New England. JAMA 1982;247:3095–120.

[30] Dunea G. Vampires. BMJ 1999;318(717):135A.

[31] Harada FA, Shwayder TA, Desnick RJ, et al. Treatment of severe congenital erythropoietic porphyria by bone marrow transplantation. J Am Acad Dermatol 2001;45:274–82.

[32] Granick JL, Sassa S, Kappas A. Some biochemical and clinical aspects of lead intoxication. In: Bodansky O, Latner AL, editors. Advances in clinical chemistry. New York: Academic Press; 1978. p. 287.

ELSEVIER
SAUNDERS

EMERGENCY
MEDICINE
CLINICS OF
NORTH AMERICA

Emerg Med Clin N Am 23 (2005) 901–908

Altered Mental Status Due to Metabolic or Endocrine Disorders

Andrew M. Bazakis, MD, FACEP[a,b,*],
Catherine Kunzler, DO[c]

[a]Synergy Medical Education Alliance, 1000 Houghton Avenue, Saginaw, MI 48602, USA
[b]Michigan State University Emergency Medicine Residency Program,
700 Cooper Avenue, Saginaw, MI 48602, USA
[c]Program in Emergency Medicine, Michigan State University College of Human Medicine,
700 Cooper Avenue, Saginaw, MI 48602, USA

"O! Now, forever
Farewell the tranquil mind; Farewell content!"
                                    -William Shakespeare, Othello

This article brings further to light some portions of the differential diagnoses for various states of mental status alteration. The term altered mental status being rather broad, the article is organized by more specific symptoms in this category including lethargy, disorientation, and seizures. It is the authors' intent not to provide necessarily a complete differential diagnosis for each of these but rather to discuss some of the often less obvious etiologies for these presentations related to endocrine and metabolic disease states. As several of the particular metabolic entities mentioned are discussed elsewhere in this issue, the discussion of these disease states is more limited than those that are not discussed elsewhere.

Fatigue

That state [of weariness or exhaustion] ... "characterized by a lessened capacity for work and reduced efficiency of accomplishment ... from the Latin fatigo meaning 'to tire'" [1]. Many emergency department (ED) patients complain of fatigue, weakness, or lack of energy. This state can be seen in many conditions such as cardiovascular disease, anemia, major depression, and others. Metabolic entities that must be considered in the

---

* Corresponding author. Synergy Medical Education Alliance, 1000 Houghton Avenue, Saginaw, MI 48602.
  E-mail address: abazakis@pol.net (A.M. Bazakis).

differential diagnosis include thyroid disease, abnormal potassium, phosphate, and calcium.

Mental status changes are found in nearly half of all patients with thyroid dysfunction because of changes in metabolism and the sensitivity of central nervous system (CNS) receptors to neurotransmitters. An early symptom of hyperthyroidism is chronic fatigue [2]. Hyperthyroidism with fatigue can be complicated and occult in presenting, with comorbid conditions commonly causing fatigue on their own, such as pregnancy or when presenting as depression in the case of apathetic or masked hyperthyroidism in the elderly [3]. In hypothyroidism, desensitized neuroreceptors, decreased glucose use, and decreased cerebral blood flow all contribute to the CNS symptoms seen in patients [2]. Fatigue is a common finding in patients with hypothyroidism; a gradual decline in activities is typical.

Electrolyte disturbances are found often in patients who complain of fatigue, although it is difficult to separate symptoms of the primary disease from those of the abnormal electrolytes. For example, hypokalemia and hyperkalemia are commonly the result of processes that result in hypovolemia, such as gastroenteritis, kidney disease, and vomiting with gastrointestinal (GI) hemorrhage. Both the hypovolemia and the abnormal potassium value can cause symptoms of fatigue. Other etiologies associated with hyperkalemia include diabetic ketoacidosis, tumor lysis syndrome, hemolysis, and more atypical scenarios such as acromegaly, vitamin D intoxication, pseudohypoparathyroidism, and phosphorus burns [4].

Many of these same etiologies affect calcium and phosphate metabolism, which share the symptoms of fatigue and weakness. When hypocalcemia is suspected, the severity of symptoms is dependent on the rapidity of the fall of serum calcium. Frequently heard complaints range from fatigue and weakness to confusion and hallucinations [5]. The signs and symptoms of hypercalcemia, noted in the mnemonic "stones, bones, abdominal moans, and psychic groans," are often a manifestation of primary hyperparathyroidism. The psychic groans refer to the neuromuscular complaints of impaired concentration and memory, confusion, stupor, coma, lethargy, fatigue, and muscle weakness [6]. Hyperphosphatemia also may present with fatigue associated with generalized weakness and sleep disturbance.

In short, these entities, and others, can present most commonly with comorbid causes for fatigue, and abnormal electrolytes should be excluded even if other causes are identified. Laboratory evaluation of the typical electrolyte panel and calcium, phosphate, and thyroid function studies are indicated in patients complaining of fatigue with the appropriate clinical picture.

Generalized weakness

According to Webster, weakness is "the state or quality of lacking or being deficient in physical strength" [7]. To differentiate weakness from fatigue is commonly a task akin to the splitting of hairs; however, weakness as a muscular phenomenon shall be discussed as opposed to the more constitutional entity of fatigue mentioned previously. Almost any electrolyte or metabolic abnormality can cause this condition. Electrolyte abnormalities causing this phenomenon include hyperkalemia, hypokalemia, hypercalcemia, hypomagnesemia, hypermagnesemia, hypophosphatemia, hyperphosphatemia, and hypernatremia. For additional consideration, there are metabolic causes such as thyrotoxicosis (including thyrotoxic periodic paralysis), hypothyroidism, acromegaly, vitamin D deficiency, Cushing's syndrome, and Addison's disease. Of particular note, hypomagnesemia is common in intensive care unit (ICU) patients, affecting up to 65% of patients, with decreased nutrition intake, hypoalbuminemia, diuretics, and some antibiotics all playing a role. Generalized weakness that progresses to tetany can be seen in patients with significant hypomagnesemia, and this should be assessed [8].

Lethargy

"A state of deep and prolonged unconsciousness, resembling profound slumber, from which one can be aroused but into which one immediately relapses, from the Greek lethargis, meaning 'drowsiness'" [1]. Etiologies to be considered in addition to the typical infectious and other etiologies include: hypernatremia, hyponatremia, hypercalcemia, hypomagnesemia, and hypoglycemia.

Although lethargy can be attributed only to a single primary disorder, careful attention may uncover a secondary metabolic abnormality associated with the primary disease state, which also may contribute to the lethargy. Hypernatremia is found with CNS trauma and intracranial hemorrhage because of the more obvious etiologies such as diabetes insipidus. In the setting of therapy with lithium carbonate, aminoglycosides, amphotericin, and colchicines, or in association with ethanol ingestion, hypernatremia should be considered as a comorbid entity for the patient presenting with lethargy. Hyponatremia can present with headache and lethargy and then can progress to obtundation, coma, and seizure [9,10].

Hypercalcemia can be seen in several scenarios and should be considered in patients taking thiazides, theophylline, and lithium carbonate. Other causes of elevated calcium include acromegaly and hyperthyroidism. Suspicion for hypomagnesemia is increased with known diuretic use, aminoglycoside therapy, cyclosporine therapy, foscarnet therapy, chronic alcoholism, and acute pancreatitis [4].

A common cause of lethargy in children between 6 months and 9 years of age is idiopathic ketotic hypoglycemia. The most common cause of hypoglycemia in children, it often presents in a child who goes without feeding for a prolonged length of time. The otherwise healthy child will be found to be hypoglycemic and have ketones in the urine. Glucose administration is the treatment of choice [11]. Once again, the identification of one etiology for the lethargic state does not necessary complete the list of possible comorbid sources for the patient's lethargic state.

Coma

Coma (derived from the same word in Greek meaning "deep sleep") is a "state of profound unconsciousness from which one cannot be roused [1]." Relevant etiologies for this state include disorders of: abnormal levels of sodium, calcium, magnesium, phosphate, and potassium, and porphyria, Wenicke's disease, and myxedema coma from profound hypothyroidism. Further discussion of these endocrine and metabolic disorders is found elsewhere in this issue. Of note, while disease states such as Wernicke's disease are not classified typically as a metabolic disorder, the correction of this thiamine deficiency only will reverse the resultant coma if the magnesium deficiency, a necessary cofactor in the metabolism of thiamine, is repleted. Coma can be a supratentorial manifestation of hypomagnesemia by itself [12]. Uncontrolled diabetes also can lead to hyperosmolar hyperglycemia, resulting in coma. In fact, severe hyperosmolar hyperglycemia has been noted by at least one author to be the most frequent cause of an altered state of consciousness in patients with uncontrolled diabetes. Often, these patients are chronically ill and have depleted stores of potassium, phosphate, and magnesium [13,14].

Seizure

Seizures, "convulsion; an epileptic fit" [1], are less typically related to metabolic or endocrine disorders, but they indicate a high level of severity. For purposes of this discussion, the term seizure is considered synonymous with the tonic–clonic (formerly known as grand mal) type of seizure. Relevant etiologies for this condition include hypernatremia (or its rapid correction), hyponatremia, hypercalcemia, hypocalcemia, hypomagnesemia, thyrotoxicosis, pyridoxine deficiency, pellagra, and hypoglycemia. The emergency physician should be aware of not only the typical electrolyte abnormalities but also the secondary causes. For example, the teenage patient seizing in the resuscitation room with a pacifier around his neck may be refractory to lorazepam therapy, because he may have syndrome of inappropriate antidiuretic hormone (SIADH) from the use of 3,4 Methylenedioxymethamphetamine (ecstasy) with concomitant free water intake in his attempt to prevent hyperthermia while at a rave party earlier that evening [15]. The alcoholic seizing patient may be experiencing ethanol withdrawal, but hypoglycemia and pellagra may be prudent to consider also. Patients presenting to the ED after trauma can have altered mental status, focal neurological deficits, or seizures that can be attributed to a head trauma when hypoglycemia is actually the cause [16].

Hypomagnesemia has been associated with various neurologic abnormalities. There are multiple case reports of patients with short gut syndrome who develop low magnesium stores and consequently have mental status changes including irritability and seizures [17]. Even years after thyroid surgery, patients can develop hypoparathyroidism. This leads to hypocalcemia, which can result in choreaform movements and seizures. Many cases have been reported in the medical literature, one presenting with low calcium as long as 61 years after surgery [18].

Dementia, delirium, and disorientation

Aberrancies of orientation are commonplace enough in their presentation to the ED with common etiologies such as drug ingestion, ethanol intoxication, concussion, medication reaction, and the like. Confusional states also can be induced by endocrine and metabolic disorders such as hypoglycemia, hypocalcemia, hypophosphatemia, Wernicke's disease, hyperthyroidism, pellagra, Cushing's disease, porphyria, and others. An electrolyte abnormality as the etiology of disorientation in an ED patient generally can be discovered by routine laboratory evaluation.

Other laboratory tests that should be considered in patients with disorientation are calcium, magnesium, and thyroid function studies. Confusion or stupor is the presenting complaint in 41% of patients with malignancies found to be hypercalcemic. It is felt that normalizing the calcium is associated with clinical improvement in mental status [19]. Hypermagnesemia inhibits parathyroid hormone (PTH) and therefore leads to hypocalcemia, a cause of delirium. Iatrogenic hypermagnesemia can be found in the setting of pre-eclampsia treatment and can lead to this hypocalcemic state [20]. There are multiple case reports of patients with short gut syndrome who develop low magnesium stores and consequently have mental status changes including irritability and seizures [17]. Finally, in one study of 1000 people with delirium, one of the most common reversible causes was thyroid disease. Thyroid function tests always should be considered in the workup for the acute state of confusion [21].

Psychosis

Psychosis is defined as "a mental and behavioral disorder causing gross distortion or disorganization of a person's mental capacity" [1]. The acutely psychotic patient often presents with primary psychiatric disease or drug ingestion as the cause for the displayed symptoms of psychosis, hallucinations, and paranoia. Hallucinations, however, also have been described in the setting of hypocalcemia, porphyria, and thyrotoxicosis [6,22,23]. Additionally, paranoia has been exhibited in the latter two of these disorders. Therefore, the assessment of thyroid function and a calcium level in the patient with new onset of psychotic symptoms would be quite reasonable. In addition, the acutely psychotic patient in the right setting may prompt an investigation into the possibility of porphyria.

One of the most common endocrine disorders with mental status changes is adrenal dysfunction. Up to 20% of patients with Cushing syndrome have been reported to have psychosis, whose presentation is often not able to be distinguished from schizophrenia. Psychosis in patients with Cushing syndrome can occur before or after treatment with corticosteroids [2]. Addison's disease also may lead to psychosis. Cortisol levels and other appropriate laboratory studies should be obtained in all psychotic patients in whom endocrinopathy is being considered.

Clinical depression

Symptoms of clinical depression have been described not only with porphyria and Wernicke's disease but also in the setting of hypomagnesemia, hypothyroidism, and hypercalcemia. Thus the fatigued, depressed patient newly on diuretics may have an electrolyte depletion problem, and the patient with weight gain and the blues would be served well to have serum thyroid studies evaluated. There are multiple supratentorial manifestations of hypomagnesemia, including apathy, delirium, and coma, along with cardiac arrhythmias and neuromuscular symptoms, making a definitive diagnosis difficult [12]. Hypercalcemia from parathyroid dysfunction can be caused by the primary disorder or the resultant elevation in calcium [2]. Finally, patients with Cushing syndrome and Addison's disease may present with severe depression. The depressive symptoms may occur before some of the more typical physical findings that would prompt evaluation for these conditions.

Anxiety and emotional lability

The anxious patient may be exhibiting the symptoms of any one of several clinical entities. Many metabolic disorders can cause anxiety, and presumption of a psychiatric disorder in a previously stable patient may lead to a missed diagnosis. Endocrinopathies are found to be the source in 25% of the patients in whom a medical disorder is identified as the cause of their anxiety [2].

The ease of use of a bedside glucometer should assure that no patient with anxiety caused by hypoglycemia is neglected. Hypoglycemia is an extremely common adverse effect of diabetes treatment. When the neurological system is low on its sole source of energy—glucose—neuroglycopenia results with symptoms such as slurred speech, blurred vision, weakness, vertigo, and concentration difficulties. Catecholamines released in association with neuroglycopenia cause anxiety, diaphoresis, tremor, and restlessness. Hypoglycemia, though most commonly caused by insulin and sulfonylureas, can occur with moderate to heavy ethanol intake. The hypoglycemia associated with ethanol use may develop 6 to 24 hours after intake, accounting for some delayed presentation of symptoms [24]. It is also of note that cognitive function may not normalize totally for 40 to 90 minutes after blood glucose levels are returned to within normal range [25].

Both excess and dearth of thyroid hormone have been blamed for anxiety and emotional lability as a part of their manifested syndromes. Hypocalcemia can cause not only neuromuscular irritability, but also emotional lability and anxiety. Screening for these disorders is indicated in patients in whom anxiety is a new complaint without concomitant social or psychological events.

Summary

Endocrine disorders and metabolic abnormalities should be considered in patients with behavior, mood, and mental status alterations. Laboratory screening for sodium, potassium, glucose, calcium, magnesium, and thyroid and adrenal dysfunction should be obtained in the ED. Even in the case of another clinically apparent source, these metabolic abnormalities should be contemplated, as they can be associated with the primary disease state.

References

[1] Stedman's Medical Dictionary. 25th edition. Baltimore (MD): Williams and Wilkins; 1990.
[2] Leigh H. Cerebral effects of endocrine disease. In: Becker KL, editor. Principles and practice of endocrinology and metabolism. 3rd edition. Philadelphia: Lippincott Williams and Wilkins; 2001. p. 1834–8.
[3] Beers MH, Berkow R, editors. The Merck Manual. West Point (PA): Merck and Company, Incorporated; 1999.
[4] Adler SN. A pocket manual of differential diagnosis. Philadelphia: Lippincott Williams and Wilkins; 2000.
[5] Juan D. Hypocalcemia. Differential diagnosis and mechanisms. Arch Intern Med 1979; 139(10):1166–71.
[6] Carroll MF, Schade DS. A practical approach to hypercalcemia. Am Fam Physician 2003; 67(9):1959–66.
[7] McKechne JL, editor. Webster's new universal unabridged dictionary. Cleveland (OH): New World Dictionaries; 1983.
[8] Zalman SA. Hypomagnesemia. J Am Soc Nephrol 1999;10:1616–22.
[9] Vellaichamy M. Hypernatremia. Available at: Emedicine.com. Accessed June 30, 2004.
[10] Goh KP. Management of hyponatremia. Am Fam Physician 2004;69(10):2387–94.
[11] Daly LP, Osterhoudt KC, Weinzimer SA. Presenting features of idiopathic ketotic hypoglycemia. J Emerg Med 2003;25(1):39.
[12] Flink EB. Magnesium deficiency. Etiology and clinical spectrum. Acta Med Scand Suppl 1981;647:125–37.
[13] Matz R. Management of the hyperosmolar hyperglycemic syndrome. Am Fam Physician 1999;60(5):1468–76.
[14] Wall BM, Kitabchi AE. Management of diabetic ketoacidosis. Am Fam Physician 1999; 60(2):455–64.
[15] Schwartz RH, Miller NS. MDMA (ecstasy) and the rave: a review. Pediatrics 1997;100(4): 705.

[16] Luber SD. Acute hypoglycemia masquerading as head trauma: a report of cases. Am J Emerg Med 1996;14(6):543–7.
[17] Leicher CR, Mezoff AG, Hymans JS. Focal cerebral deficits in severe hypomagnesemia. Pediatr Neurol 1991;7(5):380–1.
[18] Mrowka M, Knake S, Klinge H, et al. Hypocalcemic generalized seizures as a manifestation of iatrogenic hypoparathyroidism months to years after thyroid surgery. Epileptic Disord 2004;6(2):85–7.
[19] Lamy O, Jenzer-Closuit A, Bruckhardt P. Hypercalcemia of malignancy: an undiagnosed and undertreated disease. J Intern Med 2001;20(1):73.
[20] Ganzevoort JW, Hoogerwaard EM, van der Post JA. Hypocalcemic delirium due to magnesium sulphate therapy in pregnant women with pre-eclampsia. Ned Tijdschr Geneeskd 2002;146(31):1453–6.
[21] Hejl A, Hogh P, Waldemar G. Potentially reversible conditions in 1000 consecutive memory clinic patients. J Neurol Neurosurg Psychiatry 2002;73:390–4.
[22] Manifold CA. Hyperthyroidism. Available at: Emedicine.com. Accessed June 30, 2004.
[23] Frye R, et al. Acute porphyria. Available at: Emedicine.com. Accessed June 30, 2004.
[24] Binder C, Bendtson I. Endocrine emergencies. Baillieres Clin Endocrinol Metab 1992;6(1):23–39.
[25] Frier BM. Hypoglycaemia and cognitive function in diabetes. Int J Clin Pract Suppl 2001;123:30–7.

**ELSEVIER
SAUNDERS**

EMERGENCY
MEDICINE
CLINICS OF
NORTH AMERICA

Emerg Med Clin N Am 23 (2005) 909–929

The Endocrine Response to Critical Illness: Update and Implications for Emergency Medicine

Scott C. Gibson, MD, FACEP*,
David A. Hartman, MD, FACEP,
Jason M. Schenck, MD

MSU-KCMS EM, 1000 Oakland Drive, Kalamazoo, MI 49008, USA

The effect of severe trauma, disease, infection, and surgery can result in remarkable metabolic stresses on the human body. Survival of such insults depends in great part upon a functioning neuroendocrine system.

The initial response to stress results in energy conservation toward vital organs, modulation of the immune system, and a delay in anabolism. This acute response to critical illness is generally considered to be an appropriate and adaptive response that occurs in the first days after insult [1–4]. It is the phase most germane to the practice of emergency medicine. Because of its protective nature, it is also the phase that most authors suggest provides little need for medical hormonal intervention.

The body's response to protracted critical illness (weeks to months) also results in marked neuroendocrine changes. Whereas many of the chronic endocrine responses are similar to the acute phase, research is revealing that the two entities do have distinct differences [1,5,6]. The endocrine response to this prolonged critical illness can even be maladaptive. Protein breakdown and fat deposition often proceed unchecked, resulting in what has been described as a "wasting syndrome" [7,8]. In addition, a persistent hyperglycemic response and insulin resistance can ensue, and this is increasingly seen as potentially deleterious in the long run [9–15].

Although this chronic endocrine response to critical illness is of less relevance to the emergency physician than the acute phase, a working understanding of such a continuum can prove useful in identifying potential

* Corresponding author.
  E-mail address: gibsons@bronsonhg.org (S.C. Gibson).

points of intervention. There are also situations in which the patient's ability to respond appropriately to the acute critical illness has been compromised—specifically in the situation of real or relative adrenal insufficiency. Such patients may require early exogenous steroid administration to survive the critical assault. Last, the emergency physician should be aware that serologic hormonal levels can be affected differently by critical illness, depending on the phase of that illness.

This review will provide an updated overview of the neuroendocrine response to critical illness. Particular emphasis will be placed on the hypothalamus–pituitary–adrenal axis (HPA) during the acute insult. Specifically, the current evidence for "stress steroid" administration will be examined, as well as interventional glucose control during critical illness. The emergency physician will also find relevance in the alterations of thyroid hormones that occur in the face of severe illness or trauma. Such changes can seriously affect the diagnosis of thryroidal illness.

Current overview of the neuroendocrine response to critical illness

The somatotropic axis

Growth Hormone (GH) is secreted from the anterior pituitary gland under hypothalamic control. Its release is typically diurnal and pulsatile under healthy, nonstress situations [5]. The hormonal effects of GH (and its interaction with other peptides) include lipolysis, amino acid muscle deposition, anti-insulin effects, linear growth (at puberty), and overall protein anabolism [1,5,16].

In acute critical illness, the mean levels of GH become elevated, usually within hours of onset [5]. There is a rise in both peak and trough levels; however, the response may be variable [1,17,18]. Growth hormone itself directly affects fat metabolism, and rising levels lead to lipolysis and inhibited lipid uptake. GH also has direct insulin antagonizing effects.

During protein metabolism, GH normally exerts its influence indirectly through its interaction with other mediators. In a nonstress situation, this results in protein build up. The acute response to critical illness, however, has been found to inhibit this indirect, peripheral effect of GH [19–22]. The result is acute protein degradation and liberalization of amino acids.

The combination of factors exerted by the somatotropic axis in acute critical illness is generally regarded as a survival mechanism. That is, the catabolic generation of substrates such as amino acids, glucose, and free fatty acids occurs instead of anabolism.

The chronic critical illness is that phase occurring days to weeks into the insult, before recovery has begun. Growth hormone during this phase tends to show abnormal release patterns, and the total circulating GH levels are much lower than in acute illness [23–25]. The average GH levels in prolonged critical illness return toward the normal seen in the absence of stress [1]. Although the peripheral resistance to GH seen during acute critical illness resolves during this phase, the net effect of prolonged critical illness on this axis is one of a relative GH deficiency [5,24–26]. This net effect likely contributes to "the wasting syndrome." This is the syndrome noted during prolonged intensive care unit (ICU) stays in which fat deposition is prominent and protein is continually degraded. The syndrome persists until recovery from the critical illness, even when artificial nutrition is provided.

The negative consequences of "the wasting syndrome" are obvious. In addition to the insult of the critical illness, patients fail to use fatty acids as substrates [7]. They lose protein from muscle with resulting weakness and hindered recovery. This has lead researchers to investigate intervening in this axis in an attempt to blunt the deleterious effects of "the wasting syndrome." Unfortunately, in a European study of patients with prolonged critical illness, increased mortality was found in those treated with high dose GH replacement therapy [27]. Speculation as to this result is varied, and probably represents the incomplete knowledge of the whole somatotropic axis and its interplay with other endocrine axes [16]. Some have suggested that the direct administration of GH does not allow for physiologic hypothalamic feedback inhibition loops or peripheral adjustments in responsiveness to the hormone [1,5,25]. Such hypotheses have lead to additional studies using GH-secretagogues (synthetically produced substances with hypothalamus-like GH-releasing capacities) infusions [23–25]. Although preliminary, these studies suggest improvement in GH pulsatile release during chronic critical illness with maintenance of GH peripheral hormonal activity.

The thyrotropic axis

Thyroid releasing hormone (TRH) is secreted from the hypothalamus, which stimulates the anterior pituitary gland's release of thyroid stimulating hormone (TSH). TSH, in return, controls the release of thyroxine (T4) from the thyroid gland. Peripherally, T4 is converted by deiodination to T3, another active thyroid hormone.

The active thyroid hormones (T3 and T4) are regulators of cellular metabolic activity and are essential for normal cardiac, pulmonary, and neurologic function. T4 is produced almost exclusively by the thyroid gland. The majority of T3 is produced by peripheral deiodination of T4 to T3 (80%), and only 20% is produced by the thyroid gland itself. Most of the circulating T3 and T4 are bound to thyroxine-binding globulin.

In the acute phase of critical illness, changes in thyroid hormones begin to occur in as little as 30 to 120 minutes [28,29]. There is an initial drop in T3 levels that has been attributed to decreased peripheral conversion of T4 to T3 [30]. This drop in T3 levels tends to persist during critical illness; it is considered a hallmark response to a variety of critical illnesses [28,31]. In fact, studies have suggested that the magnitude of the drop in T3 directly correlates with patient mortality—the lower the T3 level, the greater the mortality risk in ill patients [32–36].

There is variability reported in the levels of T4 that occur acutely. This hormone may remain in the normal range, and there may be an early transient rise during the illness. However, in the most severely ill patients, the measured levels tend to decrease [37].

Despite this stress-induced drop in thyroid hormone levels, TSH tends to remain in the normal or low range during stress [5,6,26,31]. Under typical circumstances, a drop in T3/T4 levels would inhibit negative feedback loops, thus calling for an increase in TSH. The fact that this does not occur has been attributed to a change in the thyroid hormone set point [31]. It has also been described as a homeostatic mechanism, whose purpose is to diminish the effects of T3 within the body [16], perhaps to conserve energy expenditure [5,38]. However, this teleologic view has been recently argued [39–41].

Irrespective of these changes in thyroid hormone levels, such seriously ill patients generally do not acutely show evidence of thyroidal illness. This condition (low T3 and normal TSH levels in the face of critical illness with no clinical evidence of thyroid disease) has been termed "sick euthyroid syndrome," "low-T3 syndrome," or "nonthryroidal illness". The syndrome's implications to emergency medicine are described in further detail later in this article.

During chronic critical illness, T3 remains low, and TSH secretion, although typically measured in low-normal concentrations, loses its physiologic pulsatile pattern of secretion [26]. Because T3 contributes to the body's ability to synthesize protein, to use fats for fuel, and assists in GH functions, this chronic low T3 state has been theorized as contributing to the "wasting syndrome" of prolonged critical illness. Early studies using thyroid hormone replacement, aimed at reversing this state, have failed to show benefit [42,43]. However, recent investigations using TRH infusions (combined with GH hormones) have suggested the ability to reactivate a physiologic thyroid axis during chronic critical illness, and may indicate a future treatment option [23].

The hypothalamus–pituitary–adrenal axis

Cortisol is the predominant glucocorticoid secreted from the adrenal cortex in humans. Stress-induced cortisol release is driven indirectly by corticotropin-releasing hormone (CRH) from the hypothalamus and directly via adrenocorticotropic hormone (ACTH), which responds to the CRH stimulus. In healthy individuals, this secretion occurs in a diurnal pattern that typically involves a low trough at approximately 2 a.m. and a peak at 8 a.m.

The accepted metabolic effects of cortisol include the maintenance of normal vascular tone, vascular permeability, and distribution of total body water. Cortisol also functions to potentiate the vasoconstrictor action of catecholamines.

Acute critical illness such as trauma, burns, sepsis, anesthesia, and extensive surgery is known to induce a state of hypercortisolism. Hypercortisolism tends to be energy producing—that is, cortisol shifts energy production and substrates to vital organs and delays anabolic buildup [1,5]. This creates immediate energy sources for the "fight or flight" stress response. Energy produced becomes selectively available to the vital organs of the body. Increased cortisol in acute illness has been speculated to help mute the body's own inflammatory response to disease, protecting itself against overreaction [44]. Each of these effects of cortisol appears to be augmented by a concomitant decrease in cortisol binding proteins (thus increasing the metabolically, protein-free hormone) during acute illness [45].

Along with the rise in cortisol during critical illness, catecholamines are secreted. Epinephrine and norepinephrine have numerous essential functions in the body's stress response. The major homeostatic functions in critical illness include stimulation of heart rate, myocardial contractility, and vasoconstriction of some vascular beds (gut, skin, and skeletal muscle). These responses enable the body to maintain perfusion to vital organs in the setting of hypovolemia, sepsis, or cardiac failure. Catecholamine-mediated vasoconstriction is potentiated by cortisol, and cortisol may also be necessary for the production and secretion of the catecholamines themselves.

In addition to the rise in cortisol and catecholamines during acute critical illness, the renin–angiotensin system is stimulated and aldosterone is produced. The net effect of these responses is fluid retention, vasoconstriction, and enhanced hemodynamics.

This overall HPA response to acute critical illness, lasting hours to days, is generally considered adaptive, evolutionary, and is one of the most important coping mechanisms the body has to such stressors [1,3,6,46].

During chronic critical illness, cortisol levels remain elevated and may shift the immunologic balance further toward immunosuppression [6]. However, the normal diurnal variation is lost or blunted. As critical illness becomes prolonged, serum corticotropin (ACTH) levels drop, while cortisol concentrations remain elevated, if a properly functioning HPA axis exists.

Over time, the glucocorticoid effects of cortisol become increasingly prominent, and these effects are relied upon for ongoing hemodynamic stability [6]. Such reliance has lead to the description of a "relative adrenal insufficiency" state in some ICU patients (particularly those with septic shock) who may respond with improved outcomes when therapeutic doses of glucocorticoids are administered exogenously [47–50]. Support for such treatment is not without conflicting data and continued debate, however [51]. A detailed update on steroid replacement in critical illness and the implications of the HPA to emergency medicine follows this section.

Other axes

Given the known anabolic properties of testosterone, it makes sense that alterations in gonadal hormones might occur during times when anabolism is being discouraged. Indeed, testosterone levels are acutely lowered during stressful conditions [52–54]. Such a decrease is hypothesized to be secondary to an immediate and direct Leydig cell suppression [1,5]. As critical illness becomes prolonged, luteinizing hormone release is diminished in both men and women [52,55,56]. Hypogonadism is frequently a result of these gonadal hormonal changes, albeit a transient effect [57].

Prolactin levels also vary during critical insults, rising acutely [58] and showing blunted pulsatile secretion in the chronic phase [23]. Diminishing prolactin levels may play a role in the immunosuppression associated with prolonged critical illness, particularly when combined with dopamine infusions [5,59,60].

A summary of the hormonal changes during critical illness for each axis is shown in Table 1.

Hypothalamus–pituitary–adrenal axis in critical illness—implications for emergency medicine

Adrenal insufficiency—emergency department presentation

A 75-year-old woman with a known history of type II diabetes, congestive heart failure, and renal insufficiency presents with fever (102.4°F) and hypotension (65/30 mmHg). For the past 2 weeks she has been undergoing treatment for a urinary tract infection but has continued to decline. The patient has pyuria (> 100 white blood count [WBC]/high power field [HPF], leukocytosis (22,000 cells/L), hyponatremia (123 mEq/L), and hyperkalemia (5.7 mEq/L). Despite fluid resuscitation with 4 liters of crystalloid and appropriate broad-spectrum antibiotics, she remains hypotensive and tachycardic.

Adrenal insufficiency–pathophysiology

As discussed, an intact HPA axis is essential to the body's intrinsic stress response in acutely ill patients. Many critical illnesses result in an abnormal HPA axis response. The incidence of adrenal insufficiency in the critically ill is quite variable, and depends on the patient's underlying disease process and the severity of each patient's illness. The overall incidence of adrenal insufficiency in critically ill patients is approximately 30%, with a higher incidence of 50% to 60% in patients with septic shock [61]. In general, two subgroups of adrenal insufficiency exist—absolute adrenal insufficiency, and relative adrenal insufficiency.

Absolute adrenal insufficiency implies a malfunction of the HPA. Typically, this occurs because of prolonged glucocorticoid dependence or

Table 1
Summary of hormonal changes during critical illness

Hormone	Change during acute critical illness	Physiological effects of the acute change	Change during chronic critical illness	Physiological effects of the chronic change
GH	• Increases • Resistance to GH effects develops at tissue level	• Lipolysis • Inhibited lipid uptake by cells • Effects of insulin are antagonized • Protein degradation	• Normalizes • Abnormal secretion patterns • Relative GH deficiency	• Fat deposition in tissues • Continued protein degradation • Contributes to "wasting syndrome"
T3	• Decreases	• Minimal effects • Possibly allows energy conservation	• Remains decreased	• Contributes to "wasting syndrome"
T4	• Variable, generally decreases	• Minimal effects • Possibly allows energy conservation	• Remains decreased	• Contributes to "wasting syndrome"
TSH	• Normal or low normal	• Minimal effect • Change in thyroid "set point" (TSH normal despite drop in T3, T4)	• Normal or low normal	• Contributes to "wasting syndrome"
Cortisol	• Increases	• Energy production • Shifts energy to vital organs • Delays anabolism • Mutes inflammation • "Fight or Flight"	• Remains elevated • Diurnal variation lost	• Additional immunosuppression • Increased glucocorticoid effects
Testosterone	• Decreases	• Decreased anabolism	• Remains decreased	• Hypogonadism
Prolactin	• Increases	• Possibly stimulates inflammatory cascades	• Normalizes • Abnormal secretion patterns	• Possibly inhibits immune system

adrenal gland inactivity from disease, surgical removal, or Addison's primary adrenal insufficiency.

There is increasing evidence for a syndrome of relative adrenal insufficiency, in septic patients and other critically ill ICU cases [46–50,62–65]. As critical illness becomes prolonged, particularly in patients over the age of 50, the incidence of such relative adrenal insufficiency is markedly increased [50]. The causes of this syndrome are partially speculative, but may include such factors as head injury, adrenal hemorrhage, drugs, and inflammatory mediators [66,67].

Evidence is mounting regarding the benefit of steroid therapy in critically ill patients with relative adrenal insufficiency. Bollaert et al [48] performed a randomized double-blind placebo controlled study using glucocorticoid treatment (100 mg intravenous [IV] every 8 hours) in patients with septic shock. They showed a reversal of shock at 7 days and 28 days compared with placebo. They also showed a significant reduction in 28-day mortality (30% versus 70%, respectively) compared with placebo.

Breigel et al [49] drew similar conclusions, demonstrating improved shock reversal and decreased length of vasopressor support in those patients treated with intravenous hydrocortisone compared with placebo. Their study also suggested earlier resolution of organ dysfunction, shorter ventilator time, and shorter ICU stays.

An investigation by Annane et al [68] revealed a significant reduction in the risk of death in those patients with septic shock and relative adrenal insufficiency. Mortality was 53% in those receiving corticosteroids, compared with the placebo rate of 63%. Rivers et al looked at high risk surgical patients with relative adrenal insufficiency, again suggesting faster weaning from vasopressors and improved survival in those treated with physiologic doses of glucocorticoids [69].

Putting such evidence into clinical practice is not without its detractors. These newer studies, suggesting a benefit from physiologic, low-dose steroids must be weighed against older investigations that did not reach such conclusions using high-dose regimens, including two meta-analyses [70–74]. Opponents suggest that these conflicting outcomes, coupled with yet unfolding current evidence, merit caution before the physiologic dose therapy is put into widespread clinical practice [51].

Adrenal insufficiency—emergency department evaluation

The key to these treatment decisions revolves around identification of patients with adrenal insufficiency, and that, too, is a source of some controversy. Important clinical diagnostic clues include hemodynamic instability despite adequate fluid resuscitation and ongoing evidence of systemic inflammation without an obvious source that has not responded to empirical treatment [66,67]. Other symptoms and physical findings that may be helpful in increasing the clinical suspicion of adrenal insufficiency are listed in Box 1.

If testing is to be used, the most practical method to assess adrenal function in the emergency department (ED) is a random cortisol level. Random cortisol levels have been advocated by many in the literature to be

---

Box 1. Features suggesting corticosteroid insufficiency

Symptoms
  Weakness and fatigue
  Anorexia, nausea, vomiting
  Abominal pain
  Myalgia or arthralgia
  Postural dizziness
  Craving for salt
  Headaches
  Depression
Findings on physical examination
  Increased pigmentation
  Hypoitension (postural)
  Tachcardia
  Fever
  Decreased body hair
  Vitiligo
  Features of hypopituitarism
    Amonorrhea
    Intolerance of cold
Clinical problems
  Hemodynamic instability
    Hyperdynamic (common)
    Hypodynamic (rare)
  Ongoing inflammation with no obvious source
  Multiple-organ dysfunction
  Hypoglycemia
Laboratory findings
  Hypoantremia
  Hyperkalemia
  Hypoglycemia
  Eosinophilia
  Elevated thyrotropin levels

From Cooper MS, Stewart PM. Corticosteroid insufficiency in acutely ill patients. N Engl J Med 2003;348(8);727–34; with permission.

a more practical way to assess for adrenal insufficiency in the critically ill, especially when compared with a corticotropin stimulation test [1,61,64]. A random serum cortisol level of >25 µg/dL is thought to be normal in the severely stressed with normal adrenal function [61]. Other authors believe that adrenal insufficiency is unlikely if the random cortisol level is >34 µg/dL. Adrenal insufficiency is likely if the serum cortisol is <15 µg/dL during acute severe stress [66].

Patients that fall into the gray area (random cortisol level of 15–34 µg/dL) may require further testing to assess adrenal function. Corticotropin stimulation testing can help identify those patients where exogenous supplementary glucocorticoids would be beneficial in patients with equivocal random cortisol levels (Fig. 1). However, these tests are unlikely to be performed in the ED and are more suitable for the ICU setting, following admission.

Random cortisol testing is a relatively quick and easy way to obtain useful information on the status of the HPA axis, making it potentially informative in the ED setting (Fig. 1). The timing of random cortisol levels is not important, due to the fact that the normal diurnal pattern of cortisol secretion is disrupted during critical illness [61].

Adrenal insufficiency—emergency department management

Regarding treatment, those with clear or known absolute adrenal insufficiency should receive "stress steroids." Initial dose recommendations typically are in the range of 50 mg hydrocortisone (or equivalent), given parenterally, every 6 hours [66].

In patients where the diagnosis of relative adrenal insufficiency is established, intravenous or intramuscular steroids are generally indicated. When relative adrenal insufficiency is suspected in the acute setting, steroids may be initiated empirically at physiologic doses in hypotensive patients with presumed sepsis and failure to respond to initial treatment [66] (Fig. 2). The evidence for replacement therapy in critical illness other than sepsis is not established enough to suggest empiric treatment in such cases. However, a random cortisol test may be sent, ideally at the time of initial presentation to guide treatment decisions going forward. Dosing recommendations vary, but one proposed dosing guideline is outlined in Fig. 2.

Another strategy that can be applied, especially in situations where a random cortisol level or the corticotropin (ACTH) stimulation test cannot be done acutely, is to employ dexamethasone. Administration of dexamethasone (2 mg IV or intramuscularly) does not significantly alter the cortisol assay results and can be administered to patients pending adrenal testing [61]. Such empiric dexamethasone therapy can be initiated based on clinical suspicion in patients with signs or symptoms suggesting corticosteroid insufficiency (Box 1).

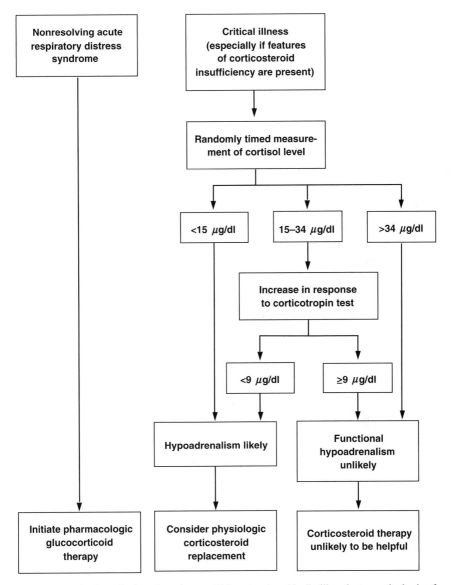

Fig. 1. Investigation of adrenal corticosteroid function in critically ill patients on the basis of cortisol levels and response to the corticotropin stimulation test. The scheme has been evaluated for patients with septic shock. It must be borne in mind, however, that no cutoff value will be entirely reliable. (*From* Cooper MS, Stewart PM. Cortisosteroid insufficiency in actuely ill patients. N Engl J Med 2003;34(8):727–34; with permission.)

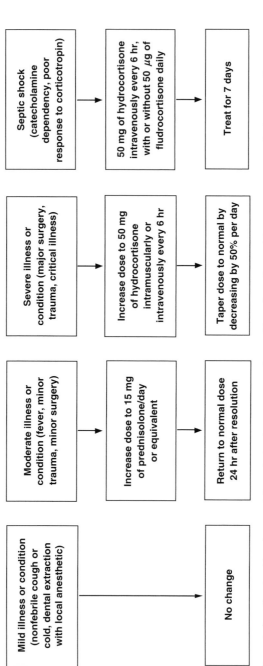

Fig. 2. Suggested corticosteroid-replacement doses during intercurrent and acute illness in patients with proven or suspected adrenal insufficiency, including those receiving corticosteroid therapy. (*From* Cooper MS, Stewart PM. Cortisosteroid insufficiency in actuely ill patients. N Engl J Med 2003;34(8):727–34; with permission.)

Emergency physicians should be aware of a drug that can alter the functioning of the HPA. Etomidate, often administered as a potent sedative or induction agent, influences adrenal function by blunting cortisol production [75,76]. Although real, the true clinical implications of this blunted response are not clear.

Glucose homeostasis—emergency department presentation

A 78-year-old man presents with vomiting and epigastric pain radiating into the back. He is found to be hypotensive (75/42 mmHg), tachycardic (122/bpm), and afebrile (98.4°F). Laboratory studies suggest a diagnosis of pancreatitis with a lipase level of 6440 U/L. The patient has no history of diabetes, but the serum glucose level is elevated (314 mg/dL).

Appropriate fluid resuscitation marginally improves the blood pressure (95/52) and tachycardia (110/bpm). The patient is to be admitted to the intensive care unit. However, the unit currently has no beds, and the patient will be boarded and managed in the ED for the next 12 hours.

Glucose homeostasis—pathophysiology

Glucose metabolism is significantly altered during times of high stress. These changes occur as an adaptive mechanism during critical illness. Counterregulatory hormones released by the body, including glucagon, epinephrine and cortisol, oppose the normal action of insulin. These hormones increase the availability of gluconeogenic substrates necessary for the body to cope with acute stressors. However, as these stressors persist, hyperglycemia becomes persistent. Evidence is mounting that suggests such persistent hyperglycemia may be associated with the development of complications and a poor prognosis in patients with critical illnesses [9–15].

There are two primary mechanisms for hyperglycemia in critical illness: enhanced hepatic glucose production (increased gluconeogenesis), and decreased peripheral glucose use (insulin resistance). Hyperglycemia associated with insulin resistance is common in the critically ill, in both diabetic and nondiabetic patients. Some suggested mechanisms for insulin resistance include impaired insulin receptor binding and signal transduction, impaired glycogen synthesis, increased hepatic glucose production, and decreased peripheral glucose uptake [9].

Glucose homeostasis—emergency department management

Malmberg et al [15] revealed a relative mortality reduction of 29% at 1 year by using insulin–glucose infusion and multidose subcutaneous insulin to obtain strict glycemic control in diabetic patients with acute myocardial infarction.

In a prospective, randomized controlled study, Van den Berghe et al showed that maintenance of serum glucose level <110 mg/dL, using intensive insulin therapy (insulin infusion), significantly improved in-hospital mortality and morbidity in the critically ill [15]. Overall in-hospital mortality was decreased by 32%, acute renal failure requiring dialysis or hemofiltration by 41%, blood-stream infections by 46%, and critical illness polyneuropathy by 44%. This study population only included 13% previously diagnosed diabetes mellitus patients.

These findings have led to the goal of strict glycemic control in most critically ill patients. This is an area of intense current investigation. The evidence is not clear on how expeditiously such intensive insulin therapy should be started and whether initiation in the ED would enhance the benefits suggested in the ICU. This is a topic ripe for research. If there is going to be a substantial delay in ICU bed acquisition, it may be reasonable to initiate such protocols in the ED setting, provided appropriate monitoring can be assured.

Intensive insulin therapy has been primarily studied in adult patients thus far, and not in the pediatric population. Thus, it is difficult to know if such recommendations will prove useful in younger, critically ill populations.

The use of an insulin infusion protocol makes it much simpler to initiate therapy. Typical protocols are aimed at maintaining glucose <110 mg/dL [14]. Such a sample protocol is shown in Fig. 3.

The thyroid axis in critical illness—implications to emergency medicine

Thyroid axis—emergency department presentation

An 83-year-old woman presents with hypothermia (89.9°F) after she fell 14 hours previous in her breezeway and could not get up. She arrives at an ED in Michigan during the month of December and is found to be shivering. As part of her evaluation, thyroid hormone levels (T3, T4) are checked and are found to be low. The TSH level is normal. The treating physician questions whether her presentation is simple exposure hypothermia or whether it might be related to hypothyroidism.

Thyroid axis—pathophysiology

Acute illness, burns or major trauma induce changes in the thyroid hormone axis within the first few hours. However, despite low T3 and T4 levels, the TSH level may be normal or even decreased. These abnormalities in the negative feedback loop of the hypothalamus, the pituitary and the thyroid gland imply a new set point and have been referred to as the sick thyroid syndrome, the low T3 syndrome, or nonthyroidal illness.

Thyroid axis—emergency department evaluation

Emergency physicians need be aware of such changes, as a measured T3 or T4 level during acute stress will typically be low. Such a drop does not, however, imply hypothyroidism. The diagnosis of preexisting thyroid disease

TARGET BLOOD GLUCOSE 100-130 mg/dl

1. Start regular insulin infusion (concentration 100 units/100cc) via pump piggyback to maintenance I.V. as follows:

Blood Glucose	IV Insulin Bolus	Initial Insulin rate: units/hr (circle one)	
		Non-diabetic patients, NIDDM or IDDM preop < 40 u/day	IDDM preop ≥ 40 u/day
120-179	0	1.0 units/hr	2.0 units/hr
180-239	0	2.0 units/hr	3.5 units/hr
240-299	4 units	3.5 units/hr	5.0 units/hr
300-359	8 units	5.0 units/hr	6.5 units/hr
> 360	12 units	6.5 units/hr	8.0 units/hr

2. Test B.G. by finger stick method or arterial line drop sample. Frequency of CBGs:
   a. Check BG every hour.
   b. When BG 100-150 with < 15 mg/dl change and insulin rate remains unchanged x 4 hr., then may test every 2 hrs.
   c. May stop every 2 hr. testing on POD #3 (see items #4 and #7 below).
   d. Check blood glucose every AC and every HS; OR   every_____ once the insulin infusion completed.

3. Insulin titration:
   For titration purposes, infusion rates should be rounded up on the pump.

Blood Glucose	Action
<75	Stop insulin; give 25 cc D50W and recheck BG in 30 minutes. When BG > 75, restart with rate 50% of previous rate.
75-100	If < 10 mg/dl lower than last test, decrease rate by 0.5 units/hr. If ≥ 10 mg/dl lower than last test, decrease rate by 50%. If neither continue current rate.
101-150	Same rate. **EXCLUSION: If the decrease in the Blood Glucose is attributable to a recent doubling of the rate (for BGs over 200), then decrease the rate by 50%. Check BG in 30 minutes.**
151-200	If lower than last test – same rate. If higher than last test – then increase rate by 0.5 units/hr.
>200	If ≥ 30 mg/dl lower than the last test - same rate. If < 30 mg/dl lower than last test (OR if higher than last test) increase rate by 1 unit/hr. AND – if > 240 mg/dl IV – bolus with regular insulin as per "Initial IV Insulin Bolus" dosage scale above (see item #1).

If BG > 200 mg/dl and has not decreased after 3 consecutive increases in insulin, then double insulin rate.
If BG > 300 for 4 consecutive readings: call MD for additional IV bolus orders.

#4 - #7 are additions for open heart surgical patients only
For all other patients follow physician orders regarding discontinuation of the infusion.

4. Start "Continuous Intravenous Insulin Protocol" during surgery and continue through 7 AM of the 3rd POD. Patients who are not taking enteral nutrition on the 3rd POD should remain on this protocol until taking at least 50% of a full liquid or soft ADA diet. The sliding scale preprinted orders should be used once the infusion is discontinued on the 3rd POD or later.

5. No concentrated sweets cardiac diet starts with any PO intake.
6. For Diabetic patients, restart the following pre-admission glycemic control medications on

_____
_____
_____

7. For Non-Diabetic patients, administer postmeal S.Q. Humalog Insulin Supplement in addition to Insulin Infusion when oral intake advanced beyond clear liquids:
   If patient:
   a. Eats 50% or less of servings on breakfast, lunch or dinner tray, then give 3 units of Novolog insulin S.Q.immediately following that meal.
   b. Eats more than 50% of serving on breakfast, lunch or supper tray, then give 6 units of Novolog insulin S.Q. immediately following that meal.
   Discontinue Novolog Insulin Supplements when Protocol completed.
   M.D. Signature_____DATE_____TIME_____

Form # 9002559 (Revised 1/04)
BRONSON CONTINUOUS INTRAVENOUS INSULIN PROTOCOL (NOT TO BE USED FOR DKA)

Fig. 3. Example protocol for glucose control during critical illness. (Reproduced with permission from Bronson Methodist Hospital, Kalamazoo, Michigan.)

in patients who are critically injured or ill is very difficult. Clues to true thyroid disease might include: hypothermia, unexplained tachycardia or bradycardia, atrial arrhythmias, lethargy, or sensitivity to narcotics or sedatives. Patients may also have a history of previous thyroid disease, radiation, or surgery. A review of previous thyroid testing results is also mandatory.

The initial test for critically ill patients with a suspicion of underlying true thyroid disease should be a TSH level. A normal TSH virtually excludes thyrotoxicosis or hypothyroidism [31]. A low TSH level may indicate hyperthyroidism or nonthyroid illness. The lower the level the more likely the diagnosis of hyperthyroidism [31]. A high TSH may indicate hypothyroidism, early nonthyroidal illness, or recovering nonthyroidal illness. Measuring T3 levels in critically ill patients is not helpful in diagnosing primary thyroid disease because of the high prevalence of the low T3 syndrome.

Thyroid axis—emergency department management

The treatment of nonthyroid illness is controversial. Two promising studies involving intravenous T3 infusion to elective coronary artery bypass graft (CABG) patients with an ejection fraction of less than 40% did improve postoperative cardiac function but did not improve mortality [77,78]. However, as previously noted, such promise must be weighed against older studies showing a lack of effectiveness of thyroid hormone administration in critically ill patients [42,43].

Effects of exogenous catecholamine administration on the endocrine system—implications to emergency medicine

Catecholamines are commonly used in the ED and ICUs. They cause vasoconstriction (alpha-receptor), tachycardia, and increased cardiac output (beta-receptors). They also augment glycogenolysis in liver and muscle to provide energy during stress. Exogenous catecholamines may also be beneficial in critical illness by modulating the cytokine response. Catecholamines beneficially affect this cytokine response by decreasing pro-inflammatory cytokines, while at the same time increasing some anti-inflammatory cytokines [79,80]. This may help in acutely ill patients by limiting the severity of their illness.

Dopamine has several potential negative effects on the endocrine system. First, it has been shown to decrease serum prolactin levels [81,82]. Prolactin is an immunomodulatory hormone involved in the stress response, and any decrease in its concentration may make critically ill patients more prone to infectious complications [82].

Second, dopamine has been shown to induce a reversible suppression of growth hormone and thyrotropin secretion in critically ill infants and children [82]. At what point these potentially deleterious endocrine effects of dopamine may clinically impact patients, is unknown.

Summary

Critical illness induces a variety of hormonal changes, which may be divided into acute and chronic phases. In general, the acute phase alterations are beneficial and adaptive. Hormonal medical interventions during this phase are generally not beneficial. However, in those patients with known, measured, or a strong suspicion of adrenal insufficiency, exogenous steroid replacement is suggested. Recent research suggests this may be especially true in septic shock.

Intensive insulin therapy to reverse insulin resistance during times of critical illness is increasingly seen as beneficial in stressed patients. Hospitals should consider institution of protocols to maintain tight glycemic control in both diabetics and nondiabetics under such stress.

Emergency physicians should be aware of the "euthyroid sick syndrome" and its implications to thyroid test interpretation. Routine testing of thyroid function in critically ill patients is unnecessary, as the result may be confusing. If true thyroid disease is suspected, TSH is the test of choice, and a normal TSH level virtually excludes thyrotoxicosis and myxedema. Low T3 levels may indicate primary thyroid disease or nonthyroidal illness.

References

[1] Van den Berghe G, de Zegher F, Bouillon R. Acute and prolonged critical illness as different neuroendocrine paradigms. J Clin Endocrinol Metab 1998;83(6):1827–34.

[2] Laloga GP. Sepsis-induced adrenal deficiency syndrome. Crit Care Med 2001;29(3):688–90.

[3] Chrousos GP. The hypothalamic–pituitary–adrenal axis and immune-mediated inflammation. N Engl J Med 1995;332(20):1351–62.

[4] Utiger RD. Decreased extrathyroidal triiodothyronine production in nonthyroidal illness: benefit or harm? Am J Med 1980;69(6):807–10.

[5] Van den Berge G. Dynamic neuroendocrine responses to critical illness. Front Neuroendocrinol 2002;23(4):370–91.

[6] Van den Berge G. Novel insights into the neuroendocrinology of critical illness. Eur J Endocrinol 2000;143(1):1–13.

[7] Streat SJ, Beddoe AH, Hill GL. Aggressive nutritional support does not prevent protein loss despite fat gain in septic intensive care patients. J Trauma 1987;27(3):262–6.

[8] Gamrin L, Essen P, Forsberg AM, et al. A descriptive study of skeletal muscle metabolism in critically ill patients: free amino acids, energy-rich phosphates, protein, nucleic acids, fat, water, and electrolytes. Crit Care Med 1996;24(4):575–83.

[9] Robinson LE, van Soeren MH. Insulin resistance and hyperglycemia in critical illness: role of insulin in glycemic control. AACN Clin Issues 2004;15(1):45–62.

[10] Stranders I, Diamant M, van Gelder RE, et al. Admission blood glucose level as risk indicator of death after myocardial infarction in patients with and without diabetes mellitus. Arch Intern Med 2004;164(9):982–8.

[11] Laird AM, Miller PR, Kilgo PD, et al. Relationship of early hyperglycemia to mortality in trauma patients. J Trauma 2004;56(5):1058–62.

[12] Krinsley JS. Association between hyperglycemia and increased hospital mortality in a heterogeneous population of critically ill patients. Mayo Clin Proc 2003;78(12):1471–8.

[13] Finney SJ, Zekveld C, Elia A, et al. Glucose control and mortality in critically ill patients. JAMA 2003;290(15):2041–7.

[14] Van den Berghe G, Wouters P, Weekers F, et al. Intensive insulin therapy in the critically ill patients. N Engl J Med 2001;345(19):1359–67.

[15] Malmberg K, Ryden L, Efendic S, et al. Randomized trial of insulin–glucose infusion followed by subcutaneous insulin treatment in diabetic patients with acute myocardial

infarction (DIGAMI study): effects on mortality at 1 year. J Am Coll Cardiol 1995;26(1): 57–65.

[16] Nylen ES, Muller B. Endocrine changes in critical illness. J Intensive Care Med 2004;19(2): 67–82.

[17] Ross R, Miell J, Freeman E, et al. Critically ill patients have high basal growth hormone levels with attenuated oscillatory activity associated with low levels of insulin-like growth factor-I. Clin Endocrinol (Oxf) 1991;35(1):47–54.

[18] Voerman HJ, Strack van Schijndel RJ, de Boer H, et al. Growth hormone: secretion and administration in catabolic adult patients, with emphasis on the critically ill patient. Neth J Med 1992;41(5–6):229–44.

[19] Bentham J, Rodriguez-Arnao J, Ross RJ. Acquired growth hormone resistance in patients with hypercatabolism. Horm Res 1993;40(1–3):87–91.

[20] Timmins AC, Cotterill AM, Hughes SC, et al. Critical illness is associated with low circulating concentrations of insulin-like growth factors-I and -II, alterations in insulin-like growth factor binding proteins, and induction of an insulin-like growth factor binding protein 3 protease. Crit Care Med 1996;24(9):1460–6.

[21] Hermansson M, Wickelgren RB, Hammarqvist F, et al. Measurement of human growth hormone receptor messenger ribonucleic acid by a quantitative polymerase chain reaction-based assay: demonstration of reduced expression after elective surgery. J Clin Endocrinol Metab 1997;82(2):421–8.

[22] Baxter RC. Insulin-like growth factor binding proteins in the human circulation: a review. Horm Res 1994;42(4–5):140–4.

[23] Van den Berghe G, de Zegher F, Baxter RC, et al. Neuroendocrinology of prolonged critical illness: effects of exogenous thyrotropin-releasing hormone and its combination with growth hormone secretagogues. J Clin Endocrinol Metab 1998;83(2):309–19.

[24] Van den Berghe G, de Zegher F, Veldhuis JD, et al. The somatotropic axis in critical illness: effect of continuous growth hormone (GH)-releasing hormone and GH-releasing peptide-2 infusion. J Clin Endocrinol Metab 1997;82(2):590–9.

[25] Van den Berghe G, Wouters P, Weekers F, et al. Reactivation of pituitary hormone release and metabolic improvement by infusion of growth hormone-releasing peptide and thyrotropin-releasing hormone in patients with protracted critical illness. J Clin Endocrinol Metab 1999;84(4):1311–23.

[26] Van den Berghe G, de Zegher F, Veldhuis JD, et al. Thyrotrophin and prolactin release in prolonged critical illness: dynamics of spontaneous secretion and effects of growth hormone-secretagogues. Clin Endocrinol (Oxf) 1997;47(5):599–612.

[27] Takala J, Ruokonen E, Webster NR, et al. Increased mortality associated with growth hormone treatment in critically ill adults. N Engl J Med 1999;341(11):785–92.

[28] Wellby ML, Kennedy JA, Barreau PB, et al. Endocrine and cytokine changes during elective surgery. J Clin Pathol 1994;47(11):1049–51.

[29] Michalaki M, Vagenakis AG, Makri M, et al. Dissociation of the early decline in serum T(3) concentration and serum IL-6 rise and TNFalpha in nonthyroidal illness syndrome induced by abdominal surgery. Clin Endocrinol Metab 2001;86(9):4198–205.

[30] Chopra IJ, Huang TS, Beredo A, et al. Evidence for an inhibitor of extrathyroidal conversion of thyroxine to 3,5,3′-triiodothyronine in sera of patients with nonthyroidal illnesses. J Clin Endocrinol Metab 1985;60(4):666–72.

[31] Fliers E, Alkemade A, Wiersinga WM. The hypothalamic–pituitary–thyroid axis in critical illness. Best Pract Res Clin Endocrinol Metab 2001;15(4):453–64.

[32] Chow CC, Mak TW, Chan CH, et al. Euthyroid sick syndrome in pulmonary tuberculosis before and after treatment. Ann Clin Biochem 1995;32(Pt 4):385–91.

[33] Vexiau P, Perez-Castiglioni P, Socie G, et al. The "euthyroid sick syndrome": incidence, risk factors and prognostic value soon after allogeneic bone marrow transplantation. Br J Haematol 1993;85(4):778–82.

[34] Maldonado LS, Murata GH, Hershman JM, et al. Do thyroid function tests independently predict survival in the critically ill? Thyroid 1992;2(2):119–23.

[35] Jarek MJ, Legare EJ, McDermott MT, et al. Endocrine profiles for outcome prediction from the intensive care unit. Crit Care Med 1993;21(4):543–50.

[36] Slag MF, Morley JE, Elson MK, et al. Hypothyroxinemia in critically ill patients as a predictor of high mortality. JAMA 1981;245(1):43–5.

[37] Docter R, Krenning EP, de Jong M, et al. The sick euthyroid syndrome: changes in thyroid hormone serum parameters and hormone metabolism. Clin Endocrinol (Oxf) 1993;39(5): 499–518.

[38] Gardner DF, Kaplan MM, Stanley CA, et al. Effect of tri-iodothyronine replacement on the metabolic and pituitary responses to starvation. N Engl J Med 1979;300(11):579–84.

[39] De Groot LJ. Dangerous dogmas in medicine: the nonthyroidal illness syndrome. J Clin Endocrinol Metab 1999;84(1):151–64.

[40] Glinoer D. Comment on dangerous dogmas in medicine–the nonthyroidal illness syndrome. J Clin Endocrinol Metab 1999;84(6):2262–3.

[41] Wartofsky L, Burman KD, Ringel MD. Trading one "dangerous dogma" for another? Thyroid hormone treatment of the "euthyroid sick syndrome. Clin Endocrinol Metab J 1999;84(5):1759–60.

[42] Brent GA, Hershman JM. Thyroxine therapy in patients with severe nonthyroidal illnesses and low serum thyroxine concentration. J Clin Endocrinol Metab 1986;63(1):1–8.

[43] Becker RA, Vaughan GM, Ziegler MG, et al. Hypermetabolic low triiodothyronine syndrome of burn injury. Crit Care Med 1982;10(12):870–5.

[44] Munck A, Guyre PM, Holbrook NJ. Physiological functions of glucocorticoids in stress and their relation to pharmacological actions. Endocr Rev 1984;5(1):25–44.

[45] Beishuizen A, Thijs LG, Vermes I. Patterns of corticosteroid-binding globulin and the free cortisol index during septic shock and multitrauma. Intensive Care Med 2001;27(10): 1584–91.

[46] Zaloga GP. Sepsis-induced adrenal deficiency syndrome. Crit Care Med 2001;29(3):688–90.

[47] Koo DJ, Jackman D, Chaudry IH, et al. Adrenal insufficiency during the late stage of polymicrobial sepsis. Crit Care Med 2001;29(3):618–22.

[48] Bollaert PE, Charpentier C, Levy B, et al. Reversal of late septic shock with supraphysiologic doses of hydrocortisone. Crit Care Med 1998;26(4):645–50.

[49] Briegel J, Forst H, Haller M, et al. Stress doses of hydrocortisone reverse hyperdynamic septic shock: a prospective, randomized, double-blind, single-center study. Crit Care Med 1999;27(4):723–32.

[50] Barquist E, Kirton O. Adrenal insufficiency in the surgical intensive care unit patient. J Trauma 1997;42(1):27–31.

[51] Ritacca FV, Simone C, Wax R, et al. Pro/con clinical debate: are steroids useful in the management of patients with septic shock? Crit Care 2002;6(2):113–6 [Epub 2002 Feb 06].

[52] Van den Berghe G, de Zegher F, Lauwers P, et al. Luteinizing hormone secretion and hypoandrogenaemia in critically ill men: effect of dopamine. Clin Endocrinol (Oxf) 1994; 41(5):563–9.

[53] Wang C, Chan V, Tse TF, et al. Effect of acute myocardial infarction on pituitary-testicular function. Clin Endocrinol (Oxf) 1978;9(3):249–53.

[54] Lephart ED, Baxter CR, Parker CR Jr. Effect of burn trauma on adrenal and testicular steroid hormone production. J Clin Endocrinol Metab 1987;64(4):842–8.

[55] Spratt DI, Cox P, Orav J, et al. Reproductive axis suppression in acute illness is related to disease severity. J Clin Endocrinol Metab 1993;76(6):1548–54.

[56] van Steenbergen W, Naert J, Lambrecht S, et al. Suppression of gonadotropin secretion in the hospitalized postmenopausal female as an effect of acute critical illness. Neuroendocrinology 1994;60(2):165–72.

[57] Woolf PD, Hamill RW, McDonald JV, et al. Transient hypogonadotropic hypogonadism caused by critical illness. J Clin Endocrinol Metab 1985;60(3):444–50.

[58] Noel GL, Suh HK, Stone JG, et al. Human prolactin and growth hormone release during surgery and other conditions of stress. J Clin Endocrinol Metab 1972;35(6):840–51.

[59] Devins SS, Miller A, Herndon BL, et al. Effects of dopamine on T-lymphocyte proliferative responses and serum prolactin concentrations in critically ill patients. Crit Care Med 1992; 20(12):1644–9.

[60] Van den Berghe G. Endocrine evaluation of patients with critical illness. Endocrinol Metab Clin North Am 2003;32(2):385–410.

[61] Marik PE, Zaloga GP. Adrenal insufficiency in the critically ill: a new look at an old problem. Chest 2002;122(5):1784–96.

[62] Soni A, Pepper GM, Wyrwinski PM, et al. Adrenal insufficiency occurring during septic shock: incidence, outcome, and relationship to peripheral cytokine levels. Am J Med 1995; 98(3):266–71.

[63] Drucker D, Shandling M. Variable adrenocortical function in acute medical illness. Crit Care Med 1985;13(6):477–9.

[64] Manglik S, Flores E, Lubarsky L, et al. Glucocorticoid insufficiency in patients who present to the hospital with severe sepsis: a prospective clinical trial. Crit Care Med 2003;31(6): 1668–75.

[65] Hatherill M, Tibby SM, Hilliard T, et al. Adrenal insufficiency in septic shock. Arch Dis Child 1999;80(1):51–5.

[66] Cooper MS, Stewart PM. Corticosteroid insufficiency in acutely ill patients. N Engl J Med 2003;348(8):727–34.

[67] Lamberts SW, Bruining HA, de Jong FH. Corticosteroid therapy in severe illness. N Engl J Med 1997;337(18):1285–92.

[68] Annane D, Sebille V, Charpentier C, et al. Effect of treatment with low doses of hydro-cortisone and fludrocortisone on mortality in patients with septic shock. JAMA 2002;288(7): 862–71.

[69] Rivers EP, Gaspari M, Saad GA, et al. Adrenal insufficiency in high-risk surgical ICU patients. Chest 2001;119(3):889–96.

[70] Cronin L, Cook DJ, Carlet J, et al. Corticosteroid treatment for sepsis: a critical appraisal and meta-analysis of the literature. Crit Care Med 1995;23(8):1430–9.

[71] Lefering R, Neugebauer EA. Steroid controversy in sepsis and septic shock: a meta-analysis. Crit Care Med 1995;23(7):1294–303.

[72] Effect of high-dose glucocorticoid therapy on mortality in patients with clinical signs of systemic sepsis. The Veterans Administration Systemic Sepsis Cooperative Study Group. N Engl J Med 1987;10;317(11):659–65.

[73] Bone RC, Fisher CJ Jr, Clemmer TP, et al. A controlled clinical trial of high-dose methylprednisolone in the treatment of severe sepsis and septic shock. N Engl J Med 1987; 317(11):653–8.

[74] Luce JM, Montgomery AB, Marks JD, et al. Ineffectiveness of high-dose methylprednis-olone in preventing parenchymal lung injury and improving mortality in patients with septic shock. Am Rev Respir Dis 1988;138(1):62–8.

[75] Donmez A, Kaya H, Haberal A, et al. The effect of etomidate induction on plasma cortisol levels in children undergoing cardiac surgery. J Cardiothorac Vasc Anesth 1998; 12(2):182–5.

[76] Boidin MP. Serum levels of cortisol in man during etomidate, fentanyl and air anesthesia, compared with neurolept anesthesia. Acta Anaesthesiol Belg 1985;36(2):79–87.

[77] Klemperer JD, Klein I, Gomez M, et al. Thyroid hormone treatment after coronary-artery bypass surgery. N Engl J Med 1995;333(23):1522–7.

[78] Mullis-Jansson SL, Argenziano M, Corwin S, et al. A randomized double-blind study of the effect of triiodothyronine on cardiac function and morbidity after coronary bypass surgery. J Thorac Cardiovasc Surg 1999;117(6):1128–34.

[79] Ligtenberg JJ, Girbes AR, Beentjes JA, et al. Hormones in the critically ill patient: to intervene or not to intervene? Intensive Care Med 2001;27(10):1567–77.

[80] Uusaro A, Russell JA. Could anti-inflammatory actions of catecholamines explain the possible beneficial effects of supranormal oxygen delivery in critically ill surgical patients? Intensive Care Med 2000;26(3):299–304.

[81] Bailey AR, Burchett KR. Effect of low-dose dopamine on serum concentrations of prolactin in critically ill patients. Br J Anaesth 1997;78(1):97–9.

[82] Van den Berghe G, de Zegher F, Lauwers P. Dopamine suppresses pituitary function in infants and children. Crit Care Med 1994;22(11):1747–53.

ELSEVIER
SAUNDERS

EMERGENCY
MEDICINE
CLINICS OF
NORTH AMERICA

Emerg Med Clin N Am 23 (2005) 931–936

Index

Note: Page numbers of article titles are in **boldface** type.

A

Acetazolamide, hyperchloremic anion gap acidoses and, 782

Addison's disease, 692

Adolescents, abuse of steroids by, 821

Adrenal emergencies, recognition and management of, **687–702**

Adrenal gland, incidentalomas of, 699
pathophysiology of, 692–694
physiology of, 691

Adrenal hyperplasia, congenital, 879–880

Adrenal insufficiency, clinical characteristics of, 692, 693
corticosteroid therapy and, 697–699
definition of, 692
etiologies of, 692–694
evaluation in, 696–697, 916–918, 919
features suggesting, 917
management of, 918–921
pathophysiology of, 914–916
presentation in, 694–696, 914

AIDS, steroids in, 822

Amenorrhea, osteopenia in, 793

Amiodarone, as cause of hypothyroidism, 653

Amiodarone-induced thyroiditis, 672

Anabolic steroids, **815–826**
abuse of, by adolescents, 821
epidemiology of, 815–816
adverse effects of, 819–820
effects on organs, 816
efficacy of use of, 818
physiology of, 816
trade names of, 819
use in medical practice, 821–823

Androstenedione, 803–804

Anion gap acidoses, elevated, ethylene glycol poisoning and, 779–780
etiologies of, 772–781
in lactic acidosis, 777–779

in salicylate toxicity, 780–781
iron and, 776–777
isoniazid and, 776
ketoacidoses and, 774–775
methanol and, 773
paraldehyde and, 775
uremia and, 773–774
hyperchloremic, acetazolamide and, 782
etiologies of, 782–784
hyperalimentation and, 781–782
in diarrhea and diuretics use, 783–784
in pancreatic fistula, 784
in ureteroenterostomy, 784
renal tubular acidoses and renal insufficiency and, 782–783

Anorexia nervosa, 792–794

Anticonvulsants, as cause of hypothyroidism, 653–654

Antidiuretic hormone, inappropriate secretion of. See *SIADH.*

Anxiety, in endocrine and metabolic disorders, 906–907

B

Bariatric surgery, nutritional consequences of, 796–797

Beta-hydroxy-beta-methylbutyrate, 802–803

Bicarbonate, in diabetic ketoacidosis, 620–621, 622
in hyperkalemia, 743

Bone, anatomy of, 703–704
and mineral metabolism, **703–721**
effects of steroids on, 817–818
metabolism of, abnormalities of, management in, 706–707
pathophysiology of, 705–706
presentation in, 705
normal, 704–705